Examination of the newborn

An evidence-based guide

Examination of the newborn

An evidence-based guide

EDITED BY

Anne Lomax RN, RM, ADM, ENB 405, ENB N96,
Cert Ed, MEd
Senior Lecturer in Midwifery, University of Central Lancashire, Preston, UK

SECOND EDITION

WILEY Blackwell

This edition first published 2015 © 2015 by John Wiley & Sons, Ltd

Registered office: John Wiley & Sons, Ltd, The Atrium, Southern Gate, Chichester, West Sussex, PO19
8SQ, UK

Editorial offices: 9600 Garsington Road, Oxford, OX4 2DQ, UK
The Atrium, Southern Gate, Chichester, West Sussex, PO19 8SQ, UK
1606 Golden Aspen Drive, Suites 103 and 104, Ames, Iowa 50010, USA

For details of our global editorial offices, for customer services and for information about how to apply for
permission to reuse the copyright material in this book please see our website at
www.wiley.com/wiley-blackwell

Library of Congress Cataloging-in-Publication Data

Examination of the newborn : an evidence-based guide / edited by Anne Lomax. – Second edition.
      p. ; cm.
   Includes bibliographical references and index.
   ISBN 978-1-118-91319-2 (paper)
   I. Lomax, Anne, editor.
   [DNLM: 1. Physical Examination–methods. 2. Evidence-Based Medicine. 3. Infant, Newborn.
4. Midwifery–methods. 5. Neonatal Nursing–methods. 6. Neonatal Screening–standards. WS 141]
   RJ255.5
   618.92′01–dc23

                                                                                          2015015027

A catalogue record for this book is available from the British Library.

Wiley also publishes its books in a variety of electronic formats. Some content that appears in print may not
be available in electronic books.

Cover image: Newborn Heartbeat ©Lokibaho/istockphoto

Set in 9.5/13pt, MeridienLTStd by SPi Global, Chennai, India
Printed and bound in Malaysia by Vivar Printing Sdn Bhd

1   2015

Contents

List of contributors, vii

Acknowledgements, ix

Introduction, xi

About the companion website, xvii

1 History taking and the newborn examination: an evolving perspective, 1
Claire Evans

2 Cardiovascular and respiratory assessment of the baby, 32
Christopher D. Bedford and Anne Lomax

3 The neonatal skin: examination of the jaundiced newborn and gestational age assessment, 71
Morris Gordon and Anne Lomax

4 Examination of the head, neck and eyes, 104
Carmel Noonan, Fiona J. Rowe and Anne Lomax

5 Examination of the newborn abdomen and genitalia, 124
Morris Gordon

6 Developmental dysplasia of the hip and abnormalities of the foot, 142
Robin W. Paton and Naomi Davis

7 Chromosomal and genetic problems: giving feedback to mothers and fathers, 171
Delyth Webb and Anne Lomax

8 Newborn behavioural aspects, 192
Jeanette Appleton

9 Examination of the newborn: professional issues in practice, 213
Norma Fryer and Claire Evans

Appendix 1 Useful website addresses, 229

Appendix 2 NIPE Information leaflet for mothers and fathers, 232

Glossary of terms, 238

Index, 241

List of contributors

Jeanette Appleton Dip COT, SROT
Developmental Care Specialist Consultancy and Training and Trainer Brazelton Centre in Great Britain, UK

Christopher D. Bedford BSc (Hons), MB ChB, DCH, MRCP, FRCPCH, MA
Consultant Paediatrician, Warrington and Halton Hospitals NHS Foundation Trust, Warrington, Cheshire, UK

Naomi Davis BMedSci, BM BS, FRCSEd (Tr & Orth)
Consultant in Paediatric Orthopaedic Surgery and Honorary Clinical Lecturer, Royal Manchester Children's Hospital, Central Manchester University Hospitals NHS Foundation Trust, Manchester, UK

Claire Evans MA Neonatal Studies, BSc (Hons)
Warrington and Halton Hospitals NHS Foundation Trust, Warrington, Cheshire, UK Seconded post as Implementation Lead with the UK NSC NIPE Programme Centre, Public Health England, London, UK

Norma Fryer MA (Health Care Ethics), Cert Ed, ADM, RM, Dip N (A), RN
Retired Senior Lecturer now working in a 'consultancy' capacity, as a Midwifery Advisor/Trainer, Member of the NMC Fitness to Practise Investigating Committee, UK

Morris Gordon MBChB, MRCPCH, PGDipMedEd, FHEA
Specialist Registrar in Paediatric Gastroenterology, Royal Manchester Children's Hospital, Manchester, UK

Anne Lomax RN, RM, ADM, ENB 405, ENB N96, Cert Ed, MEd
Senior Lecturer in Midwifery, University of Central Lancashire, Preston, UK

Carmel Noonan FRCOphth, FRCSI (Ophthal)
Consultant Ophthalmologist, Aintree University Trust, Liverpool, UK

Robin W. Paton FRCS, FRCS (Orth)
Consultant Orthopaedic Surgeon and Honorary Senior Lecturer, Orthopaedic
    Department, University of Manchester, Manchester, UK
East Lancashire Hospitals NHS Trust, Blackburn, Lancashire, UK

**Catherine Quarrell RGN, RM, BSc (Hons), DAM, MSc, PG Cert (Education), PG
    Dip with Distinction (Education)**
Senior Lecturer/Supervisor of Midwives, Birmingham City University, Birming-
    ham, UK

Fiona J. Rowe PhD, DBO
Senior Lecturer and Programme Director, Directorate of Orthoptics and Vision
    Science, University of Liverpool, Liverpool, UK

Delyth Webb MBChB, FRCPCH, MMedSci
Consultant Paediatrician, Warrington Hospital, Warrington, Cheshire, UK

Acknowledgements

Firstly I would like to thank Wiley for giving me the opportunity to produce a second edition of the book, also to all the contributors who have, yet again, dedicated time, effort and their valuable expertise to update the information. Special thanks go to Claire Evans, Chris Bedford and Jeanette Appleton who have found time in their busy schedules to update and revise their chapters and provide real-life case studies.

Many thanks go to Jill Walker and the UK National Screening Committee, Public Health England, for keeping me informed of all the up-to-the-minute changes that are taking place within the National Antenatal and Newborn Screening Programmes and for allowing me to use material from their site.

Thanks again to Dr David Clark and the American Academy of Pediatrics, for giving me access to the many images I have used for the book.

Finally, thanks to Jen at the stables for giving me help with Billy when I needed it the most. Very much appreciated.

Introduction

Anne Lomax

Frontline staff, who perform the examination of the newborn, are in an ideal position to influence health choices made by women and their families to help ensure good maternal health and, in the longer term, optimum life chances of newborn babies. Newborn screening has the potential to prevent infant deaths by detecting certain congenital anomalies or conditions that contribute to long-term illness (DH 2007a). Moreover, it can provide a valuable opportunity to advise women on health promotion issues such as nutrition and feeding smoking, sudden unexpected death in infancy and immunisation programmes.

Since the last independent review of maternity services in 1995–1996 by the Audit Commission (1997), the Department of Health has published the *National Service Framework for Children, Young People and Maternity Services* (DH 2004a). This highlighted that high-quality maternity care can ensure a healthy start for the baby and help mothers and fathers become skilled in parenting The document also set out a 10-year programme for improvement

More recently, the Royal College of Obstetricians and Gynaecologists and the National Institute for Health and Clinical Excellence (NICE) have provided expert clinical guidance in all aspects of provision of maternity care (NICE 2006, RCOG 2008). Other government initiatives have provided the platform for changes in the way NHS staff work, to reduce waiting times and deliver modern patient-centred care. These initiatives include the following: *Making a Difference* (DH 1999); *The National Plan for the New NHS* (DH 2000); *European Working Time Directive* (DH 2002) and the *NHS Changing Workforce Programme* (DH 2003). The resulting reduction in junior doctors' hours has contributed to the need for different ways of working to provide maternity care, namely, that team midwifery and more specialised services may need to be concentrated in fewer facilities. At the same time, midwifery services will need to be strengthened in the community which, it may be said, is the most appropriate setting for straightforward low-risk women (DH 2008).

Alongside this, a change in professional boundaries has been inevitable and midwives have undertaken additional training to enhance their traditional roles (DH 2000). With regard to examination of the newborn, many midwives view this as a natural extension of their traditional role (Lomax and Evans 2005).

A growing body of evidence suggests that midwives are ideal candidates to undertake this enhanced role; however, the literature does indicate that a practitioner who is adequately trained, experienced, skilled and competent is more important than professional background. Also that the standard quality and content of the examination should be consistent throughout the United Kingdom (Wolke et al 2002a, 2002b, Townsend et al 2004, Williamson et al. 2005, Hall and Elliman 2006)

Mothers and babies should have access to a practitioner who provides a flexible but informed attitude to care, designed to meet their individual needs (DH 2004b). Above all, midwives must be committed to this concept as difficult as this may be against the backdrop of a service which is still dealing with large numbers of hospital-based low-risk women.

Recently, the Midwifery 2020 document (DH 2010) emphasised the unique and essential role of the midwife in the care of both low-risk *and* high-risk women. It recognizes the important role that midwives play in communicating key public health messages to these women throughout the childbearing continuum. Midwifery 2020 calls for the inclusion of examination of the newborn, prescribing, suturing and intravenous cannulation skills to be included in pre-registration midwifery curricula in order to ensure that all newly qualified midwives are proficient in caring for women of all risks.

The UK National Screening Committee

The UK National Screening Committee (UKNSC) launched the national standards for the newborn infant examination in 2008. This was part of a wider announcement on the Child Health Promotion Programme (CHPP). The document *The Child Health Promotion Programme, Pregnancy and the First Five Years of Life* (DH 2008) is an update of standard one of the *National Service Framework for Children, Young People and Maternity Services* and sets the context for neonatal examinations. The CHPP has now been superseded by The Healthy Child Programme (HCP) (DH 2009).

In April 2013, the UK National Screening Programmes became part of Public Health England. Public Health England is the expert national public health agency working on behalf of the Secretary of State to protect health and health inequalities and promote the health and well-being of the nation. More information on Public Health England can be found here: https://wwwgovuk/government/organisations/public-health-england and also on the website that accompanies this book.

The standards set out within the UKNSC's document, *Newborn and Infant Physical Examination* (NIPE) (UK National Screening Committee 2008), are currently being reviewed and will include updated standards for both 72 hours and 6–8-week screening elements of the physical examination.

However for the purposes of this edition, the NIPE Standards document will be a reference source until updated. The document can be accessed at: http://newbornphysicalscreeningnhsuk/. As soon as the standards are re-launched, they will appear on the NIPE website and on the website that accompanies this book.

Also being reviewed is the DH National Service Specification 21 Newborn and Infant Physical Examination Screening Programme (DH 2013). The service specification will ensure consistency in approach to the newborn and infant examinations and will be used to commission and monitor provision of NIPE services across England. It represents the NIPE service that should be provided and outlines the requirements for commissioning of a safe effective screening programme. Screening programmes fall under the remit of the Section 7a Agreement (NHS 2013), which allows responsibility for commissioning some of the public health budget to be passed to NHS England (2013). It also ensures that decisions are made by those with subject expertise, that a collaborative and strategic leadership approach is adopted and that screening programme boards are in place.

Alongside this, the NIPE programme requires a robust information support system to assure quality and provide a failsafe element to the newborn examination to help detect and prevent late or missed examinations and to track babies along the screening pathway. Information sharing and provision of a sound data base is central to the continued success of the programme. The NIPE programme team is therefore in the process of formally rolling out the NIPE Programme including recommending use of the NIPE Screening Management and Reporting Tools (NIPE SMART). IT system SMART provides a consistent means of gathering important data from the newborn examination. The system can also help with audit of performance against national standards and key performance indicators and can ensure a local and national failsafe.

The features of a fully implemented and functioning newborn screening programme can be found on the NIPE website.

Most chapters in this edition have been updated and there is an addition of clinical case studies at the end of each chapter except Chapter 1. The addition of a case study here was not considered relevant. A selected topic has been applied to practice within each case study. There is also a website that accompanies this book which provides a wealth of information on all aspects of examination of the newborn.

In Chapter 1, Claire Evans has revised and updated the text which will help the practitioner gather all the necessary information prior to conducting the newborn examination. This chapter emphasises the importance of recognizing diagnostic information from the antenatal history and directs the practitioner to the optimal course of management.

Chapter 2 merges the physiology of the fetal and neonatal cardiovascular and respiratory systems with the clinical examination. Chris Bedford has updated the information on pulse oximetry in line with the new UKNSC guidelines. After consultation in 2013, the UKNSC recommended that pulse oximetry be included in the screening process for the full examination of the newborn. This practice is currently being piloted in England and the NIPE Programme Team will assess the impact of this on the screening process as a whole. The website that accompanies this book contains links to videos and other sources of information to help you examine the heart and lungs effectively. Some current information on delayed cord clamping has also been included.

Chapter 3 has been updated in terms of how we view the use of cleansing products and their affect on newborn skin. The addition of colour photos throughout the book greatly enhances text, particularly in Chapter 3.

Chapter 4 includes an updated and extended section on examination of the mouth for cleft lip and palate. The Royal College of Pediatricians and Child Health have developed guidelines for inspection of the mouth for cleft lip and palate. These are available at http://wwwrcpchacuk/. Chapter 4 also includes some updated information on tongue tie and its treatment. More information on both these topics can be found on the website that accompanies this book.

Information regarding Developmental Dysplasia of the Hip and Abnormalities of the Foot has been merged in Chapter 6. The website contains links to videos and other sources of information to help you examine the hips effectively.

Chapters 7 and 8 have been revised and updated and there are links in the appendix and on the website for you to access lots of additional evidence-based information on chromosomal abnormalities.

Chapter 9 contains information on both professional practice and safeguarding and attempts to inform the reader of some of the far-reaching changes to the Nursing and Midwifery Council (NMC 2013). The NMC is currently in the process of revising the revalidation of registrants to assess their continued fitness to practice. The NMC has also embarked on a public consultation on how revalidation can be applied in practice and is planning to develop a fair and proportionate system of revalidation by the end of 2015 (NMC 2013). The new Code was effective from 31 March 2015 and can be found at: http://www.nmc.org.uk/globalassets/siteDocuments/NMC-Publications/revised-new-NMC-Code.pdf.

References

DH (1999) *Strengthening the Nursing, Midwifery and Health Visiting Contribution to Health and Health Care: Making a Difference*. London: HMSO.

DH (2000) The National Plan for the New NHS Presented to Parliament by the Secretary of State for Health, pp. 82–87.

DH (2002) *The European Working Time Directive*. London: Department of Health.

DH (2003) *NHS Changing Workforce Programme*. London: Department of Health.

DH (2004a) *Agenda for Change: Final Agreement*. London: Department of Health.

DH (2004b) *National Service Framework for Children, Young People and Maternity Services*. London: The Stationery Office, Department of Health.

DH (2007a) *Implementation Plan for Reducing Health Inequalities in Infant Mortality: A Good Practice Guide*. Review of the health inequalities PSA target. London: Department of Health.

DH (2007b) *Maternity Matters: Choice, Access and Continuity of Care in a Safe Service*. London: Department of Health.

DH (2008) *Our NHS Our Future. The Next Stage Review, Interim Report*. London: Department of Health.

DH (2009) *The Healthy Child Programme Pregnancy and the First Five Years of Life*. London: Department for Children, Schools and Families.

DH (2010) *Midwifery 2020 Delivering Expectations*. London: Department of Health. Available from: https://wwwgovuk/government/uploads/system/uploads/attachment_data/file/216029/dh_119470pdf (accessed August 2014).

DH (2013) National Service Specification 21 Newborn and Infant Physical Examination Screening Programme. Available from: https://wwwgovuk/government/uploads/system/uploads/attachment_data/file/213168/21-NIPE-Service-Specification-121023pdf (accessed August 2014).

Hall D, Elliman D (2006) *Health for All Children*, 4th edn. Oxford: Oxford University Press.

Lomax A, Evans C (2005) Examination of the newborn: the franchise experience: integrating theory into practice *Infant Journal* **1**(2), 58–61.

NICE (2006) *Routine Postnatal Care of Women and Their Babies*. NICE Clinical Guide No 37. London: National Institute for Clinical Excellence.

NHS England (2013) NHS Public health functions agreement 2014-15 Public health functions to be exercised by NHS England NHS England 2013. Available from: https://wwwgovuk/government/uploads/system/uploads/attachment_data/file/256502/nhs_public_health_functions_agreement_2014-15pdf (accessed August 2014)

Nursing and Midwifery Council (2013) Our response to the Francis report. Available from: http://wwwnmc-ukorg/About-us/Our-response-to-the-Francis-Inquiry-Report/ (accessed August 2014).

RCOG (2008) *Standards for Maternity Care – Report of a Working Party*. London: RCOG Press.

Townsend J, Wolke D, Hayes J, Dave S, Rogers C, Bloomfield L, Quist-therson E, Tomlin M, Messer D (2004) Routine examination of the newborn; The EMREN study Evaluation of an extension of the midwife role including a randomised control trial of appropriately trained midwives and paediatric senior house officers. *Health Technology Assessment* **8**(14), 1–73.

UK National Screening Committee (2008) *Newborn and Infant Physical Examination: Standards and Competencies*. NHS. Available from: http://newbornphysicalscreeningnhsuk/ (accessed July 2010).

Williamson A, Mullet J, Bunting M, Eason J (2005) Neonatal examination: are midwives clinically effective? *Midwives RCM* **8**(3), 116–118.

Wolke D, Dave S, Hayes J, Townsend J (2002a) Routine examination of the newborn and maternal satisfaction: a randomised controlled trial. *Archives of Disease in Childhood: Neonatal Edition* **86**, F155–F160.

Wolke D, Dave S, Hayes J, Townsend J, Tomlin M (2002b) Archives of disease in childhood: a randomised controlled trial of maternal satisfaction with the routine examination of the newborn at 3 months post birth. *Archives of Disease in Childhood* **18**, 145–154

About the companion website

Do not forget to visit the companion website for this book:

www.wiley.com/go/lomax/newborn

There you will find valuable material designed to enhance your learning, including:

- Interactive multiple choice questions
- "Step By Step Guide to Examination of the Newborn" PowerPoint presentation
- Online checklists, guidelines and other resources

Scan this QR code to visit the companion website.

CHAPTER 1

History taking and the newborn examination: an evolving perspective

Claire Evans

[1] *Warrington and Halton Hospitals NHS Foundation Trust, Warrington, Cheshire, UK*
[2] *Seconded post as Implementation Lead with the UK NSC NIPE Programme Centre, Public Health England, London, UK*

KEY POINTS

- The principal aim of history taking is to screen for predictive risk indicators that may predispose the newborn to an adverse postnatal transition or presence of an abnormality that requires an appropriate and timely referral for further diagnostics.

- The newborn examination history-taking process should be mapped to the UK NSC Antenatal and Newborn Screening Programme and be used as a benchmark for screening and assessment of risk factors in the neonatal period and beyond.

- Identification of risk factors within the newborn screen examination can isolate and target health promotion issues.

Introduction

A comprehensive history taking is implicit to all health-care disciplines to aid the diagnostic consultation process and to inform the optimal course of management. The skill of history taking has changed over the decades and has adopted a wider context as a predictive diagnostic tool. In order to facilitate a more holistic approach to the examination of the newborn, a thorough evaluation of the maternal and newborn history is essential. Short-term outcomes, long-term morbidities or even mortality can be influenced by the quality of the history taking in terms of the predictive risk for some adverse clinical conditions.

This chapter outlines the context of the history profile from the maternal, perinatal and familial perspectives. It also addresses history taking as a skill and the potential barriers that may reduce the effectiveness of the process. The aim

---

Examination of the Newborn: An Evidence-Based Guide, Second Edition. Edited by Anne Lomax.
© 2015 John Wiley & Sons, Ltd. Published 2015 by John Wiley & Sons, Ltd.
Companion Website: www.wiley.com/go/lomax/newborn

of this chapter is not only to address common risk factors but also to embrace the wider context of history taking from a psychosocial and safeguarding perspective. The focus on history taking must be meaningful, achievable and valuable to the newborn examination practitioner. History taking remains the principal standard underpinning the clinical examination; disregarding the importance of history taking may lead to suboptimal practice and outcomes. Gathering a history effectively demands time and should not be rushed as it is a powerful instrument that can influence the quality of the examination.

Several national directives have raised the profile of the newborn physical examination. They stipulate the importance of a thorough and, to some degree, systematic history assessment (Skills for Health, 2004; NICE 2006a, 2006b; NHSQIS, 2004; UK NSC, 2008). In particular, the *UK NSC Newborn and Infant Physical Examination Standards and Competencies* (UK NSC, 2008) outlines a competency statement that addresses the history assessment. The NIPE Standards are currently under development for republication. Following the relaunch, the new standards will be available to view on the UK NSC NIPE Screening Programme website: http://newbornphysical.screening.nhs.uk/. However, for the purposes of this chapter, the NIPE Standards document will be a reference source until updated. This approach should encompass all relevant information from the maternal and newborn medical records, dialogue with the mother and/or father and information from clinical staff.

Objectives and characteristics of good history taking

The principal aim of the history-taking exercise is to find predictive risk indicators that may identify those newborns who are at risk of an adverse postnatal transition extending into childhood. Families with newborns who are identified as being at risk will then benefit from early detection, intervention and therapeutic options. To achieve this, the history profile must be factual, accurate, concise, informative and relevant. Discussions with the mother and father, to gather the history, can also offer a platform that targets health awareness and safety issues to promote optimal health in the neonatal period and beyond. A review of maternal and parental lifestyle habits in general, e.g. smoking, addictive behaviours and high-conflict relationships can be identified, and appropriate referrals or support can be arranged. Other health promotion issues include BCG vaccination to high-risk populations.

The quality of the history-taking process is largely dependent on the skill of the practitioner. Health-care professionals who conduct the newborn screen examination are fortunate in having pre-existing skills that are transferable. Doctors and midwives engage in history taking on a regular basis within their daily practice. However, the underlying principles of history taking follow that of all patient groups. Howard (2008) comments upon the role of history taking in establishing trust which in turn paves the way for the physical examination. Thus, the interpersonal skills of the newborn examiner can influence the quality of the history obtained. Mannerisms, eye contact, body language, patience, listening skills and empathy are all key skills that any health-care professional requires to obtain a good history. If there is any deficiency in these key skills, the level of narrative imparted by the mother or father to the health professional may be negatively affected. Stoeckle and Billings (1987), in their signature work on history taking, refer to the process as a clinical interview and the manner in which it is conducted will influence the communicative processes necessary to generate the clinical picture.

Parallels can be drawn between history taking for the newborn examination and maternal history taking throughout pregnancy (NHS QIS, 2004), which may illuminate any element of risk to the mother/infant dyad. In addition, engagement of mothers and fathers with the history-taking exercise facilitates participation in the decision-making process and the request for consent (NHS QIS, 2008). These aspects of history taking are just as relevant to the newborn.

It is important to note that in the event of any subsequent admission to hospital for the infant, the first point of reference is the history and newborn physical examination. In addition, should anything have been missed during the examination, e.g. cleft palate, a dislocated hip, then this may result in a complaint and possible litigation (see also Chapter 9). A thorough history can identify potential as well as actual risk of an aspect being overlooked, which may later impact upon neonatal and infant outcome.

Concise and thorough history taking will also assist the health-care professional to ascertain whether or not the criteria are met for the examination of a healthy newborn. Some aspects of the history may require midwives or neonatal nurses to refer the newborn to a medical colleague as a more detailed examination may be necessary. For this reason, it is vital that maternity units have local guidelines in place to support all health-care disciplines who undertake the newborn examination.

Paediatric medicine has long since considered family history as key to the clinical examination process. The family profile is informative when screening for common complex and single-gene conditions but includes isolating genetic predispositions in some families (Green, 2007). As a result, several family-history-taking checklists in the form of mnemonics have emerged to guide paediatricians. Such systems may be helpful and indeed insightful, but it cannot be fully applied to newborn history taking. However, it does highlight the importance of gathering information in an ordered manner, and, most importantly, that the family history must be placed at the centre of history taking for the newborn infant.

Building a history profile: where to start?

When building a history profile, there is a clear identifiable process to follow. Assimilation of the perinatal history can be challenging, and therefore, the first point of reference has to be the maternal medical records. However, knowing what to look for and having some order of assemblage in the gathering of information is crucial if the task is to be efficient and not time-consuming. The maternal booking history often yields the most significant information alongside the serology results. The maternal early booking history will, in the main, provide most of the baseline history. This should provide the medical and surgical history of the mother as well as the maternal well-being so far with the pregnancy. The maternal booking interview should be completed before the twelfth week of pregnancy as proposed by *Maternity Matters* (DH, 2007), the policy document on maternity care, and endorsed by the UK National Screening Committee (NSC, 2007). Early booking will maximise a woman's exposure to, and choice of, the screening programmes available, thus identifying those women and families who need interventional support with lifestyle choices.

Reliance upon the maternal medical records alone will not provide all the information needed. It is, therefore, necessary to question the mother and/or father on family history in order to extract the risk factors that parallel the national standards (UK NSC, 2008). The core elements of the national standards for the newborn screen examination have provided a structure for risk assessment through history taking.

The UK NSC Antenatal and Newborn Screening Programme should be used as the benchmark screening tool for the newborn screen examination (see Table 1.1). The maternal antenatal screen will provide a framework of investigative results for the examiner that will provide the foundation for the history profile. The *Newborn and Physical Examination Standards and Competencies* document (UK NSC, 2008) found at: http://newbornphysical.screening.nhs.uk/ provides a structure within competency statement 1, which outlines the aspects to be considered when assimilating the history profile. Table 1.2 outlines the content of Competency 1 and can be used as a point of reference.

Evaluation of maternal medical records: biophysical information

The maternal socio-demographic and biophysical details should be assessed. Age must be noted, particularly in the teenage primigravida, as additional health promotion and education by the examiner may be necessary upon completion of the examination. Early and recent evidence suggests that upper and lower margins of maternal age are adversely related to prenatal and perinatal outcome (Haines et al., 1991; Viegas et al., 1994; Battin and Sadler, 2010). However,

Table 1.1 Key elements of the National Antenatal and Newborn Screening Programme.

	Timing	Biophysical details
Serology investigations		
Blood profile to include group, rhesus and antibodies status and haemoglobin	At booking Antibodies and haemoglobin repeated at 28 weeks	Approximately 15% of the population are rhesus-negative (Salem and Singer, 2009). Anti-D immunoglobulin is offered to all rhesus-negative women at 28 weeks' gestation to prevent haemolytic disease in the newborn. Maternal antibodies can also cause haemolytic disease.
Sickle cell	As early as possible preferably by 10 weeks' gestation	Inherited genetic condition resulting in the red blood cell forming a sickle cell shape. There are variants of this disease which impacts on the severity. In cases where women are healthy carriers, the baby's father should be offered screening. The risk of an affected infant is 1:2 where both parents are carriers (NHS ANSP, 2008).
Thalassaemia	As early as possible preferably by 10 weeks' gestation	Inherited genetic condition which affects the production of red blood cells. The genes that make haemoglobin are altered causing anaemia. This condition takes two forms: alpha and beta (Ryan et al., 2010).
Hepatitis B	At booking	Some populations of women are at high risk of Hepatitis B infection (HBsAG positive). Transmission of the virus is through sexual contact, vertical transmission or contaminated blood, e.g. needle sharing. Transmission to the fetus can be transplacental. Vaccination of the newborn must be offered to HBsAG positive women and their partners (DH, 2003).
HIV	At booking	HIV infection is a retrovirus that causes an alteration of the immune system. The virus infects the CD4 cells or the helper T cells which lower the body's cell-mediated immunity. Infection with HIV-1 can progress to AIDS (Carpenter et al., 2009).
Syphilis	At booking	Sexually transmitted disease with a risk of transplacental transmission.

(continued overleaf)

Table 1.1 (*Continued*).

	Timing	Biophysical details
Rubella	At booking	Viral infection with risk transplacental transmission.
First trimester combined test	11 + 2 – 14 + 1	Combined screening test with combination of age, blood profile, nuchal scan measurement and other factors.
Ultrasonography		
Nuchal translucency	11–14 weeks (Part of combined test)	Nuchal translucency measurement greater than 3.5 mm in early pregnancy. This finding is significant as associated with cardiac and syndromic pathology. This finding is also part of the 'combined' screening test for trisomy 21.
Quadruple test	14 + 2 – 20 + 0 weeks	Biochemistry tests, which include AFP, BHcG, oestriols and inhibin A.
Fetal anomaly	18 – 20 + 6 weeks	This scan can detect certain gross structural anomalies but does have its limitations. Approximately 45% of cardiac defects can be detected at this particular time.
Newborn and Infant Physical Examination (NIPE) National Standards	Within first 72 hours of birth Repeated at 6–8 weeks of age	Full physical and behavioural examination of the newborn incorporating the four core condition-related screening standards – developmental dysplasia of the hip, examination of the eye, congenital heart defects and undescended testes.

Data sources: NSC (2007, 2008); NHS, Greater Manchester Public Health Network (2009).

Table 1.2 How Competency 1 of the *Newborn Physical Examination Standards and Competencies* (UK NSC, 2008) can be used to create a history profile.

		Creating a history profile			
Maternal biophysical data	**Antenatal screening results**	**Pregnancy and labour history**	**Family history**	**Psychosocial factors**	**Newborn**
Health status	Serology reports	Incidence of infection and bacteria isolate	History of diabetes	Smoking	Resuscitation at birth and response
Cardiac disease	Rhesus status	Pathologies	Intergenerational Conditions	Substance use	Mode of feeding
Renal disease	Ultrasound scan	Pre-eclampsia	Inborn errors of metabolism	Alcohol dependency	Passage of urine and meconium
Hypothyroidism	profile	Placental insufficiency, etc.		Depression	
Depression	Diagnostic investigations			High-conflict	
Nutritional status and BMI		Mode of delivery and presentation	First-degree relative	Relationship	General health since birth
		Pre-labour length of membranes rupture	with CHD	Safeguarding issues with siblings	
			First-degree relative with DDH	Social services involvement with family	Parental concerns
					Symptomatic of illness

Bornstein et al. (2006) explore this relationship, concluding that varied age groups have differing parenting abilities. Nevertheless, the teenage mothers may require more intensive health promotion advice for themselves, possibly their partners and their newborn infants.

There is a new general health agenda emerging within society in relation to lifestyle and in particular to maternal diet and weight profile. A raised body mass index (BMI) can influence general health and may also indicate the family unit's dietary habits. A positive relationship exists between a raised BMI and complications of pregnancy including diabetes, hypertensive disease and thromboembolic disorders (Bhattacharya et al., 2007; CEMD, 2002; CMACE/RCOG, 2010). Pregnancy outcome can be affected, resulting in macrosomia, shoulder dystocia at delivery and hypoglycaemia of the newborn (Sebire et al., 2001; Kalk et al., 2009; Khashan and Kenny, 2009). Maternity units must have a policy in place for the prevention, detection and treatment of neonatal hypoglycaemia to identify those newborns most at risk.

Previous obstetric histories can provide information regarding maternal well-being and pregnancy outcome, which may be of relevance. Particular notice should be taken of the health of existing siblings. Where there has been a previous sudden infant death syndrome (SIDS) sibling, this must be noted. It is good practice to offer the option of an ECG being performed on the new sibling to rule out any risk of cardiac conduction disorders, e.g. prolonged QT syndrome or Wolff–Parkinson–White syndrome. The newborn would also be on the Care of the Next Infant scheme with the provision of an apnoea monitor prior to discharge.

The medical history can reveal conditions such as maternal hypothyroidism, cardiac disease, blood disorders, e.g. idiopathic thrombocytopenia, haemophilia Von Willebrand disease or maternal depression. The surgical history may not have such a direct impact upon risk for the newborn but does add to the completeness of the history-taking process for the health-care professional.

The intrapartum history is important in terms of identifying risk factors for the newborn. Taking note of the mode of delivery is important as this in itself may impact upon the health of the newborn. If shoulder dystocia presented during the second stage, the infant must be thoroughly examined by a senior paediatrician for evidence of an Erb's palsy, a clavicle fracture or sternomastoid muscle damage. An examination in the immediate post-delivery period by a paediatrician should be part of the maternity service local shoulder dystocia management guideline.

Breech presentation carries a strong correlative risk of Developmental Dysplasia of the Hip and is, therefore, a nationally recognised risk factor. Breech presentation at birth irrespective of mode of delivery or clinically diagnosed in pregnancy after 36 weeks' gestation or if external cephalic version performed for breech presentation irrespective of gestational age at delivery requires referral of the newborn in line with the national NIPE Standards (UK NSC, 2008).

Table 1.3   Maternal medical records: summarised alert indicators.

Maternal medical records: alert indicators
Ultrasound scans:

- Polyhydramnios
- Oligohydramnios
- Dilated renal pelves
- Intrauterine growth restriction
- Suspected chromosomal or syndromic aberrations
- Other significant ultrasound screening findings
- Congenital heart defect

Abnormal combined or quadruple test result
HIV positive serology status
Hepatitis B and C
Haemoglobinopathy
Maternal antibodies
Maternal pyrexia in labour
Prolonged fetal tachycardia
Pre-labour prolonged rupture of membranes
Meconium-stained liquor
Maternal Group B streptococcal infection
Breech presentation
Maternal disease state: type 1 and type 2 diabetes, autoimmune disorders, e.g. systemic lupus
    erythematosus
Maternal substance use
Maternal alcohol dependency
Thrombocytopenia

A precipitate delivery may cause facial congestion, which can be misdiagnosed as cyanosis. An instrumental delivery may result in the newborn suffering a degree of head trauma, such as bruising, which may require analgesia and can increase the risk of hyperbilirubinaemia (see Table 1.3 and also Chapter 3).

Meconium-stained liquor (MSL) can be problematic for a minority of newborns and, therefore, must be noted from the delivery summary. The presence of MSL is associated with an increased mortality and morbidity, accounting for 2% of perinatal deaths (NICE, 2007). It is relatively common with an occurrence of 15–20% in term pregnancies (NICE, 2007). Although meconium aspiration syndrome is relatively rare, some of these infants may seem well at delivery but rapidly develop signs of respiratory compromise as a result of aspiration. NICE (2007) advocate close observation of the newborn with MSL present at delivery in the immediate postnatal period.

Newborn examiners must be continuously on the alert for possible risk factors for early-onset neonatal sepsis. Early-onset sepsis in the newborn is a significant contributor to mortality statistics. One of the most common bacterial isolates is group B haemolytic streptococcus (GBS) that carries a mortality of 6% in term infants and 18% in preterm infants (NICE, 2007). Maternal infection during the antenatal period must be actively treated with antibiotic therapy. Treatment with antibiotics for the newborn may also be required but is risk dependent or if the newborn is symptomatic. Ohlsson and Shah (2009) inferred that intrapartum antibiotic therapy does reduce the risk of early-onset GBS in the newborn. Ungerer et al. (2004) reported mortality as high as 50% in untreated infants.

In the case of pre-labour prolonged rupture of membranes, the length of time must be noted (NICE, 2012). The risk of early-onset GBS infection in the new-born is greater in women with PROM (RCOG, 2003; NICE, 2007). In the absence of any other symptoms, true maternal pyrexia in labour must never be ignored. In addition, there was no strong evidence to recommend antibiotic prophylaxis for newborns of women with PROM in labour (NICE, 2012).

Conversely, the symptomatic newborn must commence antibiotic therapy and admission to the neonatal unit for further diagnostics. Every newborn must be treated on an individual basis, depending on the risk factors presenting. Multiple risk factors will necessitate newborn screening for infection and the commencement of antibiotic prophylaxis until blood culture results become available. Local policy on the prevention and detection of early-onset sepsis in the newborn must reflect the red flag and non-red flag risk indicators as detailed in the NICE guidance for antibiotics for early-onset neonatal infection (NICE, 2012) available at http://www.nice.org.uk/guidance/CG149/resources. The NICE guidance advocates the avoidance of routine antibiotic therapy. It is estimated that 90% of newborns with early-onset sepsis will be symptomatic within 12 hours of birth (NICE, 2007). Therefore, all newborns with risk factors for early-onset infection must receive close observation and documentation of an observations regime. The newborn examiner must ensure that the observations are documented and reviewed within the context of the examination and assessment of the overall health of the newborn.

The newborn of the diabetic mother, irrespective of diabetes type, will require blood glucose monitoring. The newborn examiner must review the blood glucose results prior to conducting the examination. Local policy will dictate the monitoring intervals for such newborns. Suboptimal results will require more active management of hypoglycaemia that may necessitate admission to the neonatal unit.

The UK NSC Antenatal Screening Programme

The UK NSC Antenatal Screening Programme components (Table 1.1) aim at helping the examiner through the investigations and results and signpost the relevant information within the maternal medical records. Familiarisation with the key components of the programme will enhance this process.

The maternal prenatal serology results must be evaluated, particularly the rhesus status. A maternal rhesus-negative status or the presence of antibodies should alert the examiner to the possibility of rhesus incompatibility and the risk of early-onset pathological hyperbilirubinaemia with the first 24 hours of life. A sibling of the newborn with neonatal jaundice requiring phototherapy carries a significant risk (NICE, 2010). Further information on neonatal jaundice management guidelines can be found on the NICE website: http://www.nice.org.uk/guidance/CG98. Surveillance of the newborn should be increased, particularly in the case of an early discharge to the community. The maternal rubella status should be noted as postnatal maternal vaccination may be required.

The human immunodeficiency virus (HIV), hepatitis B and hepatitis C status should be reviewed in all cases. However, such infections may be more likely alongside evidence of maternal substance misuse.

A family history of metabolic disease must also be noted particularly following the incident alert with medium-chain acyl-coenzyme A dehydrogenase deficiency (MCADD) (NPSA, 2011). If MCADD is known within the family, then the newborn will require early special rapid bloodspot testing at 24–48 hours of age prior to the standard bloodspot screen in 5–7 days. Further information on bloodspot screening can be obtained from the UK NSC Bloodspot website: http://newbornbloodspot.screening.nhs.uk/ and the British Inherited Metabolic Disease Group at: http://www.bimdg.org.uk/site/index.asp.

Fetus in focus

Ultrasonography in pregnancy is part of the UK NSC Fetal Anomaly Screening Programme (FASP) where two key ultrasound scans are offered as a minimum standard (UK NSC FASP 2010). The first scan is the early dating scan. It is, therefore, important to note the gestational age of the newborn from the earliest ultrasound scan result prior to conducting the examination.

The second is the 18–20-week fetal anomaly scan. Additional serial scans will be performed if and when an abnormality is detected, either with the fetus or with the intrauterine environment, e.g. liquor volume or placental positioning. Fetal growth estimation is the primary parameter assessed. Evidence of intrauterine growth restriction is not an uncommon finding at this stage. There may be evidence in the maternal history that may indicate why the infant is small for gestation age. There may be a pre-existing maternal medical condition that has adversely contributed to placental function resulting in a poor fetal growth profile. Fetal growth restriction may be a feature of an underlying chromosomal abnormality or some other pathology, e.g. transplacental viral transmission or the effect of a toxic substance, e.g. alcohol excess in pregnancy. Further information on the UK NSC FASP Programme can be obtained from the website: http://fetalanomaly.screening.nhs.uk/.

The UK NSC FASP (2010) has set a benchmark for the condition that should be screened for during this particular anomaly scan. Whilst it is useful in many cases, it is prudent to accept that this scan does have its limitations; therefore, the focus lies with a standard for 11 structural conditions where the specificity for detection is greater than 50% (UK NSC FASP, 2010). Conditions screened for are given as follows:

- Anencephaly
- Open spina bifida
- Cleft lip
- Diaphragmatic hernia
- Gastroschisis
- Exomphalos
- Serious cardiac anomalies
- Bilateral renal agenesis
- Lethal skeletal dysplasia
- Edward's syndrome (trisomy 18)
- Patau's syndrome (trisomy 13)
  Adapted from the UK NSC Fetal Anomaly Screening Programme

The presence of other findings is significant and, as such, is reportable by the ultrasonographer as listed subsequently.

- Nuchal fold (>6 mm)
- Ventriculomegaly (atrium >10 mm)
- Echogenic bowel (with density equivalent to bone)
- Renal pelvic dilatation (AP measurement >7 mm)

Fetal renal pelvic dilatation will require serial scan monitoring throughout the pregnancy. However, it is particularly important to note this during history taking and to arrange follow-up ultrasound scans and urology clinic referral for the newborn.

The presence of oligohydramnios must alert the examiner to the possibility of the following:

- Prolonged rupture of membranes earlier in the pregnancy
- Urinary tract anomaly or uropathy
- Fetal growth restriction (Baxter et al., 2010)
- Intrauterine infection

Conversely, polyhydramnios will alert the examiner to consider the following:

- Duodenal atresia or stenosis (Rajiah, 2009)
- Oesophageal atresia
  (See also Chapter 5)

Exposure to the effects of intrauterine teratogens has been investigated and publicised over recent decades, but arguably the most common causes of such exposure are smoking and excessive alcohol consumption during pregnancy. Smoking is the most common substance dependency, yet the most preventable. Reduction in maternal smoking during pregnancy remains high on the public health agenda through smoking cessation initiatives as part of maternity care (NICE, 2010). Clinical guidance can be found on the NICE website:

http://www.nice.org.uk/nicemedia/live/13023/49346/49346.pdf. There is compelling evidence highlighting the adverse effects of maternal smoking in both the antenatal and postnatal periods (La Souef, 2000; Gilliland et al., 2001; Landau, 2001; Stocks and Dezateux, 2003; British Medical Association, 2004; Bradley et al., 2005). The adverse health implications for the newborn and older children are numerous and can impact on mortality and morbidity.

Perhaps the most significant, devastating and indeed most publicised adverse effect of parental smoking is the increased risk of SIDS (McMartin et al., 2002; Anderson et al., 2005; Matturi et al., 2006; Sellwood and Huertas-Ceballos, 2008). The hypothesis surrounding this causal relationship is multifactorial ranging from respiratory infection susceptibility to altered respiratory control mechanisms (Hofhuis et al., 2003). This positive association cannot be underestimated nor ignored; therefore, the prevention of SIDS is high on the maternity services' health education agenda for the newborn examination.

Smoking cessation merits a much higher profile during the antenatal and immediate postnatal period and must be addressed thoroughly at the time of the newborn examination.

Fetal alcohol exposure from excessive maternal consumption is associated with dysmorphic features and varied neurodevelopmental and behavioural disorders ranging from fetal alcohol syndrome to fetal alcohol spectrum disorders (Disney et al., 2008). Maternal alcohol consumption is often associated with an existing suboptimal social environment (Dawson, 2003). The newborn can also suffer withdrawal symptoms from prenatal alcohol exposure, which may result in seizure activity (Lall, 2008).

Admittance to alcohol consumption during pregnancy in excessive amounts is often retrospective (Jacobson et al., 2002); therefore, intervention and preventative strategies must be put in place for subsequent pregnancies. Disney et al. (2008) reports on the long-standing evidence (Olson et al., 1997; Roebuck et al., 1999) to support altered neurobehavioural abilities in infancy through to antisocial behaviour and attention deficit disorders in children from small amounts of alcohol during pregnancy (Jacobson et al., 2002; Sayal, 2007; Sayal et al., 2009). Enquiries into maternal alcohol and units consumed are made by midwives at the prenatal booking interview. For some newborns, the cessation of alcohol use, even early in the first trimester, may be too late.

Maternal substance-misuse signals a probable newborn withdrawal process and a challenge to the health-care team in establishing the exact nature of the drugs taken. In the first instance, the newborn examiner must establish what illicit drugs have been taken in pregnancy and the immediate pre-labour period. However, obtaining an accurate substance use history is often fraught with imprecise maternal disclosures. Such behaviour can be linked to the social stigmatisation of drug misuse and the fear of the newborn being placed in foster care. Sensitive, but direct, further maternal questioning may be required, especially in cases of polysubstance use.

The withdrawal timelines for the common illicit substances have been well documented over recent years. Withdrawal from opiates and heroin can be evident in the newborn within hours of birth, whilst the effects of exposure to cocaine and amphetamine begins within 48 hours of birth (Wang 2010) (Wang, 2010) and withdrawal from methadone does not occur until 48–72 hours of age (Leggate, 2008) but it can be as long as 7–14 days before withdrawal is evident (Lall, 2008; Wang, 2010). The longer half-life of methadone is known to prolong and increase the severity of the withdrawal symptoms. Neonatal abstinence syndrome (NAS) is often considered the foremost adverse condition for the newborn of the substance-misuse mother; however, the effects upon fetal brain development have far more significant and long-lasting consequences. Substance use in the first 20 weeks of pregnancy can cause disruption in the cytogenesis and cell migration processes. In the subsequent weeks of pregnancy, cell differentiation and overall brain growth can be disturbed (Wang, 2010), including midline defects and congenital heart defects (Mone et al., 2004).

NAS indicates multisystem involvement, resulting in a cascade of symptoms. Fetal growth is disrupted, resulting in growth restriction which can independently place the newborn at greater risk of co-morbidity (Smith et al., 2006). Normal neurobehavioural function is altered resulting in a display of central nervous system instability, abnormal feeding behaviour, respiratory compromise and gastrointestinal symptoms (Volpi-Wise, 2005; Hamden, 2009). Seizure activity can manifest as a late-onset symptom of diazepine withdrawal.

NAS can occur with prescribed maternal medication. Morphine-based analgesia for long-term protracted pain management and psychotropic drugs for mental illness are the most common. The social context of the mother requiring morphine for long-term pain in many cases differs from that of the illicit substance user. Nonetheless, a sensitive approach is required with these parents when reiterating information about the clinical presentation of NAS, as they will have already received information in the prenatal period.

Where maternal substance use is known, it may be prudent for midwives and neonatal nurses to refer the examination to a senior paediatrician as the newborn will require a more thorough examination to assess for withdrawal symptoms.

Risk factors and the newborn examination

Intergenerational traits may indicate an inheritance risk to the newborn. History taking may elicit such conditions (see Chapter 7). However, they may have already been identified in prenatal period, particularly the haemoglobinopathies, e.g. thalassaemia or sickle cell disease. The UK NSC Antenatal Screening Programme performs well in such cases. Additional risk factors can be isolated through application of the *NIPE Standards and Competencies* (NSC, 2008). Table 1.4 presents the four screening components from the NIPE Standards document and demonstrates conditions that carry a predictive risk, as well as other conditions that may have a positive family trait.

It can be argued that some elements of the newborn screening agenda perform poorly in terms of predictive risk based on clinical examination alone. The newborn screen examination does have its limitations. The most common example is current screening techniques for congenital heart defects (CHD) (see also Chapter 2). It is estimated that 50% of CHDs are not detected in the newborn period (Wren et al., 2007; Sharland, 2010). Despite prenatal cardiac screening as part of the fetal anomaly scan and the clinical cardiovascular assessment at the newborn screen examination, current methods of detection do not compete on merit as an effective screening tool. This is particularly the case for critical duct-dependent anomalies (Abu-Harb et al., 1994; Green and Oddie, 2008; Ewer et al., 2012). Sharland (2010) confers that the majority of congenital cardiac anomalies lie within low-risk factions. However, a positive family history does correlate with a higher incidence (Romano-Zelekha et al., 2001).

The use of pulse oximetry as an additonal tool in the newborn and screening examination may improve the detection rate of critical CHD for some newborns. There is compelling and increasing evidence to support the use of pulse oximetry as an adjunct to the newborn examination (Knowles et al., 2005; Thangaratinam et al., 2012; Valmari, 2007; Ewer et al., 2012), thereby increasing the sensitivity of this screening tool overall.

Increased risk of cardiac anomalies related to newborn

- *Sibling*: Recurrence of 2–3% in a subsequent sibling increasing to a 50% recurrence rate in three affected siblings.
- *Parental cardiac anomaly*: 2–5% risk to infant.
- *Maternal diabetes*: 2% risk to infant particularly in uncontrolled diabetes.
- *Drug related teratogens*: For example, phenytoin, 2% risk to infant (adapted from Sharland, 2010).
- *Intrinsic fetal anomalies*: Incidence increased in the presence of other fetal structural or chromosomal anomalies, e.g. the triad of trisomies 21, 18 and 13.
- *Transplacental viral transmission*: Increased risk of CHD.
- *Parental consanguinity*: Increased risk of CHD (Ramegowda and Ramachandra, 2006; Khalid et al., 2006).
- Psychotropic drugs: Teratogenic and newborn effects, e.g. paroxetine may increase the risk of ventricular septal defect, lithium may increase the risk of Ebstein's anomaly.

Other common traits within families are atopy and asthma (Moore et al., 2004; Wadonda-Kabondo et al., 2004). These conditions can be of concern to parents and are often raised at the time of the newborn examination. Devereux et al. (2002) reported that maternal environmental factors could influence the fetal immune system and thus neonatal immunity resulting in an increased risk

Table 1.4 Predictive risk factors with potential impact upon newborn outcome.

The four NIPE Screening elements and others	Risk factors	Specific condition	Intergenerational trait status
Examination of the hips	First-degree relative with DDH Risk factors: persistent breech presentation or breech delivery Local policy risk factors, e.g. oligohydramnios, severe talipes, multiple birth	Developmental dysplasia of the hips	Positive
Examination of the eyes	First-degree relative with congenital eye condition	Congenital cataracts if associated with syndromes Glaucoma retinoblastoma	Positive
Examination of the heart	First-degree relative with CHD Major CHD on fetal anomaly scan Previous SIDS	Congenital heart defect Cardiac conduction mechanism disorders, e.g. prolonged QT syndrome, Wolf–Parkinson–White syndrome	Positive (dependent on cause)
Examination of the testes	Isolated finding	Unilateral or bilateral undescended testes – bilateral very significant	Positive
Significant others	Siblings First-degree relative Intergenerational	Chromosomal aberrations Genetic disorders Structural anomalies Syndromes Inborn errors of metabolism	Positive
	First-degree relative First-degree relative (sibling)	Severe congenital hearing deficit Jaundice treated with phototherapy	Positive Positive
	First-degree relative	Atopy: Dermatitis Eczema Epidermolysis bullosa	Positive
	First-degree relative	Asthma	Positive (multi-factorial variables – genetic, environmental)
	Intergenerational	Haemoglobinopathies, e.g. thalassaemia, sickle cell disease	Positive
	First-degree relative	Tongue tie	Positive
	Intergenerational	Marfan syndrome	Positive
	Intergenerational/first-degree relative	Myasthenia gravis	Positive

of atopy and asthma. Similarly, Moore et al. (2004) cited ethnicity, gender, gestational age at birth and family history, particularly maternal, as factors influencing the development of atopic dermatitis within the first 6 months of life. Such findings can confirm the genetic disposition of these disorders.

The NIPE Screening Monitoring and Reporting Tool (SMART) IT system provides a field containing the seven national risk factors mapped to the UK NSC Antenatal and Newborn Screening Programme. The NIPE Standards stipulate that 'family history' should be confined to a first-degree relative (UK NSC, 2008). Additional local risk factors, e.g. BCG vaccination requirement, maternal GBS infection, sibling with jaundice at birth, can be added to the risk factor menu for each individual maternity unit (see Introduction). The system provides data collection for audit purposes and the provision of key performance indicator (KPI) data against the NIPE national standards screening elements for quality assurance purposes and local performance monitoring. Most importantly, the system provides a 'failsafe' process to ensure that mothers and fathers are offered the newborn screen examination to avoid reportable incidents of 'missed' examinations.

The safety net for additional screening remains with the examiner at the time of the newborn physical examination to determine any further element of risk with the clinical assessment.

The psychosocial and safeguarding agenda

Parental psychosocial influences and adverse lifestyle choices have consistently demonstrated an impact upon the outcome for newborn infants, throughout childhood and into adulthood in terms of psychopathology morbidity (Hien and Honeyman, 2000; Maughan et al., 2001; Dawson, 2003; Disney et al., 2008) and mortality in extreme cases (Victoria Climbié Inquiry (Lord Laming Chair, 2003)). There are extensive and varied socio-demographic variables incorporated, which indicate the complexity of the subject matter (see the website that accompanies this book for more information on safeguarding). Co-morbidities exist between smoking, alcohol and substance misuse, domestic violence, maternal depression and adverse social environments, which place the newborn at a greater risk of maladaptive behaviours in childhood and adulthood that can replicate that of the parents (Leonard et al., 2007). Therefore, the aim of social support and intervention strategies in the prenatal period and beyond is to break the cycle. Previous discussions in this chapter surrounding all forms of substance addiction leave the newborn examiner in no doubt as to why women with such addictions require targeting in the immediate postnatal period as much as the antenatal period. See Table 1.5 for a summary of fetal and newborn outcome adverse effects related to lifestyle.

Maternal depression will be of significant interest to the newborn examiner. The use of psychotropic drugs can have an effect upon the newborn in relation to withdrawal symptoms (NICE, 2007; Wang 2010). In comparison to withdrawal

Table 1.5 Summary of defined and national risk factors.

Antenatal and Newborn Screening Programme risk factors	Additional defined risk factors
First-degree relative with DDH or hip problem in infancy or childhood	Maternal GBS positive status in current pregnancy/risk of early-onset neonatal infection
Breech presentation at birth or after 36 weeks gestation	Meconium-stained liquor present in labour
First-degree relative with a congenital heart defect	Risk of haemolytic disease in the newborn
First-degree relative with a congenital eye condition	Sibling with neonatal jaundice requiring phototherapy
Major cardiac defect detected on ultrasound scan	Neonatal BCG vaccine required
Major abnormality detected on ultrasound scan	
Maternal Hepatitis B, HIV, syphilis or rubella infection	
Family history of metabolic disease particularly MCADD	

behaviours in the newborn from illicit substances, the effects from antidepressant medication, particularly the selective serotonin reuptake inhibitors (SSRIs), are perhaps better defined (Sanz et al., 2005; Wang, 2010). The NICE Antenatal and Postnatal Mental Health guideline quick reference guide (National Collaborating Centre for Maternal Health, 2007) provides a useful table which contains the pertinent drug therapy for each psychopathological condition. This is very helpful to the newborn examiner who is perhaps unsure of the significance of such drugs taken during pregnancy. In summary of this document, the following drugs do have a known teratogenic effect upon the embryo in the first trimester:

- *Lithium*: Increased risk of fetal cardiac anomalies including Ebstein's anomaly. High levels in breast milk.
- *Valproate*: Increased risk of neural tube defects, altered cognitive development in childhood.
- *Carbamazepine*: Increased risk of neural tube defects, major fetal malformations including gastrointestinal tract and cardiac anomalies.
- *SSRIs*:
  - *Paroxetine*: Fetal cardiac anomalies
  - *Fluoxetine*: Lowest known risk during pregnancy but high levels in breast milk
- *Benzodiazepines*: Cleft palate and other fetal anomalies, 'floppy baby' syndrome in the neonate.
- *Tricyclic antidepressants (TCAs)*: For example, amitriptyline has the lowest level of risk in pregnancy.
  Adapted from NICE (2007).

Within the antidepressant medication range, the SSRIs demonstrate the lowest level of risk in terms of withdrawal in the newborn period (Wang, 2010). Nevertheless, paroxetine, which is an SSRI, does cause mild withdrawal symptoms, which include jitteriness and signs of respiratory distress (Sanz et al., 2005;

Murray et al., 2007). Sanz et al. (2005) reported a higher incidence of withdrawal from paroxetine compared to fluoxetine (Prozac). Paroxetine is also associated with a higher incidence of ventricular septal defects (Stiskal et al., 2001; Health Canada, 2005).

The newborn examiner must firstly establish when the mother commenced the medication, and, secondly, check if the mother is still taking medication. There is an associated risk to the mother if she has abruptly stopped taking the medication at any point without seeking medical advice. This is particularly relevant in the immediate postnatal period and may predispose her to active postnatal depression. If the mother is still taking medication, then the newborn must have a thorough neurological examination. There is some debate as to whether withdrawal from antidepressant medication in the newborn is more of a toxicity reaction (NICE, 2007; Wang, 2010) to the drug as opposed to active drug withdrawal, which would increase the severity and prolong the severity of the symptoms.

Maternity services may have local guidelines in place for postnatal observation on newborns of mothers who have been prescribed antidepressant medication in pregnancy particularly during the latter stages.

In summary, the newborn examiner has the opportunity to observe the behavioural interactions between a mother and her newborn at the time of the newborn examination. Any concerns about abnormal attachment behaviour must be relayed to the midwife caring for the mother and newborn, in the first instance. The level of concern may necessitate the activation of the 'Safeguarding' pathway.

Public policy, with reference to Safeguarding, has rapidly changed the landscape of history taking. Having been brought into sharp focus on a national scale over the last 20 years since the advent of the Cleveland Report (1988) and the Children's Act of 1989, this issue is high on the agenda within maternity and paediatric services (DH, 2004). Evaluation of the family psychosocial background is an important facet of the newborn examination as it is at any other time in childhood. It is the responsibility of the newborn examiner to raise any concerns that have not already been addressed with the Safeguarding named midwife. Once this process is activated, the safety of that newborn will become paramount.

Paternal information is often viewed as a lesser priority. However, the father's date of birth is an important demographic in tracing any previous safeguarding issues or domestic violence should concerns be raised. With the date of birth, the police protection services can investigate any previous convictions or concerns. With the movement of some population groups around the country and the fluidity of family units within society, male partners may move from one family unit to another and not disclose any information about previous relationships, e.g. SIDS, congenital anomalies or previous child deaths. It is also important to know the names and dates of birth of other siblings even when not biologically belonging to the mother of the new infant.

It is vital that all aspects of Safeguarding are considered and applied during the history-taking process for the newborn screen examination. All significant information must be made available and shared between health professionals including neonatal and paediatric community teams and other multidisciplinary organisations involved in the protection of children. Lack of communication has been cited as a common and sadly repetitive failing of the 'Safeguarding Children' systems (*The Victoria Climbié Inquiry Report*) (House of Commons Health Committee, 2003; CEMACH, 2008; Haringey Local Safeguarding Children Board, 2008; CQC, 2009; NPSA, 2009).

Parental dialogue and involvement with the newborn assessment process

Women and their partners may already have concerns about their newborn at the start of the examination. These concerns may have a physical or behavioural focus. The history-taking process must include discussion with the mother and father, if present, prior to commencing the examination and invited to share those concerns. Some of these concerns may be delayed until the examination is completed. The dialogue regarding family history or worries demonstrates a collaborative approach to the examination and many mothers and fathers welcome the opportunity to engage with this aspect of their newborn's care. The history-taking interview for some parents can be therapeutic as they have a staff member who is more than willing to listen.

History taking following the NIPE Standards (UK NSC, 2008) for the examination of the newborn can be used to gain more information from the mother and father if present as detailed in Table 1.6. If the mother or father was adopted, then gaining a thorough family history will be problematic; therefore, a sensitive approach will be required.

The involvement of mothers and fathers in such conversations will not only engage them with the examination but also engender an early sense of responsibility for their newborn. Blake (2008) advocates the empowerment of women to examine their newborns, thereby making an active contribution to the assessment of the neonate. This level of participation can enhance the women-centred care experience for many mothers as well as helping to lessen the incidence of abnormalities which are missed at the newborn screen examination. Many women and their partners examine their newborn in detail and can often be the authority on many aspects of their newborn's external appearance and behaviour.

The culture within maternity care services requires implementation of the concept by Blake (2008) from a health promotion perspective. In the first instance, a time line exists within those initial stages of newborn care and surveillance where mothers and fathers must assume responsibility for the

Table 1.6 Maternal/paternal lifestyle and psychosocial influences.

Lifestyle	Fetal effect	Potential neonatal and childhood outcome
Smoking	Spontaneous abortion Altered placental morphology Chronic hypoxia Intrauterine growth restriction (IUGR)	Abnormal newborn neurobehaviour Increased risk of infant irritability Hypertonia Childhood behavioural problems Lowered immunity SIDS, RSV infection Lower respiratory tract infections Altered pulmonary function Childhood asthma Increased risk of tobacco dependency in adulthood
Alcohol use	Fetal alcohol syndrome (FAS) IUGR	FAS Fetal alcohol disorder spectrum Behavioural problems
Substance misuse	Risk of transplacental transmission of Hepatitis B and C Congenital anomalies Symmetrical IUGR Prematurity Meconium liquor	Neonatal Abstinence syndrome
High-conflict relationships: domestic abuse	Intrauterine death Increased risk of acute obstetric complications which impact on newborn outcome	Child abuse Cognitive psychological impairment Childhood depression
Parent in care system		Increased risk of infant in care system Increased risk of child neglect

Data sources: Hien and Honeyman (2000), Maughan et al. (2001), Dawson et al. (2003), Disney et al. (2008).

welfare of their newborn. Therefore, they must be advised of the signs of illness and indicators for concern prior to discharge. This could have the following advantages:

- Possible earlier detection of CHD in the postnatal period.
- Probable earlier recognition of illness and a medical review by the general practitioner sought more promptly.
- Potential to prevent sudden infant death syndrome in infants with subtle symptoms of illness.

Currently, maternity services facilitate early and very early discharge options for mothers and newborns; therefore, parental awareness of the signs of illness and points of contact must be reprioritised within the health promotion agenda for the newborn screen examination.

Parental concern during the examination in relation to the cosmetic aspects of any minor findings and is often of great significance to them. The practitioner

Table 1.7   Common parental concerns at the newborn examination.

Syndactyly
Polydactyly
Feeding issues, e.g. vomiting
Mild talipes previously undiagnosed on ultrasound scan
Tongue tie
Skin tags
Sinuses
Birthmarks
Pseudo-menstruation
Moulding
Caput
Cephalhaematoma
Birth trauma markings
Intergenerational eczema, dermatitis and asthma
Intergeneration conditions and syndromes
Congenital abnormalities in first-degree relatives

must be able to recognise what is a minor variant in comparison to possible clinical dysmorphology. There are some physical findings, which may be a familial trait, e.g. syndactyly or polydactyly. See Table 1.7 for a list of common parental concerns found at the newborn screen examination. The practitioner must keep an open mind to the possibility of 'subtle' dysmorphic findings indicating a possible syndrome in the presence of other abnormal clinical features. There may be a contextual basis for this result, e.g. familial; therefore, examiners must assess the complete prenatal and postnatal history before seeking a senior paediatric option or expert review.

Interpretation of the information

Aside from the psychosocial skills of history taking, the ability of the examiner to interpret the information being given in a relevant way is just as significant. The history profile is only as good as the facts that are given and acknowledged as pertinent. The mother and father of the newborn may not recognise the significance of the questions being asked specific to family history. Some may be unaware of intergenerational traits within the family or of its significance to the newborn if there was. Romitti (2007) commented on the accuracy of reporting family history by relatives. Interestingly, some mothers did not always disclose that they had a previous child with a birth defect, and also the nature of the defect was not always accurately named. Socio-demographic variables did influence the accuracy of detail given. However, factual details from the family are often confounded by their own understanding of the condition and their description of the condition or defect when medical terminology is not used. Indeed, they may not be clear on the exact position of the affected member in the family tree. It is not uncommon for a mother or father to contact other family members at the time of the newborn screen examination to obtain more information about conditions within the family.

As with many families who do have a positive trait for congenital anomalies or conditions, constructing the aetiology of the family from the environmental or genetic predisposition is often difficult. If a detailed family history is needed in the case of a positive intergenerational trait, then it may be desirable for the examination to be conducted by a senior paediatrician.

Importance of location for the newborn physical examination

The location of the examination is crucial to the quality of the history-taking discussion with the mother or both parents. The postnatal ward is not a benign environment as the majority are bustling and noisy and not conducive to a history interview. Women may not disclose sensitive information in this environment for fear of being overheard by other patients and health-care workers. Disclosure of domestic violence within the high-impact family relationship can be prohibited due to lack of privacy. Indeed, the presence of the father or other family members may also prevent disclosures of abuse. Patient confidentiality is paramount within the health service. Equally, noise is a distracting feature for both the examiner and the mother. The maternity services of the future may need to revise the existing provision for the examination of the newborn to accommodate an environment that provides privacy and quietness.

Electronic as well as written documentation should acknowledge and reflect that a detailed history has been taken. The use of a history sheet to record the pertinent history themes and significant risk factors can be used. The history sheet can then be placed in the newborn's medical records as evidence of the history-taking process.

Limitations to history taking

This chapter has addressed the elements of the history-taking assessment in order to inform the newborn screen examination. However, there are obstacles that may present and complicate the process. The two most common problems are time and the environment. These two elements alone can have a significant impact upon the quality and outcome of the history-taking exercise. The workload pressures endured by many newborn examiners impact upon the time available to perform the examination (Table 1.8).

Table 1.8   Limitations to effective history taking.

Time constraints in relation to excessive workload
Inappropriate questions
Questioning technique, e.g. manner
Misrepresentation of facts given about family history
Environment in which history is being obtained, e.g. noise
Confidentiality
Lack of privacy
Suppression of disclosure due to partner presence
Equality and diversity issues, e.g. language barriers, understanding, cultural diversity, disability, maternal
  deafness
Misinterpretation of information given

There are other barriers that can compromise the quality of history taking. The questioning technique, manner and general communication skills of the examiner can compromise the level of information imparted by the mother or both parents who may interpret the line of questioning as invasive, particularly at a sensitive time after childbirth. Conversely, they may have something to hide and fear probing questions. The language barrier has become an increasing problem for many minority groups. All maternity units have access to interpretation services and the 'Screening Tests for You and Your Baby' booklet is available in a variety of languages. Mothers with hearing disabilities must also be accommodated with a sign language representative.

The evidence base to support the varied facets of the newborn examination may be developing, but examination of the newborn practitioners must continue to acknowledge the importance of an evidence base to underpin and validate practice. Therefore, practitioners must engage with current empirical evidence and embrace the research process. As the body of midwives and neonatal nurses who are trained to conduct the newborn screen examination is relatively small, in comparison to our medical colleagues, it is important that we contribute to the evidence in order to take practice initiatives forward.

Conclusion

Good history taking has always underpinned effective medicine. However, the nature of the history profile has changed through the incorporation of government directives and a public policy agenda. The UK NSC Antenatal and Newborn Screening Programme can be mapped to the history-taking process to help guide the practitioner towards gathering the relevant information. Whilst the maternal obstetric, surgical and medical history remains firmly implicit with the history-taking process, the psychosocial agenda now reflects the challenges facing families coupled with today's parental lifestyle choices. It can be strongly argued that parental psychosocial influences can impact directly upon not only the newborn period but also childhood and indeed adulthood. The newborn physical examination provides a platform to address some of these issues so that interventional measures can be implemented at an early stage. This may go some way to help direct parents and safeguard the vulnerable newborn, thereby protecting the health of a future generation. History taking remains an active element of the newborn examination. Without it, the clinical validity of the newborn examination itself could indeed be negligible.

This chapter provides an overview and context of the changing and dynamic nature of history taking as part of the newborn physical examination. The following websites will provide additional specific information and resources:

Clinical Condition	Useful website
Congenital heart defect	http://www.nhs.uk/conditions/congenital-heart-disease/Pages/Introduction.aspx
	http://www.bhf.org.uk/healthcare-professionals.aspx?sc_id=FrontNAV-Healthcare
	http://newbornphysical.screening.nhs.uk/
	http://pathways.nice.org.uk/pathways/structural-heart-defects?fno=1
Developmental dysplasia of the hips	http://newbornphysical.screening.nhs.uk/
	http://www.steps-charity.org.uk/
Eye conditions	http://newbornphysical.screening.nhs.uk/
	http://www.rnib.org.uk/?gclid=CJOErMnopsACFSXKtAodUEcAWg
	http://www.nhs.uk/Conditions/Cataracts-childhood/Pages/Introduction.aspx
	http://www.nhs.uk/Conditions/retinoblastoma/Pages/Introduction.aspx
	http://www.childrenwithcancer.org.uk/News/retinoblastoma?gclid=CPKz6l3ppsACFabLtAodbBwANA
Undescended testes	http://www.nhs.uk/conditions/undescendedtesticles/Pages/Introduction.aspx
	http://www.nlm.nih.gov/medlineplus/ency/article/000411.htm
BCG vaccination	http://www.nidirect.gov.uk/bcg-vaccination
	http://www.nhs.uk/Conditions/vaccinations/Pages/bcg-tuberculosis-TB-vaccine.aspx
Metabolic diseases	http://www.bimdg.org.uk/site/index.asp
NICE and national guidance documents	
Antenatal and postnatal mental health: Clinical management and service guidance	https://www.nice.org.uk/Guidance/CG45
Antibiotics for early-onset neonatal infection: Antibiotics for the prevention and treatment of early-onset neonatal infection	http://www.nice.org.uk/guidance/CG149

Neonatal jaundice	http://pathways.nice.org.uk/pathways/neonatal-jaundice?fno=1
CHD	http://pathways.nice.org.uk/pathways/structural-heart-defects?fno=1
Reducing differences in the uptake of immunisations	http://www.nice.org.uk/guidance/PH21
Drug misuse – opioid detoxification	http://www.nice.org.uk/guidance/CG52
UK NSC Antenatal and Newborn Screening Programmes	http://fetalanomaly.screening.nhs.uk/
	http://infectiousdiseases.screening.nhs.uk/
	http://sct.screening.nhs.uk/
	http://cpd.screening.nhs.uk/nipe
	http://newbornphysical.screening.nhs.uk/
	http://newbornbloodspot.screening.nhs.uk/
	http://hearing.screening.nhs.uk/

References

Abu-Harb M, Hey E, Wren C (1994) Death in infancy from unrecognised heart disease. *Archives of Disease in Childhood* **71**, 3–7. Available from: www.fn.bmj.com (accessed July 2014).

Anderson ME, Johnson DC, Batal HA (2005) Sudden infant death syndrome and prenatal maternal smoking: rising attributed risk in the back to sleep era. *BMC Medicine* **3**, 4. Available from: http://www.biomedcentral.com/1741–7015/3/4 (accessed July 2014).

Battin M, Sadler L (2010) Neonatal intensive care utilization and neonatal outcome of infants born to women aged 40 years and over in New Zealand. *Acta Paediatrics* **99**(2), 219–224. Available from: http://onlinelibrary.wiley.com/doi/10.1111/j.1651-2227.2009.01581.x/epdf (accessed February 2015).

Baxter JK, Sehdev HM, Breckenbridge MD (2010) Oligohydramnios. eMedicine Radiology. Available from: http://emedicine.medscape.com/article/405914-overview (accessed July 2014).

Bhattacharya S, Campbell DM, Liston WA, Bhattacharya S (2007) Effect of Body Mass Index on pregnancy outcomes in nulliparous women delivering singleton babies. *BMC Public Health* **7**, 168.

Blake D (2008) Assessment of the neonate: involving the mother. *British Journal of Midwifery* **16**(4), 224–226.

Bornstein MH, Putnick DL, Suwalsky JTD, Gini M (2006) Maternal chronological age, prenatal and perinatal history, social support and parenting of infants. *Child Development* **77**(4), 875–892.

Bradley JP, Bacharier LB, Bonfiglio J, Schechtman KB, Strunk R, Storch G, Castro M (2005) Severity of respiratory syncytial virus bronchiolitis is affected by cigarette smoke exposure and atopy. *Pediatrics* **115**, e7–e14

British Medical Association (2004) *Smoking and Reproductive Life; The Impact of Smoking on Sexual Reproductive and Child Health*. London: Board of Science and Education and Tobacco Control Resource Centre.

CareQuality Commission (2009) Review of the involvement and action taken by health bodies in relation to the case of Baby P. CQC. https://www.whittington.nhs.uk/document.ashx?id=1660 (accessed February 2015).

Carpenter RJ, Hale BR, Chan Tack M (2009) Early symptomatic HIV infection. *eMedicine*. Available from: http://reference.medscape.com/article/211873-overview (accessed February 2015).

CEMACH (2008) *Why Children Die: A Pilot Study*. London: CEMACH. Available from: www.cemach.org.uk.

CEMD (2002) *Why Mothers Die 1997–1999*. London: RCOG.

Cleveland Report (1988) *Report of the Inquiry into Child Abuse in Cleveland 1987*. Cmd 412. London: HMSO.

CMACE/RCOG (2010) *Joint Guidance: Management of Women with Obesity in Pregnancy*. London: Centre for Maternal and Child Enquires and Royal College of Obstetricians and Gynaecologists.

Dawson DA (2003) Methodological issues in measuring alcohol use. *Alcohol Research and Health* **27**, 18–29 http://pubs.niaaa.nih.gov/publications/arh27-1/18-29.htm

Department of Health (2004) National Service Framework for Children, Young People and Maternity Services. www.dh.gov.uk/en/healthcare/nationalserviceframewroks/childrenservices/childrenservicesinformation/dh_4089111 (accessed February 2015).

Devereux G, Barker RN, Seaton A (2002) Antenatal determinants of neonatal immune responses to allergens. *Clinical Experimental Allergy* **32**(1), 43–50.

DH (2007) *Maternity Matters: Choice, Access and Continuity of Care in a Safe Service*. London.HMSO Department of Health Available at: http://dera.ioe.ac.uk/9429/1/dh_074199.pdf (accessed August 2014).

Disney EAR, Iacono W, McGue M, Tully E, Legrand L (2008) Strengthening the case: prenatal alcohol exposure is associated with increased risk for conduct disorder. *Pediatrics* **122**, e1225-e1230.

Ewer AK, Furmston AT, Middleton LJ, Deeks JJ, Daniels JP, Pattison HM, Powell R, Roberts TE, Barton P, Auguste P, Bhoyar A, Thangaratinam S, Tonks AM, Satodia P, Deshpande S, Kumararatne B, Sivakumar S, Mupanemunda R, Khan KS (2012) Pulse Oximetry as a screening test for congenital heart defects in newborn infants: a test accuracy study with evaluation of acceptability and cost-effectiveness. *Health Technology Assessment* **16**(2), 1366–5278. Health Technology Assessment HTA Programme.

Gilliland, FD et al. (2001) Effects of maternal smoking during pregnancy and environmental tobacco smoke on asthma and wheezing in children *American Journal of Respiratory Critical Care Medicine*, **163**(2), 429–436.

Green RF (2007) Summary of working group meeting on use of family history information in pediatric primary care and public health. *Pediatrics*, **120**, S87–S100. http://www.pediatrics.org/cgi/content/full/120/supplement_2/s87 (accessed 16 February 2010).

Green K, Oddie S (2008) The value of the postnatal examination in improving child health. *Arch. Dis. Child. Fetal Neonatal Ed.* **93**: F389-F393.

Haines CJ, Rogers MS, Leung DH (1991) Neonatal outcome and its relationship with maternal age *Australian and New Zealand Journal of Obstetrics and Gynaecology* **31**(3), 209–212.

Hamden AH (2009) Neonatal Abstinence Syndrome. *eMedicine*. Available http://emedicine.medscape.com/article/978763-overview (accessed February 2015).

Haringey Local Safeguarding Children Board (2008) *Serious Case Review. Child A. Executive Summary*. London: Haringey Local Safeguarding Children Board.

Health Canada (2005) Important safety information on Paxil (paroxetine) and increased risk of cardiac defects following exposure during first trimester of pregnancy: for health professionals. GlaxoSmithKline, Inc. Available from: www.hc-sc.gc.ca (accessed July 2014).

Hien D, Honeyman T (2000) A closer look at the drug abuse: maternal aggression link. *Journal of Interpersonal Violence* **15**, 503. Available from: http://www.gsk.ca/english/docs-pdf/PAXIL_PregnancyDHCPL_E-V4.pdf (accessed February 2015).

Hofhuis W, de Jongste JC, Merkus PJFM (2003) Adverse health effects of prenatal and postnatal tobacco smoke exposure on children. *Archives of Disease in Childhood* **88**, 1086–1090. Available from: www.archdischild.com (accessed 20 January 2011).

House of Commons Health Committee (2003) *The Victoria Climbié Inquiry Report*. London: Stationery Office http://www.publications.parliament.uk/pa/cm200203/cmselect/cmhealth/570/570.pdf (accessed July 2014).

Howard FM (2008) History-taking and interview techniques and the physician–patient relationship. *Global Library of Women's Medicine* **1756–2228**. DOI: 10.3843/GLOWM.10411. Available from: http://www.glowm.com/index.html?p=glowm.cml/section_view&articleid=410 (accessed July 2014).

Jacobson SW, Chiodo LM, Sokol RJ, Jacobson JL (2002) Validity of maternal report of prenatal alcohol, cocaine, and smoking in relation to neurobehavioral outcome. *Pediatrics* **109**, 815–825. Available from: www.pediatrics.org (accessed July 2014).

Kalk P, Guthman F, Krause K, Delle K, Godes M, Gosing G, Halle H, Wauer R, Hocher B (2009) Impact of maternal mass index on neonatal outcome. *European Journal of Medical Research* **14**(5), 216–222.

Khalid Y, Ghina M, Fadi B, et al. (2006) Consanguineous marriage and congenital heart defects: a case–control study in the neonatal period. *American Journal of Medical Genetics. Part A* **140**(14), 1524–1530.

Khashan AS, Kenny LC (2009) The effects of maternal body mass index on pregnancy outcome. *European Journal of Epidemiology* **24**(11), 697–705.

Knowles R, Griebsch I, Dezateux C, Brown J, Bull C, Wren C (2005) Newborn Screening for congenital heart defects: a systematic review and cost-effectiveness analysis. *Health Technology Assessment HTA Programme* **9**(44).

La Souef PN (2000) Pediatric origins of adult lung diseases. 4. Tobacco related lung diseases begin in childhood. *Thorax* **55**, 1063–1067.

Lall A (2008) Neonatal abstinence syndrome. *British Journal of Midwifery* **16**(4), 220–223.

Landau LI (2001) Parental smoking: asthma and wheezing illnesses in infants and children. *Paediatric Respiratory Reviews* **2**, 202–206.

Leggate J (2008) Improving pregnancy outcomes: mothers and substance misuse. *British Journal of Midwifery* **16**(3), 160–165.

Leonard NR, Gwardz MV, Cleland CM, Vekaria PC, Ferns B (2007) Maternal substance use and HIV status: adolescent risk and resilience. *Journal of Adolescence* **3**, 389–405. Available from: www.sciencedirect.com (accessed July 2014).

Matturi L, Ottaviani G, Lavezzi AM (2006) Maternal smoking and sudden infant death syndrome: epidemiological study related to pathology. *Virchows Archiv* **449**(6), 697–706. Available from: www.springerlink.com/content/p50475078hpl0128 (accessed July 2014).

Maughan B, Taylor C, Taylor A (2001) Pregnancy smoking and childhood conduct problems: a causal association? *Journal of Child Psychology and Psychiatry* **42**(8), 1021–1028.

McMartin KI, Platt MS, Hackman R, et al. (2002) Lung tissue concentrations of nicotine in sudden infant death syndrome (SIDS). *Journal of Pediatrics* **140**, 205–209.

Mone SM, Gillman MW, Miller TL, Herman EH, Lipshultz SE (2004) Effects of environmental exposures on the cardiovascular system: prenatal period through adolescence. *Pediatrics* **113**(3), 1058–1069. Available at: http://pediatrics.aappublications.org/content/113/Supplement_3/1058.full (accessed August 2–14).

Moore M, Rifas-Shiman MPH, Rich-Edwards JW, Kleinman KP, Camargo CA, Gold D, Weiss ST, Gillman M (2004) Perinatal predictors of atopic dermatitis occurring in the first six months of life. *Pediatrics* **113**, 468–474. Available from: http://www.pediatrics.org/cgi/content/full/113/3/468 (accessed 12 January 2010).

Murray KC, Millar K, Pearson M (2007) Perinatal/neonatal n presentation. *Journal of Perinatalogy* **27**, 517–518.

National Collaborating Centre for Maternal Health (2007) *Antenatal and Postnatal Mental Health: The NICE Guideline On Clinical Management and Service Guidance*. London: NICE, for the British Psychological Society and the Royal College of Psychiatrists. www.nice.org.uk.

National Patient Safety Agency (2011) Rapid Response Report – keeping newborn babies with a family history of MCADD safe in the first few hours and days of life. Safety Alert 2. Available from: http://www.nrls.npsa.nhs.uk/resources/?EntryId45=132858 (accessed August 2014)

NHS ANSP (2008) Sickle cell and thalassaemia. Information for midwives. Available from: http://www.screening.nhs.uk.

NHS FASP (2010) Update on NIPD (Non-Invasive Prenatal Diagnosis. Available from: www.fetalanomaly.screening.nhs.uk (accessed July 2014).

NHS, Greater Manchester Public Health Network (2009) The Greater Manchester Down's Syndrome Screening Programme. Available from: www.northwest.nhs.uk (accessed July 2014).

NHS QIS (2008) Best practice statement: routine examination of the newborn. Available from: www.nhshealthquality.org (accessed July 2014).

NHSQIS (2004) Best Practice Statement: Routine Examination of the Newborn. Available from: www.nhshealthquality.org (accessed July 2014).

NICE (2006a) Routine Postnatal Care of Women and Their Babies. NICE clinical guideline 37. National Institute of Health and Care Excellence. Available from: www.nice.org.uk/CG037 (accessed July 2014).

NICE (2006b) Therapeutic Amnioinfusion for Oligohydramnios during Pregnancy (Excluding Labour). IPG 192. National Institute of Health and Care Excellence. Available from: www.nice.org.uk/guidance/IPG192 (accessed July 2014).

NICE (2007) *Intrapartum Care: Care of Healthy Women and Their Babies During Childbirth. Clinical Guideline.* London: RCOG Press. Available from: http://www.nice.org.uk/nicemedia/live/11837/36275/36275.pdf (accessed July 2014).

NICE (2010) Quitting smoking in pregnancy and following childbirth. Quick reference guide. National Institute of Health and Care Excellence. Available from: http://www.nice.org.uk/nicemedia/live/13023/49346/49346.pdf (accessed July 2014).

NICE (2012) NICE Clinical Guidance for Antibiotics for Early-Onset Neonatal Infections. National Institute of Health and Care Excellence. Available from: http://www.nice.org.uk/guidance/CG149/resources (accessed August 2014).

NPSA (2009) *Review of Patient Safety for Children and Young People.* London: NHS.

Ohlsson A, Shah VS (2009) Intrapartum antibiotics for known maternal Group B streptococcal colonization. *Cochrane Database of Systematic Reviews* **3**, CD007467. DOI: 10.1002/14651858. CD007467.pub2. Available from: http://mrw.interscience.wiley.com/cochrane/clsysrev/articles/CD007467/pdf_standard_fs.html (accessed July 2014).

Olson H, Streissguth A, Sampson P, Barr H, Bookstein F, Theide K (1997) Association of prenatal alcohol exposure with behavioural and learning problems in early adolescence. *Journal of the American Academy of Child and Adolescent Psychiatry* **36**(9), 1187–1194. Cited by Disney et al. (2008), Op cite.

Rajiah P (2009) Polyhydramnios. *eMedicine Radiology.* Available from: http://emedicine.medscape.com/article/404856-overview (accessed February 2015).

Ramegowda S, Ramachandra NB (2006) Parental consanguinity increases congenital heart diseases in South India. *Annals of Human Biology* **33**(5–6), 519–528.

RCOG (2003) Prevention of Early Onset Neonatal Group B Streptococcal Disease. Available from: http://www.rcog.org.uk/womens-health/clinical-guidance/prevention-early-onset-neonatal-group-b-streptococcal-disease-green- (accessed July 2014).

Roebuck TM, Mattson SN, Riley EP (1999) Behavioural and psychosocial profiles of alcohol-exposed children. *Alcoholism, Clinical and Experimental Research* **23**(6), 1070–1076 cited in Disney et al. (2008). Op cit.

Romano-Zelekha O, Hirsh R, Blieden L, Gree MS, Shohat T (2001) The risk of congenital heart defects in offspring of individuals with congenital heart defects. *Clinical Genetics* **59**, 325–329.

Romitti PA (2007) Utility of family history reports of major birth defects as a public health strategy. *Pediatrics* **120**, s71–s77. Available from: http://www.pediatrics.org/cgi/content/full/120/supplement_2/s71 (accessed July 2014).

Ryan K, Bain B, Worthington D, James J, Plews D, Mason A, Roper D, Rees DC, de la Salle B, Streetly A (2010) Significant haemoglobinopathies: guidelines for screening and diagnosis. *British Journal of Haematology* **149**, 35–49.

Salem L, Singer KR (2009) Rh incompatibility. *eMedicine*. Available from: http://emedicine.medscape.com/article/797150-overview (accessed February 2014).

Sanz EJ, Delas-Cuevas C, Kiuru A, Bate A, Edwards R (2005) Selective serotonin receptor uptake inhibitors in pregnant women and neonatal withdrawal syndrome: a data analysis. *Lancet* **365**(9458), 482–487.

Sayal K (2007) Alcohol consumption in pregnancy as a risk factor for later mental health problems. *Evidence-Based Mental Health* **10**, 98–100.

Sayal K, Heran J, Golding J, Alati R, Smith GD, Gray R, Emond A (2009) Binge pattern of alcohol consumption during pregnancy and childhood mental health outcomes: longitudinal population-based study. *Pediatrics* **123**(2), E289–E296. Available from: http://pediatrics.aapublications.org/cgi/contnent/abstract/123/2/e289 (accessed July 2014).

Sebire NJ, Jolly M, Harris JP, Wadsworth J, Joffe M, Beard RW, Regan L, and Robinson S (2001) Maternal obesity and pregnancy outcome: a study of 287,213 pregnancies in London. *International Journal of Obesity & Related Metabolic Disorders: Journal of the International Association for the Study of Obesity* **25**(8), 1175–1182.

Sellwood M, Huertas-Ceballos A (2008) Review of NICE guidelines on routine postnatal infant care. *Archives of Disease in Childhood. Fetal And Neonatal Edition* **93**, F10–F13. Available from: www.fn.bmj.com (accessed July 2014).

Sharland G (2010) Fetal cardiac screening: why bother? *Archives of Disease in Childhood. Fetal And Neonatal Edition* **95**, F64–F68. Available from: www.fn.bmj.com (accessed July 2014).

Skills for Health (2004) *National Workforce Framework for Maternity and Care of the Newborn*. London: Department of Health. Available from: https://tools.skillsforhealth.org.uk/suite/show/id/23 (accessed July 2014).

Smith LM, LaGasse, Derauf C, Grant P, Shah R, Arria A, Huestis M, Haning W, Strauss A, Grotta SD, Liu J, Lester BM (2006) The infant development, environment and lifestyle study: Effects of prenatal methamphetamine exposure, polydrug exposure, and poverty on intrauterine growth. *Pediatrics* **118**, 1149–1156. Available from: http://www.pediatrics.org/cgi/content/full/118/3/1149 (accessed July 2014).

Stiskal PA, Kulin N, Koren G, Ho T, Ho S (2001) Neonatal paroxetine withdrawal syndrome. *Archives of Disease in Childhood. Fetal And Neonatal Edition* **84**, F134–F135. Available from: http://fn.bmj.com/content/84/21 (July 2014).

Stocks J, Dezateux C (2003) The effects of parental smoking on lung function and development during infancy. *Respirology* **8**, 266–285.

Stoeckle JD, Billings JA (1987) A history of history-taking. *Journal of General Internal Medicine* **2**(2), 119–127.

Thangaratinam S, Brown K, Zamora J, Khan KS, Ewer AK (2012) Pulse Oximetry:screening for critical congenital defects in asymptomatic newborn babies: a systematic review and meta analysis. *Lancet* **379**(9835), 2459–2464.

UK NHS Fetal Anomaly Screening Programme (2010) http://fetalanomaly.screening.nhs.uk/ (accessed February 2015).

UK NSC (2006a) Fetal Anomaly Ultrasound Screening Flow Chart. Available from: http://www.screening.nhs.uk/fetalanomaly/home.htm (accessed 15 July 2014).

UK NSC (2006b) Statement on Soft Markers on the 18–20 Week Anomaly Scan. Available from: http://www.screening.nhs.uk/downs/risk_recalculation_lepdf (accessed 15 July 2010).

UK NSC (2007) *Consent and Standards for Fetal Anomalies during Pregnancy 2007*. London: UK NSC.

UK NSC (2008) *Newborn and Infant Physical Examination: Standards and Competencies*. London: UK NSC. Available from: www.screening.nhs.uk/home.htm (accessed August 2014).

Ungerer RLS, Lincetto O, McGuire W, Saloojee HH, Gülmezoglu AM (2004) Prophylactic versus selective antibiotics for term newborn infants of mothers with risk factors for neonatal infection. *Cochrane Database of Systematic Review* **4**: CD003957. DOI: 10.1002/14651858. CD003957.pub2. Available from: http://www2.cochrane.org/reviews/en/subtopics/82.html (accessed July 2014).

Valmari P (2007) Should pulse oximetry be used to screen for congenital heart disease? *Archives of Disease in Childhood. Fetal And Neonatal Edition* **92**(3), F219–F224. Available from: www.fn.bmj.com (accessed July 2014).

Victoria Climbié Inquiry (Lord Laming Chair) (2003) Summary and Recommendations. HMSO.

Viegas OAC, Leong WP, Ahmed S, Ratham SS (1994) Obstetric outcome with increasing maternal age. *Journal of Biosocial Science* **26**, 261–267. Available from: http://journals.cambridge. org/action/displayAbstract;jsessionid=CED579E77A4611A7BA14B2F5C3D97E0A. tomcat1?fromPage=online&aid=1640316 (accessed July 2014).

Volpi-wise M (2005) Neonatal Abstinence Syndrome. Available from: http://bach.fhs.usyd.edu. austu/hse/iec/volpiwisem/html (accessed July 2014).

Wadonda-Kabondo N, Sterne JAC, Golding J, Kennedy CTC, Archer CB, Dunnill MGS (2004) Association of parental eczema, hayfever, and asthma with atopic dermatitis in infancy: birth cohort study. *Archives of Disease in Childhood* **89**, 917–921. Available from: www.adc.bmj.com (accessed July 2014).

Wang M (2010) Perinatal drug abuse and neonatal drug withdrawal. *eMedicine*. Available from: http://emedicine.medscape.com/article/978492-overview (accessed February 2015).

Wren C, Reinhardt Z, and Khawaja K (2007) Twenty-year trends in diagnosis of life-threatening neonatal cardiovascular malformations. *Archives of Disease in Childhood. Fetal And Neonatal Edition* **93**, 33–35. Available from: www.fn.bmj.com (accessed July 2014).

CHAPTER 2

Cardiovascular and respiratory assessment of the baby

Christopher D. Bedford[1] and Anne Lomax[2]

[1] Warrington and Halton Hospitals NHS Foundation Trust, Warrington, Cheshire, UK
[2] Department of Midwifery, University of Central Lancashire, Preston, UK

KEY POINTS

- Understanding the development of the heart and lungs in fetal life is central to the practitioner's effectiveness in recognition of abnormalities in transition to extrauterine life.

- Significant cardiac lesions may not be apparent at the first neonatal examination.

- An infant who is not feeding well or is not 'quite right' should be examined closely as it may be the first manifestation of congenital heart disease.

- All infants with chromosomal abnormalities should have an early echocardiogram.

- Post-ductal oxygen saturation at the time of the neonatal examination aids detection of congenital heart disease.

Introduction

It is essential that health-care practitioners involved in examination of the newborn understand the fetal development of the lungs and cardiovascular system and related circulatory and pulmonary events that occur during the transitional period from fetal to postnatal life. The majority of full-term healthy babies will have no difficulty during this time, but practitioners must be able to recognise evidence of smooth transition both in the first few hours following birth and for several weeks after. Informed assessment of physiological well-being and timely referral of any deviation is crucial in order to implement the most appropriate intervention.

Development of the lungs

The lungs and trachea develop as an outpouching of the foregut in the neck (Figure 2.1). This pouch grows down into the chest dividing into the bronchi

---

Examination of the Newborn: An Evidence-Based Guide, Second Edition. Edited by Anne Lomax.
© 2015 John Wiley & Sons, Ltd. Published 2015 by John Wiley & Sons, Ltd.
Companion Website: www.wiley.com/go/lomax/newborn

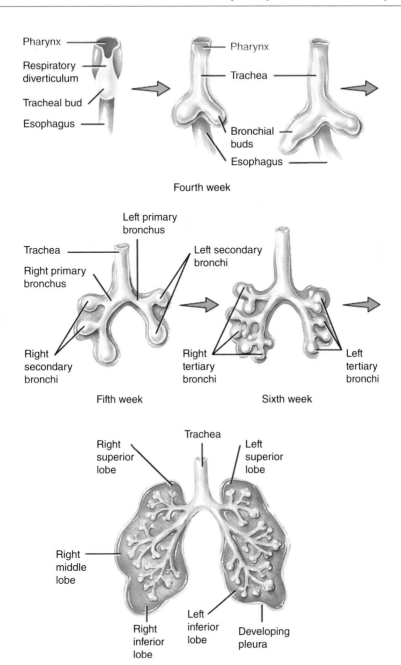

Fourth week

Fifth week   Sixth week

Eighth week

Figure 2.1 Development of the lungs. Source: Tortora and Derrickson (2009). Reproduced with permission of John Wiley & Sons.

and the smaller airways. By birth, all the divisions of the bronchiole tree have occurred and the lung surface area develops with the formation of the alveoli. This continues after birth. The cells of the surrounding mesoderm provide the blood vessels and supporting tissues. The trachea and bronchi are supplied by bronchial arteries from the dorsal aorta whilst the lung is supplied by the pulmonary arteries. Oxygenated blood from the lungs returns to the heart via the pulmonary veins. Two pulmonary veins from each lung enter the left atrium. Partial or total anomalous venous drainage occurs when one or more of the pulmonary veins fail to connect to the left atrium but join up with the systemic circulation either above or below the diaphragm.

Breathing movements occur *in utero* from about 10 weeks (Blackburn, 2007). The lungs are a source of amniotic fluid. From 24 weeks onwards, the pneumocytes lining the lungs start to produce surfactant. Prior to birth, the breathing stops and the production of amniotic fluid from the lung ceases, it is thought that the nature and function of the epithelial cells lining the alveoli undergo a change. Up to a few weeks before delivery, the epithelial cells carry out a secretory function that contributes to the already present amniotic fluid. Near to term, the same cells begin to absorb the fluid in preparation for the first breaths (Askin, 2009a). Reabsorption of lung fluid speeds up during labour and it is thought that a significant amount is removed this way before the first breath is taken. This process is aided by a surge of catecholamines occurring just before labour commences. At term, the lungs contain about 50 ml of fluid, about a quarter of this fluid is thought to be expelled as the chest wall is compressed during passage through the birth canal (Bhutani, 1997, Rudolph et al., 2003). After delivery, half is absorbed by the pulmonary lymphatics and the rest by the pulmonary capillaries. The amount of remaining lung fluid helps to partially distend the alveoli so that the opening pressure of the first breath can effectively expand the lungs.

Development of the heart

A study of the development of the heart helps to explain the origin of congenital heart disease (CHD). By the third week, the embryo is no longer able to exist on the passive diffusion of oxygen and nutrients alone. Blood vessels form in the mesoderm and the heart develops from two longitudinal strands or cords that canalise to form two endothelial tubes, which fuse to form a single primitive heart tube. The heart has two layers, the inner becomes the endocardium and the outer becomes the myocardium and the epicardium. From the twenty-first day, myocardial contractions occur in waves from what will be the atria to the truncus arteriosus.

The heart tube enlarges and by alternating dilatations and contractions, there is normal folding to the right. Separation of the atrioventricular canals, atria and

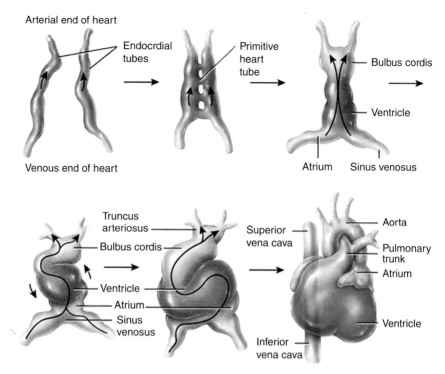

Figure 2.2 Development of the heart. Source: Tortora and Derrickson (2009). Reproduced with permission of John Wiley & Sons.

ventricles occurs around the middle of the fourth week and is completed by the end of the fifth week (Figure 2.2). Endocardial cushions bulge out from the centre of the dorsal and ventral walls and fuse in the centre of the heart tube. Lateral atrioventricular cushions form the heart tube walls and the endocardial cushions form the mitral and tricuspid valves. The atrium is divided by the septum primum and the septum secundum. A hole, the ostium primum, is left in the septum primum. Part of the septum primum degenerates to create a second hole, the ostium secundum. The ostium primum then closes and the septum secundum grows down to cover but not close the ostium secundum. This is the foramen ovale.

The ventricular septum separates the ventricle into the right and left ventricles a week after atrial separation. The final closure occurs once the truncus separates into the aorta and the pulmonary artery. The truncus arteriosus begins partition during the fifth week. The spiral septum fuses with the ventricular septum at the end of the seventh week. The aortic and pulmonary valves form from outgrowths of the endocardium. During early development of the embryo, neural crest tissue migrates into the future head and neck region. It forms six pairs of arched elevations called branchial or pharyngeal arches. These are penetrated by arteries called aortic arches. They connect the dorsal aorta to the truncus arteriosus. The six pairs of aortic arches change into the blood vessels of the head and neck. The fourth left arch becomes the arch of the aorta, whilst the sixth left and right arches become the left and right pulmonary arteries. The conducting system of the heart develops from the fifth week onwards and is functional by the tenth week, and sinus rhythm is apparent from 16 weeks.

As can be visualised, failure at any point will lead to abnormalities in the anatomy. For instance, if the endocardial cushions fail to join in the centre, this will lead to an atrioventricular defect with both atrial and ventricular septal defects (VSDs) and abnormal atrioventricular valves. If the spiral separation of the truncus arteriosus occurs abnormally, then the pulmonary artery will come off the left ventricle and the aorta off the right ventricle and the fetus will have transposition of the great vessels.

Transition to extrauterine life

During pregnancy, the placenta carries out thermal, metabolic, endocrine and immunological functions on behalf of the fetus. Following delivery, the neonate must make complex physiological changes in order to carry out these functions for itself. Major circulatory and pulmonary changes occur within the first few moments of extrauterine life but adaptation continues throughout the postnatal period. The relative resilience of the neonate during this time means that it may be difficult to recognise any underlying pathology. Practitioners need to be able to discriminate effectively between the benign clinical symptoms associated with smooth transition and the more serious pathological changes that require immediate intervention (Askin, 2009b).

Fetal circulation

In fetal life, the lungs are collapsed and fluid filled. As a consequence, pulmonary circulation is constricted, resulting in a circuit that provides a high resistance to incoming flow of blood. Respiratory gaseous exchange cannot, therefore, take place. Blood flow to the lungs is minimal in the fetus consisting of approximately 8% of the total cardiac output and utilised only to maintain lung growth and development (Mercer and Skovgaard, 2002). Thus, oxygenated blood from the placenta has to pass through the heart and into the systemic circulation without entering the lungs. It is able to do this because of four temporary anatomical structures (Figure 2.3):

- **The umbilical vein (UV)**, which brings oxygenated blood to the fetus from the placenta.
- **The ductus venosus (DV)**, which allows blood from the umbilical vein to enter into the inferior vena cava (IVC).

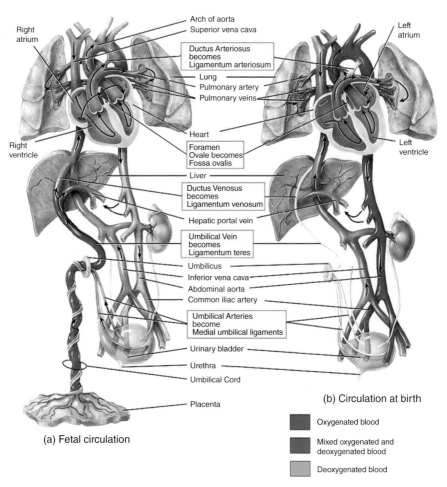

Right
atrium

Arch of aorta
Superior vena cava

Ductus Arteriosus
becomes
Ligamentum arteriosum

Lung
Pulmonary artery
Pulmonary veins

Heart

Foramen
Ovale becomes
Fossa ovalis

Liver

Ductus Venosus
becomes
Ligamentum venosum

Hepatic portal vein

Umbilical Vein
becomes
Ligamentum teres

Umbilicus
Inferior vena cava
Abdominal aorta
Common iliac artery

Umbilical Arteries
become
Medial umbilical ligaments

Urinary bladder

Urethra

Umbilical Cord

Placenta

Right
ventricle

Left
atrium

Left
ventricle

(b) Circulation at birth

(a) Fetal circulation

■ Oxygenated blood

■ Mixed oxygenated and
deoxygenated blood

□ Deoxygenated blood

Figure 2.3 Fetal and postnatal circulation. Source: Tortora and Derrickson (2009). Reproduced with permission of John Wiley & Sons.

- **The foramen ovale (FO)**, which acts as a pathway for fetal blood to flow directly from the right to the left-hand side of the heart.
- **The ductus arteriosus (DA)**, a muscular artery, which allows oxygenated blood to pass from the main pulmonary artery to the trunk of the aorta.

Blood from the placenta returns to the fetus via the umbilical vein. Approximately 80% of this richly oxygenated blood is diverted to the liver via the portal circulation. The rest is diverted through the ductus venosus, which allows blood from the umbilical vein to enter the IVC. Once in the IVC, the relatively well-oxygenated blood combines with deoxygenated blood coming from the lower half of the fetal body and some mixing occurs. However, as a result of its higher kinetic energy, the more richly oxygenated umbilical venous blood travels faster and, together with the slower moving deoxygenated blood, forms two streams in the IVC (Askin, 2009a). Once in the right atrium, most of the oxygenated blood is directed through the flap-like foramen ovale, which connects the two atria and acts as a flow distributor for the faster flowing stream (Kiserud, 2005). The direction of flow is also aided by the higher pressures that exist within the right ventricle due to the closed pulmonary circuit (Askin, 2009a). The faster stream then enters the left atrium where it mixes with a small amount of deoxygenated blood returning from the pulmonary veins. It then passes through the mitral valve and into the left ventricle. The blood is then ejected into the ascending aorta. In this way, the brain (via the carotid arteries) and the heart (via the coronary arteries) are able to receive well-oxygenated blood as a priority. A relatively small amount (approximately 10%) flows on through to the descending aorta (Blackburn, 2007).

The slower flowing column of inferior vena caval blood joins the blood draining from the superior vena cava in the right atrium and is directed through the tricuspid valve into the right ventricle. From here, this stream of blood is directed into the pulmonary artery where high resistance from the closed pulmonary circuit causes the majority of volume to be shunted across the ductus arteriosus into the descending aorta. Only a small amount (approximately 8% of the total cardiac output) is allowed to travel to the pulmonary bed to perfuse the lungs to support growth and development. In the descending aorta, the larger volume of right ventricular blood is joined by the small amount from the ascending aorta (Rudolph, 2009). Blood flows via the descending aorta to the low resistance systemic circulation and is returned to the placenta to be re-oxygenated via the two umbilical arteries.

Postnatal circulation

At birth, the cardiac output is redistributed. As the placenta separates, the volume of fetal blood it contained is now available to the neonatal circulation. Thus, the previously low resistance systemic volume is increased. The administration of oxytocic drugs together with early clamping of the umbilical cord at delivery is thought to interfere with the transfusion of blood from the placenta to the neonate. The resulting shortfall in volume transfer is considered to have an adverse effect on perfusion of the capillaries surrounding the alveoli in the pulmonary circulation. Adequate alveolar expansion, and consequently effective gaseous exchange, is therefore thought to be impaired (Mercer and Skovgaard cited in Davies and McDonald, 2008).

With the onset of respiration, blood flow to the pulmonary circuit is increased and expansion of the now air-filled alveoli causes the pulmonary vascular bed to dilate. This has the effect of lowering the high pulmonary vascular resistance that existed in fetal life.

Cessation of the placental circulation abolishes blood flow through the umbilical vein. Consequently, the reduction in blood flow through the ductus venosus causes it to constrict within minutes of birth. By 1 week of life, permanent closure of the ductus venosus has usually occurred in most full-term infants (Avery et al., 2005). After closure, the umbilical vein becomes the ligamentum teres and the ductus venosus becomes the ligamentum venosum.

Clamping of the cord and increase in blood flow through the pulmonary artery to the oxygenated lungs have the effect of lowering the pressure in the right side of the heart. An elevated blood flow to the lungs increases pulmonary venous return with the effect of raising the pressure on the left side of the heart. This closes the flap-like structure of the foramen ovale, and thus the two atria become separate. At this stage, the foramen ovale is not completely closed and a small right-to-left shunt may exist for several days, anatomical closure may take up to 9 months after birth (Blackburn, 2007). This structure then becomes known as the fossa ovalis. Closure of the ductus arteriosus at birth is stimulated by increasing oxygen levels. The duct becomes more and more sensitive to the constricting effect of oxygen in the weeks before birth. Moreover, around term, the duct begins to lose its sensitivity to the dilating effect of prostaglandin. High levels of prostaglandins and relatively low levels of oxygen allow the ductus arteriosus to remain open in utero. After birth, increased blood flow to the lungs facilitates increased prostaglandin metabolism and it is this combination of factors that cause the levels to fall (Askin, 2009a). The duct begins to close within a short time after delivery; however, shunting of blood through the duct can be present for several hours after birth and may present as a benign murmur on clinical examination. Usually, the ductus arteriosus has closed in full-term infants by 96 hours of age, obliteration of the duct can take up to 3–4 weeks. The ductus arteriosus then becomes a fibrous strand known as the ligamentum arteriosus. A patent ductus arteriosus following birth allows deoxygenated blood to cross from the right to left side of the heart. This can cause cyanosis and an audible murmur. All murmurs in the neonate must be reported and investigated immediately (Kenner and Wright Lott, 2007). Postnatally, the umbilical arteries are no longer required to transport blood and following closure become the lateral umbilical ligaments (Figure 2.3).

Delayed cord clamping in full-term healthy infants

The practice of delayed cord clamping has attracted renewed interest over the past decade.

In fetal life, the lungs are fluid filled and so it is thought that only about 10% of the total blood volume of the fetus is needed for their perfusion. At birth, air replaces the lung fluid as the baby takes its first breath. The pulmonary circulation then requires approximately four times that amount in order to prime the pulmonary circulation and open the alveoli ready to take over gaseous exchange from the placenta (Coggins and Mercer, 2009). Lung fluid is drawn from the alveolar pockets by osmosis as the small capillary network around each alveolus is filled (Mercer and Erickson-Owens, 2012).

The common practice of early cord clamping within a few seconds of birth is now thought to deprive the neonate of up to 20–40 ml/kg bodyweight of blood volume necessary to support the expanding pulmonary circulation (Palethorpe et al., 2010).

When this process is delayed by up to 3 minutes, or when pulsations cease, the placenta will continue to provide oxygen-rich blood to the baby for as long as the cord remains intact and pulsates; this ensures transfer of this much needed extra blood volume to the newborn. Moreover, in a randomised controlled trial in 2011, Andersson et al. concluded that delayed cord clamping improved ferritin levels with a benefit of between 4 and 6 month supply of iron and thus decreased the risk of iron deficiency anaemia (Andersson et al., 2011). Along with transfer of extra red blood cells, there is also transfer of haematopoietic stem cells; this contributes to improved tissue repair and strengthens the immunological system in the neonate.

The main benefits of delayed cord clamping can be found in the Cochrane review of 2013 'Effect of timing of umbilical cord clamping of term infants on maternal and neonatal outcomes' (McDonald et al., 2013).

The Resuscitation Council Guidelines (2010) have updated their guidance on delayed cord clamping, the guideline changes state that 'For uncompromised babies, a delay in cord clamping of at least 1 minute from the complete delivery of the infant is now recommended. As yet there is insufficient evidence to recommend an appropriate time for clamping the cord in babies who are severely compromised at birth. For babies requiring resuscitation, resuscitative intervention remains the priority' (Resuscitation Council Guidelines 2010, p119).

Mercer et al. have reviewed the practice of resuscitating the baby with the cord intact. They advance a theory that the pulsating cord can physiologically deliver much needed blood volume (and with it oxygen) from the placenta to the compromised infant, prolonging its function of gaseous exchange and thus supporting the baby through the resuscitation event (Mercer and Erickson-Owens, 2012). The authors go on to assert that any perceived risks of delayed cord clamping such as over-transfusion, hyperbilirubinaemia or polycythaemia have not been supported by recent research. More recently, the Royal College of Obstetricians and Gynaecologists published a Scientific Impact Paper in February 2015 which outlines a summary of the physiology of placental transfusion and reviews the evidence related to the timing of umbilical cord clamping (RCOG 2015).

Respiratory considerations

In order for effective respirations to be established at birth, the lungs need to be mature with adequate quantities of surfactant present within the alveoli. Pulmonary vascular resistance needs to be lowered to allow increased blood flow to the lungs for gaseous exchange. Fluid within the alveoli needs to be effectively cleared and replaced with air. Neurologic stimulus must ensure initiation and support of continuous respiration following birth (Avery et al., 2005).

Prior to birth, only about a tenth of the cardiac output goes through the lungs. As the lungs are inflated, the pulmonary circulation expands and the resistance to blood flow falls. As previously discussed, blood preferentially goes through the pulmonary arteries, returning oxygenated blood returns via the pulmonary veins to the left atrium and closes the foramen ovale. The rising oxygen concentration in the blood causes the muscular ring of the ductus arteriosus to contract and thus reduce then stop blood flow through the ductus arteriosus.

Once the baby is born, it starts to breathe. The first few breaths gradually inflate the lungs and over the next few hours, all parts of the lungs are aerated. However, high inspiratory pressures are needed to overcome the viscosity of the fluid-filled airways, the surface tension of the lung fluid and the resistance of the chest wall. The surfactant in the surface fluid of the lungs reduces the surface tension and stops the airways collapsing on expiration. As the alveoli inflate, the amount of surfactant per surface area diminishes and the surface tension rises, deflated alveoli have large amount of surfactant per surface area and low surface tension. Thus, there is natural balancing of alveoli size countering the effect of Laplace's law $P = 2T/r$, where P is the pressure, T is the tension in the wall of the sphere and r is the radius. Less pressure is needed to keep open larger spheres than smaller ones.

The first breath, therefore, requires pressures approximately 10–15 times higher than for subsequent breaths. Following these events, the work of breathing becomes easier. The first breaths help force the remaining fluid from the alveoli into the interstitial space where it is carried away by the lymphatic system (Alvaro and Rigatto, 2005). Any residual alveolar fluid is drained away over a period of 5–6 hours following birth.

Increased pulmonary blood flow also influences alveolar expansion. As mentioned previously, Mercer and Skovgaard (2002) reviewed the work of Jaykka, who proposed that increased pulmonary blood flow is essential to fill the network of capillaries that are attached by elastic fibres to the outside of each alveoli. Adequate blood volume would, therefore, pull the alveoli open, thus enhancing lung compliance and with it gaseous exchange. The onset of respiration is also stimulated by sensory elements such as cold, light noise and pain, as well as an accompanying rise in carbon dioxide levels.

As the lungs become responsible for gaseous exchange, the respiratory centre becomes more responsive to the resulting chemical changes and arterial oxygen levels rise and carbon dioxide levels fall over the first few days of life (Blackburn, 2007). Respirations are irregular during the first 15 minutes with respiratory rates between 60 and 80 breaths per minute (bpm). Respirations should quickly settle to between 30 and 60 bpm within the first 30 minutes (Thureen et al., 2004).

Impact of hypoglycaemia, hypoxia and hypothermia on transitional events

After birth the newborn must adapt to changes in environmental temperature and to the effects of heat loss by conduction, convection, radiation and evaporation. Even in the full-term healthy infant evaporative heat losses are high at delivery, particularly if the neonate is not properly dried after birth. Moreover, the neonate has a high surface area to body weight ratio, which also encourages heat loss. The newborn must overcome this by rapidly mobilising glucose sources in order to create heat. This process must be initiated rapidly after birth as subsequent cooling can have an adverse effect on the health of the newborn. Heat production in the newborn at this time is thought to increase twofold (Rudolph et al., 2003).

The primary mechanism of heat production in the neonate is through metabolism of brown fat or non-shivering thermogenesis as the newborn's capacity to create heat by shivering is very limited. Brown fat makes up approximately 6% of the neonate's total body weight and is well suited to create heat because of its capacity to metabolise glucose for energy production. Major locations for brown fat storage in the newborn are upper back and neck, mediastinum and around the kidneys (Boxwell, 2010). In fetal life, non-shivering thermogenesis is inhibited by placental factors. Clamping the umbilical cord at birth allows metabolism of brown fat and, therefore, heat production to take place. Cold receptors in the neonatal skin detect reductions in environmental temperature. The sympathetic nerve pathway is stimulated by norepinephrine which in turn activates brown fat metabolism. Brown fat contains a high store of triglycerides, which are broken down during the metabolic process to produce glycerol and fatty acids. It is the oxidisation of fatty acids that produces heat. This process is dependent on the presence of oxygen and glucose. So, as the body temperature falls, the consumption of oxygen and glucose increases, with further cooling, oxygen requirements will exceed the levels available in room air and the neonate will become cyanosed. Tachypnoea will develop as the neonate attempts to raise its oxygen levels.

The ambient temperature at which the neonate's oxygen consumption and metabolic rate are at a minimum is designated the 'thermal neutral range'. Within this thermal environmental range, the newborn does not need to generate additional heat through metabolic activity and can maintain a core temperature of between 36.5 and 37.3 °C with only minimal effort required (Blackburn, 2007). At delivery, therefore, midwives must provide an appropriate thermal environment to ensure that prolonged cooling does not occur.

Blood glucose levels in the neonate at birth are approximately 70–80% of maternal levels (Milcic, 2008), but maternal transfer of glucose ceases with clamping of the umbilical cord. Glucose is the main energy source needed for most metabolic pathways of the body, so the neonate must rapidly utilise its own glucose stores and be capable of producing additional glucose if adequate levels are to be maintained after birth. Hepatic glucose stores that were laid down in the last trimester of pregnancy are used up within a few hours as neonates are born into a relatively cold environment where, in particular, evaporative heat losses are high. Additionally, the neonatal brain is a significant consumer of available glucose because of the large head to body weight ratio (Rudolph et al., 2003). Within 1 hour of birth, glucose stores have dropped significantly but, in normal transition, begin to rise again by 3 hours of age. This happens because of an accompanying fall in insulin to help preserve glucose levels. In addition, the healthy full-term neonate can utilise alternative energy sources to ensure that fuel demands of the neonatal brain are adequately met. These physiological responses and consequent rise in blood glucose happen even if the newborn has not been fed (Ward-Platt and Deshpande, 2005).

A definition of acceptable glucose levels for the full-term healthy baby cannot be easily determined due to lack of research evidence in current literature. Blood glucose levels of 1.2–2.0 mmol/L or less in full-term neonates less than 24 hours old (2.2–2.8 mmol/L after 24 hours) have been put forward as the lowest levels acceptable before clinical intervention should be considered (Perrson, 2009).

Even full-term healthy newborns can develop hypothermia and consequently a degree of hypoxia. Practitioners must be aware of the importance of thermal and glycaemic maintenance at the time of birth and their interrelationship with hypoxic events. This interrelationship is probably best demonstrated through consideration of the energy triangle (Figure 2.4) (Aylott, 2006).

We have already acknowledged that hypothermia in the neonate will lead to rapid depletion of glucose stores and consequently an increase in oxygen consumption. Ultimately, demand for extra oxygen will outstrip the supply available

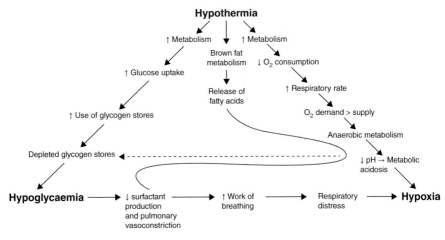

Figure 2.4 Integrated physiology underpinning the neonatal energy triangle. Source: Adapted from Aylott (2006). Reproduced with permission from Elsevier.

in room air leading to anaerobic metabolism of glucose. As a result, a state of metabolic acidosis will ensue. The existing hypoglycaemia along with this acidotic state will cause constriction of the pulmonary blood vessels and affect normal production of the surfactant in the alveoli. This will in turn exacerbate the respiratory problems by interfering with gaseous exchange and lowering arterial oxygen levels even further. Unattended, a rapid downward spiral of events will occur, and it is possible, in these adverse circumstances, that fetal circulatory channels could reopen allowing deoxygenated blood to flow directly from the right to the left side of the heart and into the aorta. This condition is known as persistent pulmonary hypertension of the newborn (PPHN) and can occur in both term and pre-term infants. In this situation, immediate intervention is necessary to ensure survival (Askin, 2009a). Prevention of excessive cooling after birth is, therefore, crucial. Maintenance of the thermal neutral range and initiation of early feeding in these first few hours will reduce the infant's energy expenditure and help ensure an uneventful transition to extrauterine life.

Prevention, anticipation and recognition of problems are key to ensuring a smooth transition from fetal to postnatal life. The importance of obtaining a comprehensive history of the mother and baby cannot be underestimated and has been outlined in Chapter 1. The practitioner must have a working knowledge of the underlying physiology of the neonate in order to recognise problems and respond appropriately. Neonates who manifest mild temporary transitional problems in the early stages may behave in exactly the same way clinically as those with more serious underlying illnesses. For instance, in cases of early infection, the neonate may manifest hypoglycaemia, hypoxia and hypothermia, giving rise to symptoms such as cyanosis, pallor, respiratory distress, hypotonia, poor handling and feeding (Aylott, 2006; Askin, 2009b). Early intervention and prompt referral in such cases are crucial, and effective referral pathways must be in place in order to facilitate this.

Examination of the cardiovascular and respiratory systems

The role of cardiovascular examination of the newborn is to detect CHD. The flow through the vascular system changes considerably over the postnatal period, and a single examination will not pick up all defects, so the infant's heart should be examined a number of times during the first weeks of life. With many infants leaving hospital within a few hours of birth, the mother and father need ready access to health professionals if they have concerns about their child. The astute practitioner will be alert to the features both in the history and in the examination that point to the potential diagnosis of CHD. Early detection and hence early treatment of serious CHD improve both the mortality and the long-term morbidity of the infant.

Table 2.1 Incidence of CHD.

Lesion	Mean incidence per million live births
Ventricular septal defect (VSD)	3,570
Patent ductus arteriosus (PDA)	799
Atrial septal defect (ASD)	941
Atrioventricular septal defect (AVSD)	348
Pulmonary stenosis (PS)	729
Aortic stenosis (AS)	401
Coarctation of the aorta (CoA)	409
Tetralogy of Fallot (ToF)	421
Transposition of the great arteries (TGA)	315
Hypoplastic right heart (HRH)	222
Tricuspid atresia	79
Ebstein's anomaly	114
Pulmonary atresia	132
Hypoplastic left heart (HLH)	266
Truncus arteriosus	107
Double outlet right ventricle (DORV)	157
Single ventricle	106
Total anomalous pulmonary venous drainage (TAPVD)	4
All cyanotic	1,391
All CHD	9,596
Bicuspid aortic valve	13,556

Adapted from Hoffman and Kaplan (2002). Reproduced with permission from American College of Cardiology Foundation.

Incidence

The incidence of CHD is between 8 and 10 per 1,000 births. A lot of the variation between studies is in the inclusion of minor defects, such as small muscular VSDs, which close spontaneously during infancy. Of more significance is the incidence of severe CHD, which will require expert cardiology care, which is between 2.5 and 3 per 1,000 live births, and moderate severe forms that account for another 3 per 1,000 live births (Hoffman and Kaplan, 2002). The frequency of the different types of malformation is given in Table 2.1.

Presentation

A retrospective study by Wren et al. (1999) from the North East England of babies born between 1987 and 1994 found that more than half with CHD were missed by routine neonatal examination and more than a third by the 6-week examination. Even when signs of a possible cardiac abnormality were found, there was a significant delay before a definitive diagnosis was made. They recommended that babies with a murmur at neonatal or 6-week examination should be referred for early paediatric cardiological evaluation.

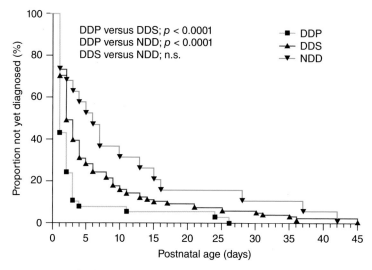

Figure 2.5 Proportion of infants with undiagnosed heart defects against postnatal age. Adapted from Mellander and Sunnegårdh (2006). Reproduced with permission from John Wiley & Sons.

A Swedish study (Mellander and Sunnegårdh, 2006) reviewed babies born between January 1993 and July 2001 who had surgical or catheter-based intervention before the age of 2 months. Out of a birth cohort of 351,483, the study had 310 babies that fitted their criteria of a critical heart defect. Almost 20% were diagnosed after their discharge from hospital. This proportion increased with time from 12.5% between 1993 and 1995 to 26.2% in 1991–2001. Changes in maternity practice meant that 26.8% of all newborns were discharged before 72 hours in 1993 and this increased to 51% in 2001. However, the proportion of infants with unrecognised critical heart defects who were discharged before 72 hours did not increase over the study period, so this was not an explanation for the rise. Figure 2.5 shows the proportion of infants with undiagnosed heart defects against postnatal age.

An American study (Schultz et al., 2008) again reviewing babies who had critical CHD and particularly significant physiological compromise (severe metabolic acidosis, seizure, cardiac arrest or laboratory evidence of renal or hepatic injury before invasive intervention) found that a third with potentially preventable significant physiological compromise were discharged home before a diagnosis of CHD had been made. Interestingly, almost 50% of their babies who had critical CHD had been diagnosed prenatally.

Heart sounds

As the heart beats, a number of noises are created. The first heart sound is created by the closure of the tricuspid and mitral valves. The second sound is from the closure of the aortic and pulmonary valves; the aortic valve closes before the

Table 2.2   A six-point scale is used to describe murmurs.

Grade of murmur	Description
1	Just audible
2	Comfortably audible
3	Loud
4	Loud with a thrill
5	Audible with stethoscope edge on the chest
6	Audible without a stethoscope or with the stethoscope not touching the chest wall

pulmonary valve leading to splitting of the second sound. This splitting varies with the respiratory cycle. Two other sounds are described and can be heard at the cardiac apex. They are generally of low volume and not usually audible. The third sound is caused by rapid ventricular filling in diastole and the fourth sound from ventricular filling upon atrial contraction. Loud third and fourth sounds are indicative of underlying cardiac problems.

Murmurs

Heart murmurs are produced by turbulent blood flow. If a fluid flows through a narrowed path, then it speeds up and the flow changes from a smooth linear flow to a turbulent jet. This creates a noise. An analogy would be the quiet flow of slow moving river to the babbling noise of a fast flowing stream. Blood flow through the heart is not completely smooth and with sufficient amplification, it would be possible to hear murmurs during systole in all children. Murmurs are described by their loudness, their timing in the cardiac cycle, and their position on the chest wall, what they sound like and, finally, where the murmur radiates to.

A six-point scale has been used to describe murmurs: grade 1 is just audible, grade 2 is comfortably audible and grade 3 is loud. If the murmur can be felt on the chest wall as a thrill, which is a vibrating sensation under the examiner's hand, then the murmur is grade 4. A grade 5 murmur is audible with the stethoscope edge on the chest and a grade 6 murmur is audible without a stethoscope or with the stethoscope not touching the chest wall (Table 2.2).

Murmurs occurring during the ventricular contraction are called systolic; they occur between the first and second heart sounds. Murmurs occurring during ventricular relaxation are diastolic and occur between the second and the first heart sounds. The majority of murmurs occur when the ventricular contraction is at its strongest and the blood flow is at its peak. They typically occur in the middle of systole and are called ejection systolic murmurs. A murmur that occurs right throughout systole often obscuring the sound of the heart sounds is called a pansystolic murmur. This is usually due to a VSD. They are not heard at birth but become apparent over the first few weeks as the left ventricular pressure increases. They are usually detected at 6–8-week check.

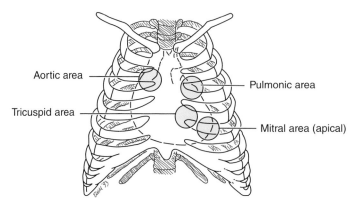

Figure 2.6 Four auscultatory areas of the heart. Reproduced with permission of Elizabeth Weadon Massari.

Murmurs occurring in diastole are uncommon and are almost invariably due to a heart anomaly. In young infants and toddlers, it is sometimes possible to hear a continuous low grade rumbling in the intraclavicular area (the area underneath the clavicles). This is heard when the child is sitting and is due to blood returning to the heart through the jugular and subclavian veins. The sound disappears if the child is lying down or the venous return is briefly blocked by gentle pressure over the jugular vein. It is of no clinical significance.

The position of maximal loudness of the murmur on the chest wall should be noted. This gives information as to where the murmur is being generated. The main areas are the pulmonary, aortic, left sternal edge and apex (Figure 2.6). The noise of the murmur will also be heard in the direction of the blood flow, so, for instance, the murmur created by aortic stenosis will also be heard over the carotids in the neck. A pulmonary stenotic murmur will be heard at the back under the left scapula.

Finally, the murmur can be described by its tone. Innocent murmurs are usually quiet and have a humming pleasant tone. Significant murmurs have a harsher, rougher sound. The typical sound of a VSD is of a harsh loud pansystolic noise at the left sternal edge, which is also audible all over the chest wall.

Other sounds

Other sounds described are the opening snaps due to an abnormal aortic or pulmonary valve being forced open. They occur just before the ejection systolic murmur of the blood flowing through the narrow valve. They are usually only heard with confidence by the experienced examiner in older children and adults.

Tools

The stethoscope is an important tool, and it is worth investing in one of good quality (Figure 2.7). The business end or head usually has two parts. The flat part

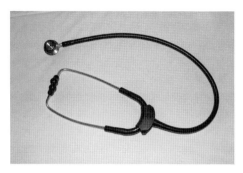

Figure 2.7 Paediatric stethoscope.

is called the diaphragm and transmits high-frequency sounds best. The open part is the bell. It needs to be in contact all around its edge in order to fully transmit sounds. It transmits low-frequency sounds best. If it is pressed hard against the skin, then the tautened skin will make it act more like a diaphragm. However, pressing hard will be uncomfortable for the patient and should be avoided. The head usually swivels so that either the diaphragm or the bell is connected via the tubing to the earpieces.

The head of the stethoscope comes in three sizes – neonatal, paediatric and adult. The paediatric head is best for examination of the newborn. The neonatal is only suitable for very small premature infants and the adult covers too much of the infant's chest.

The tubing from the head to the earpieces comes in a range of sizes but can be shortened if necessary. If a tube is too long, it leads to attenuation of the sound and if too short, the examiner is uncomfortably close to the patient. A good stethoscope has thicker tubing, which transmits the sound better.

Finally, the earpieces should be angled slightly forward so they point in the direction of the examiner's ear canal. Alternative earpieces can be bought and the examiner should choose a pair that fit comfortably in the ear.

The stethoscope should be cleaned between each patient according to the manufacturer's instructions. A good stethoscope will last for years but parts can be replaced as they wear out.

Electronic stethoscopes are now available at a reasonable price and may suit some clinicians. They have switches to alter the frequency range in a manner similar to changing from the bell to the diaphragm.

I personally examine with the bell, but if a murmur is heard, then I listen with both the bell and the diaphragm.

Examination
History
Similar to all clinical encounters, the history is very important. Perusal of the maternal case notes, supplemented and amplified with interrogation of the

mother for details of family history, maternal health, previous pregnancies and medication history. Details of the present pregnancy are required, including results of antenatal tests, illnesses during pregnancy and medication taken around conception and during pregnancy (see also Chapter 1).

Enquiries should be made as to the well-being of infants and how are they feeding. Poor or slow feeding or if the infant has to stop at frequent intervals during a feed to rest can be a sign of heart failure. It is important to ask the mother and father if they have any concerns about the infant. First-time mothers and fathers may have no or very little experience and be reluctant to express concerns because of a fear of appearing excessively ignorant. However, their observations of changes in the infant's behaviour and health may be clue to underlying problems.

Examination

In the ideal situation, the infant will be clean, awake but quiet and thus a systematic examination can be easily undertaken. However, this is not often the case, so the child has to be examined in an opportunistic manner, and if necessary, the examiner may have to return later to complete the examination.

The first part of the examination is to look at the infant. Do they look normal? Dysmorphic features may be a sign of a syndrome such as trisomy 21 (see also Chapter 7). Many syndromes have an association with CHD (Table 2.3). Is the infant behaving normally? Sleeping peacefully, moving all limbs normally? What colour is the infant's face? Cyanosis is difficult to detect clinically especially in pigmented individuals. The ambient lighting and the reflection of light from surrounding surfaces can alter the infant's colour. If there is any doubt about whether the infant is even mildly cyanosed, then it is important to measure the oxygen saturation both pre- and post-ductally using a pulse oximeter. If there has been a difficult delivery, there may be bruising and congestion of the infant's face making it look quite blue.

Once infants are undressed, their breathing should be observed. The rate should be counted over a minute as infants' breathing is irregular. The work of breathing can be seen from signs of recession, use of accessory muscles, nasal flaring and grunting (see the following section on respiratory examination). Cardiac problems lead to secondary respiratory effects.

The best pulse to feel is the brachial at the antecubital fossa. The radial pulse is often difficult to feel in newborns. The rate should be counted over 10 seconds; the rate varies from 110 to 160. The pulse should be regular, but there may be a periodic slowing and quickening in time with the respiratory cycle. This is normal and is called sinus arrhythmia and is a physiological response to the variation in blood returning to the heart during the respiratory cycle. If there is doubt about the rhythm, then it helps to listen to the heart as the ears are more sensitive to rhythm than the fingertips. If there is still doubt, then an electrocardiogram (ECG) should be done and a prolonged recording of Lead II should be done.

Table 2.3 Some syndromes associated with CHD.

Syndrome	Generic defect	Incidence	Cardiac abnormality
Down's syndrome	Trisomy 21	Affected by screening	Cardiac defects in 40–60%. Includes VSD, AVSD, ASD, TOF, PDA (Tubman et al., 1991)
Edward's syndrome	Trisomy 18	1 in 6,000	Includes VSD, ASD, PDA
Patau's syndrome	Trisomy 13	1 case per 8,000–12,000	Cardiac defects occur in 80% of ns. Includes PDA, VSD, ASD, dextrocardia
Cri du chat syndrome	Deletion of 5p, 5p15.3 and 5p15.2	1 in 50,000	Includes VSD, ASD, TOF, PDA
Wolf–Hirschhorn syndrome	Deletion of 4p, including 4p16.3	1 in 20,000 to 1:50,000	ASD, VSD, persistent left superior vena cava, valve abnormalities, complex cardiac defects (Lurie et al., 1980; Mass et al., 2008 and Zollino et al., 2008)
DiGeorge syndrome	Deletion of 22q11	1 per 2,000–4,000	Cardiac defects are observed in 74–80% of patients Any conotruncal heart defect can occur. In infancy, TOF, truncus arteriosus, and interrupted aortic arch are more common; VSD, pulmonary atresia plus VSD and other conotruncal defects are seen in cases diagnosed after age 2 years Rare cardiac anomalies include vascular ring anomaly, TGV with VSD, coarctation of the aorta, ASD, PS, hypoplastic left heart and PDA
Turner's syndrome	XO	1 in 2,000 of female infants	Coarctation of the aorta, bicuspid aortic valve
Beckwith–Wiedemann syndrome	Abnormalities in the distal region of 11p	1 in 15,000	Various (Greenwood et al., 1977)
William's syndrome	Deletion of 7q11.23	1 in 7,500–20,000	Mostly supravalvular aortic stenosis. Other arteries can be narrowed
Miller–Dieker syndrome	Deletion of 17p13	1 in 85,500	Various (Pilz, 2003)
Holt–Oram syndrome	Mutation of TBX5 gene	1 in 100,000	75% have a cardiac abnormality, usually a VSD or ASD. Cardiac conduction defects
Noonan syndrome	Four disease-causing genes (PTPN11, SOS1, RAF1 and KRAS) have been identified	1 in 1,000–2,500	50% have CHD, typically stenotic or dysplastic pulmonary valve. Hypertrophic cardiomyopathy in up to 30%
VACTERL syndrome	Unknown	1 in 6,250	VSD or ASD

The examiner should note the strength or volume of the pulse; a weak central pulse is indicative of poor cardiac output. Finally, an experienced examiner can often gain information from the character of the pulse. A pulse that decays very rapidly is a sign of a rapidly falling arterial pressure due to flow into a low pressure system such as would occur with a patent ductus arteriosus (Lundell, 1983; Zanardo et al., 2008).

The peripheral circulation of the infant should be assessed. Gentle pressure should be applied with a fingertip on the skin over the upper sternum. This pushes the blood out of the capillaries and veins and once the finger is removed, a pale area is left. The area should regain its colour in less than 2 seconds. Delay longer than this is due to reduced blood flow to the skin as a consequence of poor blood flow to the skin because of reduced body temperature, fever with a high core (rectal, oral or aural temperature) but cool limbs and skin or reduced cardiac output due to dehydration, low blood volume or cardiac failure. The same test can be applied to the big toe or one of the fingers but newborn infants often have blue feet and hands for the first few days.

The examiner should next examine the heart. A hand should be gently placed over the chest and the point of maximal impulse should be found. This is the apex beat and reflects the left ventricle. It should be felt in the fifth intercostal space in the midclavicular line. An apex beat displaced to the left can be a sign of left ventricular hypertrophy or dilatation. A rumbling sensation under the hand at systole is called a thrill and is due to a loud murmur. Finally, the ball of the hand should be placed on the lower sternum. If the right ventricle is beating harder than normal, then a strong pulse can be felt; this is called a right ventricular heave or parasternal heave. However, all these signs are very rare and unlikely to be seen in the first days of life.

In older children and adults, some clinicians recommend percussing the boundaries of the heart to detect dilation or hypertrophy or displacement. It is of limited benefit and a CXR and/or echocardiography is of more use.

Many students and indeed practitioners are uneasy about examining the heart and fear that they will miss murmurs. If they do hear a murmur, they find it difficult to describe it. However, if the examination is done in a logical and thorough manner, then significant abnormalities are unlikely to be missed. When auscultating the heart sounds, try and recognise the individual sounds separately.

Start listening at the apex, then the left sternal edge, pulmonary, aortic and tricuspid areas. At each area, identify the first heart sound, then the second sound. If an additional sound is heard, then note when it occurs in relation to the first and second sounds. Is it loud and is it a pleasant or unpleasant sound? Where is it loudest and where else is it heard?

There are a number of pitfalls; firstly, noisy infant breathing can sound like a heart murmur. Babies breathe irregularly and have periods of fast breathing followed by a pause. If you are unsure whether the noises are cardiac or respiratory, then wait until the infant is breathing quietly and then have another listen.

Secondly, if there are lots of noises to hear and you are getting confused, then stop listening, examine another system and then have another listen.

Finally, the infant should be turned on to its right side and the heart should be examined for murmurs along the route of the aorta on the left side of the spine from the interscapular area to below the ribs. Coarctation of the aorta may be detectable by the turbulent blood flow through the narrowed area.

Remember, the cardiac examination is to see if the infant needs further examinations and tests. The NIPE guidelines have a developmental standard that all babies with a suspected cardiac abnormality have pulse oximetry and an expert review within 24 hours (NIPE, 2008) (for NIPE process map, see Figure 2.8). For medical and non-medical practitioners, this means a senior medical review. The last part of the cardiac examination is to palpate the femoral pulses. This part of the examination is to detect abnormalities of the descending aorta, such as coarctation of the aorta. This can only be easily done with a quiet infant. If the infant is crying and moving its legs vigorously, then it is almost impossible. If the infant cannot be pacified easily, then the examiner should return later when settled. The legs should be gently extended at the hips and the tips of the examiner's forefingers should be placed at the midpoint between the anterior iliac spine and the pubic ramus on the inguinal crease (Figure 2.9).

The pulse should be easily palpated. If not, then take a few seconds break and have another attempt. Ensure that the fingers are only gently touching the area so as not to occlude the artery and that you are feeling in the right place. If they still cannot be palpated, then ask a colleague to examine for the pulses. Coarctation of the aorta occurs in 0.4 per 1,000 infants (Hoffman and Kaplan, 2002) and is a narrowing of the aorta in the area where the ductus arteriosus joins. Coarctation can be pre-ductal, ductal or post-ductal. In pre-ductal and ductal coarctations, the pulse may be normal until the ductus closes when the femoral pulses will become weak or disappear. The ductus up to this point is supplying blood to the lower body. If the blood supply to the lower body after closure of the ductus is inadequate, then the tissues of the legs will become hypoxic and an excess of lactic acid will be formed. The resultant acidosis affects whole body including the heart and will lead to organ failure. This will be manifested by failure to feed, mottling of the skin, cool peripheries, abnormal breathing and gradual loss of consciousness. A post-ductal coarctation will present as weak or absent femoral pulses depending on the degree of restriction to blood flow. Coarctation with mild restriction to flow may present later in childhood or in adult life either with a murmur or as a cause of hypertension.

A significant cardiac abnormality will affect the function of the other systems. Cardiac or circulatory failure will cause an increase in the respiratory rate and depth of breathing. Heart failure leads to retention of fluid. In adults, this is usually manifested as oedema in the dependant parts such as the feet and ankles but in children this does not occur but the liver is enlarged and will be felt well below the costal margin. Also, in adults with heart failure, the jugular venous

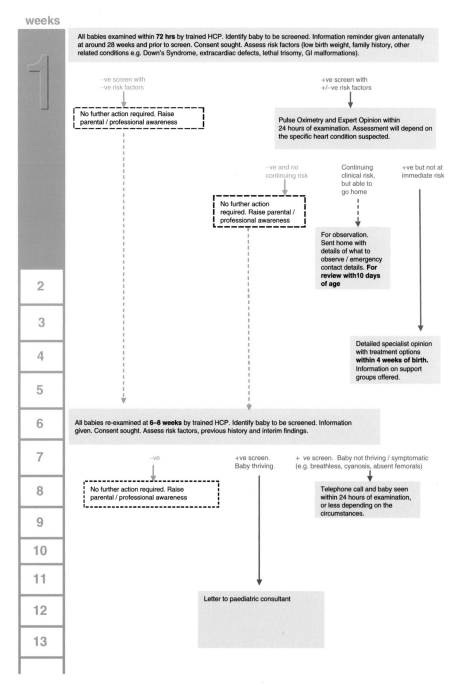

Figure 2.8 NIPE Process Map. Congenital heart disease. Source: NIPE (2008). Reproduced with kind permission of HMSO.

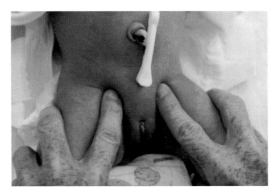

Figure 2.9 Palpating femoral pulses.

pressure is increased and can be easily demonstrated with the patient sitting at a 45° angle. In infants, though the venous pressure is raised, their short chubby neck makes detection of a raised jugular venous pressure very difficult.

In an infant with sepsis, cardiac or circulatory failure or respiratory failure, the adrenal glands produce excess adrenaline (epinephrine). This leads to arterial constriction and greatly reduced blood flow to the skin. The infant will appear deathly white.

Detection of an abnormality

The aim of the examination of the newborn is to detect abnormalities. If a cardiac abnormality is detected, then there must be a local protocol on how this is taken further. This should involve further investigation including post-ductal pulse oximetry and reassessment by another examiner. An echocardiogram should be organised. If this cannot be done within a reasonable time and the child is well with a normal saturation, then it should be done within a few days. The mother and father should be told what to do if their infant becomes unwell; poor feeding, change in colour, breathlessness, etc.

Investigations

Blood pressure

The measurement of the blood pressure is not routinely done as part of the examination of the healthy newborn. It should be measured in all sick infants and where cardiac disease is suspected. Automated oscillometric machines have been shown to give reliable measurements in neonates (Dellagrammaticas and Wilson, 1981, Baker et al., 1984). However, in severely ill neonates and premature infants, machines can be inaccurate (Dannevig et al., 2005). A range of cuffs are available to fit the upper arm, thigh and lower leg. The flush method of measuring blood pressure is no longer used; the use of a Doppler machine to detect blood flow in conjunction with a sphygmomanometer is possible but the measurement takes longer.

The measurement of four-limb blood pressure to detect differences between upper (pre-ductal) and lower (post-ductal) limb values and hence detect coarctation of the aorta has been rejected as a screening tool by a number of authors. Wilson (1999) showed that in infants with coarctation, there was not a significant difference between upper and lower limb measurements, probably due to flow through a patent ductus arteriosus. Crossland et al. (2004) found in a study of 40 infants with normal aortas that 16% had a 20 mmHg difference in blood pressure between upper and lower limbs. They calculated that using four-limb blood pressure for screening, 300 infants would need to have further investigations to detect the one with an abnormality.

If there is any concern that an infant has a coarctation of the aorta, then the infant should be referred to a cardiologist for an urgent opinion.

Pulse oximetry

The development of the pulse oximeter has been an important advance in medicine. It is a non-invasive way of measuring the oxygenation of patients. As described previously, the clinical detection of cyanosis is difficult and conversely babies with acrocyanosis or facial congestion may look cyanosed but are adequately oxygenated.

Pulse oximeters firstly measure the absorption of two different wavelengths of light. The absorption of light by oxygenated haemoglobin is different from that of deoxygenated haemoglobin. Secondly, the background absorption of light by capillaries, veins and body tissue can be subtracted from the pulsatile absorption of arterial blood (Hill and Stoneham, 2000). Pulse oximeters give the percentage oxygen saturation of the pulsatile component, the heart rate and an indication of the pulsatility of the reading. This last reading is useful as a low pulsatile signal or an irregular pattern suggests that the oxygen saturation reading will be inaccurate. The probe should be recited or adjusted until a good signal is obtained.

The arterial oxygen tension in the normal fetus is approximately 20 mmHg, equivalent to an oxygen saturation of 60% (Rabi et al., 2006). Following birth, the oxygen saturation rises over 5–15 minutes to over 90%. The post-ductal measurement takes longer (Toth et al., 2002; Mariani et al., 2007).

The measurement should be made both on the right hand (pre-ductal) and on a foot (post-ductal). The normal reading should be 95% or greater. There can be problems getting satisfactory readings because of poor peripheral blood flow or excessive movement. Infants with no other physical signs or symptoms who have a low reading should have measurements repeated an hour or so later. Infants who have physical signs or symptoms should have further investigations organised.

Electrocardiography

The ECG measures the surface electrical activity of the muscles of the heart. The adult configuration of limb and ventricular leads are used with the addition of V4r to give further assessment of the right heart.

The ECG is particularly useful for infants with irregular heartbeats. It has been used in the past in the investigation of murmurs but the ECG can be normal even in the presence of an abnormal heart.

The interpretation of the ECG is straightforward but reference to tables of normal values according to the child's age is required.

Echocardiography

This is the gold standard for the detection of CHD. It is now widely available in most hospitals. The basic techniques are relatively easy to learn though much practice and experience is needed to become a skilled operator. It is not yet practical or financially viable to do an echocardiogram on every newborn baby (Knowles et al., 2005). An echocardiogram will also detect clinically insignificant abnormalities and if done within the first few days of life, flow will be seen through a patent ductus arteriosus and patent foramen ovale (Alenick et al., 1992).

Follow-up

All infants detected on the newborn examination with a murmur or signs suggestive of CHD should be examined by a practitioner with the skills and experience to determine whether an immediate cardiac assessment is required or whether an early referral to an appropriate clinic would be more suitable.

The NIPE (2008) standards require that all infants should have a physical examination for CHD within 72 hours of birth. Infants who are screen positive and considered to be at continuing risk of clinical deterioration need to have pulse oximetry and expert review within 24 hours. The timing of the subsequent review depends on the clinical assessment and the likelihood of deterioration. However, the aim is that all infants who are screen positive have a definitive diagnosis made within 4 weeks.

Screening

Antenatal ultrasound examination

Most pregnant women have an obstetric ultrasound in the second trimester between 18 and 20 weeks looking for anomalies. The heart is screened during this procedure with either a four-chamber view or a four-chamber and outflow tract view. Many lesions can be detected (Table 2.4) but not all abnormalities

Table 2.4 Abnormalities seen on a four-chamber view.

Abnormality	Comment
Hypoplastic left heart syndrome	
Atrioventricular septal defect	80% of complete AVSDs are associated with Down's syndrome as are 40–50% of partial AVSDs
Large VSDs	Usually associated with other cardiac or extracardiac abnormalities, particularly trisomy
Hypoplastic right ventricle	Usually seen in association with tricuspid atresia or pulmonary atresia with intact ventricular septum
Right atrial dilatation	Ebstein's anomaly or pulmonary atresia with intact ventricular septum
Right ventricular dilatation	Occurring with coarctation of the aorta or severe tricuspid regurgitation
Left ventricular dilatation	Found in some cases of critical aortic stenosis
Double inlet left ventricle	Where both atrioventricular valves enter the left ventricle. The right ventricle is usually hypoplastic
Dilated cardiomyopathy	Dilated heart with poor ventricular function and atrioventricular valve regurgitation
Hypertrophic cardiomyopathy	May be associated with Noonan's or other syndromes. Sometimes familial
Rhabdomyomata	Appear as discrete masses in either or both ventricles. Commonly associated with tuberose sclerosis

Adapted from Roberts and Kitchiner (2004). Reproduced with permission from Elsevier.

Table 2.5 Common cardiac abnormalities not detected on a four-chamber view.

Abnormality	Comment
Transposition of the great arteries	
Double outlet right ventricle	Where both the aortic and the pulmonary valves arise from the same (usually) right ventricle
Tetralogy of Fallot	
Pulmonary atresia with a VSD	
Common arterial trunk	
Absent pulmonary valve syndrome	
Coarctation or interruption of the aortic valve	

Adapted from Roberts and Kitchiner (2004). Reproduced with permission from Elsevier.

are apparent on a four-chamber view (Table 2.5). More detailed fetal scanning can be done if other anomalies (such as nuchal translucency) are detected on scan or there is a high risk of trisomy 21 on the antenatal blood screening test. Major CHD was found in 7% of fetuses with an increased nuchal translucency (Clur et al., 2008). Other soft markers such as echogenic bowel, mild ventriculomegaly, echogenic focus in the heart and choroids plexus cyst are associated with an increase risk of aneuploidy (an abnormality involving a chromosome

Table 2.6   Indications for fetal echocardiography.

Indication	Comment
Suspicion of cardiac abnormality	Abnormal four-chamber view
	Non-immune foetal hydrops
	Cardiac arrhythmia
Extracardiac anomalies	Other congenital abnormality (e.g. exomphalos, congenital diaphragmatic hernia, tracheo-oesophageal fistula, bowel obstruction, renal anomalies)
	Increased nuchal translucency
Chromosomal anomalies	Aneuploidy
	Mother or partner with 22q11 deletion
Risk factor for congenital heart disease	History of congenital heart disease in a first-degree relative
	Parental consanguinity
	Maternal disease (e.g. lupus, diabetes, phenylketonuria
	Exposure to teratogens (e.g. alcohol, lithium, viruses, anticonvulsant drugs)
	Tuberose sclerosis in a first-degree relative.
	Multiple monochorionic pregnancy
Abnormal foetal growth	Intrauterine growth retardation

number that is not an exact multiple of the haploid number, i.e. trisomy 21) (van den Hof and Wilson, 2005). A single umbilical artery, enlarged cisterna magna and pyelectasis are only associated with an increased risk of a non-chromosomal abnormality when seen in isolation (van den Hof and Wilson, 2005). An isolated single umbilical artery has a higher association with renal anomalies (Srinivasan and Arora, 2004) though some authors (Persutte and Hobbins, 1995; van den Hof and Wilson, 2005) note that there is also an association with CHD and recommend that the fetus also has a fetal echocardiogram. Gossett et al. (2002) in a study suggest that a fetal echocardiogram is not required where normal four-chamber and outflow tract views have been obtained. Other indications are shown in Table 2.6.

Detailed fetal echocardiography is time-consuming and is commonly available only at tertiary centres. Studies have not shown that routine antenatal ultrasound is at present a cost–effective and reliable method of detecting CHD in the low-risk fetus (Bricker et al., 2000).

Screening pulse oximetry

In 1995, Katzman suggested that pulse oximetry should be used routinely to detect respiratory or cardiac problems in the newborn infant (Katzman, 1995). Since then, there have been a number of studies looking at the effectiveness of measuring oxygen saturation in newborn infants to detect CHD (Richmond et al., 2002; Koppel et al., 2003; Reich et al., 2003; Granelli et al., 2009; Riede et al., 2010). The premise being that the detection of mild cyanosis in seemingly well infants would lead to further investigation and treatment before the closure of the ductus arteriosus and subsequent rapid deterioration. In addition to the studies there have been a number of reviews of the subject (Griebsch et al., 2007; Thangaratina et al., 2007; Valmari, 2007; Mahle et al., 2009).

Gnanalingham et al. (2001) in a small study took post-ductal measurements at a mean of 1.7 hours (range 30 minutes to 6 hours) and found a mean saturation of 96.6 (3.8)%. In 31, (2%) cases, saturation was 90% or less, 13 of whom had clinical problems. Richmond et al. (2002), in a larger study, again measured post-ductal saturations between 2 hours of age and discharge. Just over 5% of their infants had a measurement below 95%; this reduced to 0.9% after a second measurement after an interval.

The Tennessee Task Force (Liske et al., 2006) agreed that universal screening should not be implemented at the time because of concerns about the false-positive rate, the questionable reliability of the technology and the inability to generate a reasonable cost–benefit analysis. A health technology appraisal by Knowles et al. (2005) looking at clinical examination alone, pulse oximetry and screening echocardiography concluded that clinical examination alone performed poorly, the addition of pulse oximetry was promising and whilst screening echocardiography had the highest detection rate, it was too costly. They recommended further research into pulse oximetry and to evaluate antenatal screening strategies. A systematic review by Thangaratina et al. (2007) looking at eight suitable studies found pulse oximetry to be a highly specific tool with very low false-positive rates. However, further prospective studies were needed to assess its sensitivity.

Gnanalingham et al. (2001) and Knowles et al. (2005) noted that a number of infants with low oxygen saturations had no cardiac abnormalities but had other problems including group B streptococcal infection, transient tachypnoea of the newborn, which had not been recognised at the time of the measurement. Further assessment because of the low saturation led to their diagnosis.

The National Institute for Health Research Health Technology Assessment programme funded a study of the use of pulse oximetry to detect CHD (The PulseOx study). This was run through the University of Birmingham, UK (Ewer et al., 2011). Between six maternity units in the West Midlands, they screened 20,055 asymptomatic newborn babies (gestation >34 weeks) by measuring oxygen saturation in the right hand (pre-ductal) and either foot. A saturation of <95% in either limb or a difference of >2% (if both ≥95%) was considered abnormal. If a clinical examination was unremarkable, the test was repeated 1–2 hours later. If the examination was abnormal or the repeat oximetry was abnormal, then the test was positive and the infant had an echocardiogram. All infants were followed up to 12 months of age by the use of regional and national registries and clinical follow-up.

Fifty-three infants had major congenital heart disease (24 critical) though 35 were suspected from an antenatal scan to have CHD. Sensitivity of pulse oximetry was 75% (95% confidence interval 53.29–90.23) for critical cases and 49.06% (35.06–63.16) for all major congenital heart defects. There were 169 (0.8%) false-positive results of which six cases had significant CHD and 40 had other illnesses that required urgent medical intervention. Pulse oximetry did not identify 41 infants with CHD (6 critical, 21 serious and 14 significant). Sensitivity of the test was highest in the first 12 hours.

Zhao et al. (2014) ran a large study in Shanghai which screened 122,738 consecutive newborn infants between 6 and 72 hours of age. Pulse oximetry alone had a sensitivity of 77.4% (95% CI 70.4–83.4); the addition of a clinical examination increased the sensitivity to 93.2% (95% CI 87.9–96.2%). The false-positive rate was 2.7% for clinical assessment alone and 0.3% for pulse oximetry alone.

There is now enough evidence that pulse oximetry aids in the detection of CHD and should be part of the newborn examination (Ewer, 2014). However, like all screening tests, it will miss some cases. After consultation in 2013, the UKNSC recommended that pulse oximetry be included in the screening process for the full examination of the newborn. This practice is currently being piloted in England and the NIPE Programme Team will assess the impact of this on the screening process as a whole. More information on this can be found on the NIPE website: http://newbornphysical.screening.nhs.uk/

Postnatal screening echocardiography

This is the gold standard for detecting cardiac abnormalities. A study from Northern Ireland (Sands et al., 2002) randomised low-risk infants before delivery to screening echocardiogram or routine clinical examination. Infants were screened at 48 hours by a trained ultrasonographer. Each group had over 4,800 infants, 124 of the scanned and 50 of the controls were identified as having significant congenital heart defects before hospital discharge. A further 27 infants in the control and one scanned infant were found in a minimum of a 3-year follow-up to have no life-threatening defects.

A health technology assessment by Griebsch et al. (2007) concluded that screening echocardiography was expensive and had a 5% false-positive rate. At present, screening all infants with an echocardiogram is not financially viable but an early echocardiogram should be available for all infants who need it.

The examination of the heart and circulation in the infant should not be approached with trepidation. The aim is to detect whether from the history or the examination there is any suggestion that the child may have CHD. A definitive diagnosis is not required from the screening examination, but if the screen is positive, then referral for further investigation is required.

It has been shown that not all congenital cardiac defects are detectable clinically on the newborn examination; however, pulse oximetry has been shown to be of value in detecting some life-threatening abnormalities before the infant is unwell. Health professionals need to remain vigilant in looking for signs and symptoms of CHD developing in all newborn infants.

Examination of the respiratory system

The aim of the examination of the respiratory system is to detect abnormalities of the chest and lungs. The majority of serious respiratory problems will be apparent to the examiner unlike the cardiovascular system where serious congenital abnormalities may not initially have any obvious physical signs.

Examination of the chest

History
The mother's case notes should be examined for pertinent information, particularly any abnormalities of the chest seen on antenatal ultrasound. However, any major abnormality such as a congenital diaphragmatic hernia should have been communicated to the paediatric team and arrangements made for delivery in a centre experienced in the resuscitation, stabilisation and subsequent surgical repair of the abnormality (see also Chapter 2).

Enquiries should be made of the mother and her attendants as to whether the baby is breathing normally and whether it is feeding well.

Examination
The baby should be pink centrally. Most newborns have poor circulation in their hands and feet for the first few days, so these may look dusky. Cyanosis is notoriously hard to detect and if there is any doubt about an infant's colour, then it should be measured with a pulse oximeter.

The infant should be breathing fairly regularly at a rate up to 60 bpm. In a study of sleeping term newborn babies, Cross (1949) recorded rates of between 14 and 51 bpm with an average of 29 bpm. Some periodic breathing is normal with periods of rapid breathing followed by a short pause of no longer than 10 seconds. Most of the movement occurs in the abdomen as infant breathing is primarily diaphragmatic. There should be no or very minimal sternal recession. Chest movements should be symmetrical.

The breath sounds should be auscultated anteriorly and posteriorly at the upper, mid and lower areas as well as in the midaxillary line, comparing one side against the other. Tracheal and bronchial sounds will be heard close to the sternum.

The breath sounds should be vesicular. These are soft, low pitched and have a rustling quality. When listening closer to the midline, the sounds of bronchial and tracheal airflow will be heard. These are coarser and higher pitched. The best way of hearing normal breath sounds is to listen to your own chest (Assuming you do not have underlying lung disease!).

Abnormalities

Nasal flaring occurs where the baby has to breathe harder than normal. The nostrils open wider during inspiration.

The infant chest wall is pliable because the ribs are still growing and the anterior portions are made of cartilage. There is also not much muscle between the ribs (intercostals spaces) and above the clavicle (supraclavicular area). If the lungs are stiff and difficult to inflate as in respiratory distress syndrome, pneumonia, etc., then the chest wall will be more compliant than the lungs. On inspiration, there will be a dipping in of the intercostal spaces and supraclavicular area. This is called intercostal and supraclavicular recession, respectively. With stiffer lungs, the ribs will bend in and the sternum will appear to dip downwards. This is called sternal recession. In normal infants, there is often a mild degree of intercostal recession. This is even more obvious in a premature infant because the chest wall is so compliant.

In lung disease, the respiratory rate increases. If the lungs are particularly stiff, then the infant may breathe quickly and shallowly. When the infant is getting exhausted by the effort of breathing, the rate will slow and they may have periods of not breathing for longer than 20 seconds (apnoea). They are accompanied by slowing of the heart (bradycardia). These infants need urgent medical attention (brief self-correcting bradycardias and transient apnoeas are often seen in premature infants and, assuming the infant is well, are due to immaturity of the control mechanisms).

Grunting is the sound made as the infant breathes out against a partially closed glottis. The physiological effect is to prevent airway collapse during expiration. It typically occurs in respiratory distress syndrome, transient tachypnoea of the newborn and pneumonia.

Abnormal breath sounds include wheezing, usually expiratory, due to narrowing of the large airways. Wheezing is rarely heard in the newborn and is more usually heard with bronchiolitis, viral chest infections and asthma. The sound is similar to a whistling. The expiratory phase in wheezing is longer than usual as it takes longer to exhale because of the reduced airflow. The other common abnormal sound is crepitations or crackles. This is where there is more fluid in the lungs and airways than normal. It is associated with chest infections.

Babies and infants with an obvious lobar pneumonia on chest X-ray may have normal breath sounds on auscultation. However, they will have other signs such as raised respiratory rate, some recession and not feeding well.

Infants with abnormal chest signs should have pulse oximetry done, oxygen given if oxygen saturation is below 95% and medical help summoned.

Investigations

Pulse oximetry is very useful in assessing lung disease. Oxygen saturation should be above 95% in room air.

Almost all lung diseases will show up as an abnormality on a chest radiograph. As with all radiographs, the film should be checked to see that the right patient has been examined, that the sides are clearly labelled and the study is of sufficient quality (such as positioning, all areas of the lung seen and appropriate exposure) to use. Poor films should be repeated. With the introduction of digital films, it is possible to get an opinion from a radiologist or a senior paediatric colleague even if they are off site. The request and interpretation of X-rays is not part of the routine examination of the newborn.

Transillumination of the chest wall. In infants with a suspected pneumothorax, a cold light (fibre optic source) can be applied to the chest wall and the area of transillumination noted. This is compared to the opposite side. If there is a larger enough pneumothorax, then the area transilluminated will be larger on the side with the pneumothorax. Where there is a large pneumothorax, then the whole hemithorax will be illuminated. This is a rapid test and can be used as confirmation of clinical findings prior to the emergency relief of a tension pneumothorax. Infants with a tension pneumothorax deteriorate rapidly and need decompression of the pleural cavity urgently. Getting a chest X-ray would involve an unacceptable delay. Tension pneumothoraces are associated with ongoing lung disease and the infant is usually on a ventilator or continuous positive airways pressure.

The measurement of blood gases is useful for assessing the severity of the lung disease and the infant's response. The significant measurements are the pH, pCO_2 and pO_2. The bicarbonate and base excess results are calculated by the machine. The arterial blood sample gives the most accurate result but taking blood from an artery is painful for the patient (of any age) and is not without complications. A well-taken arterial sample will give an accurate value for the oxygen content of the blood. However, this is less important, now we can measure oxygen saturation with a pulse oximeter. Venous and capillary samples are easier to get but if there is poor peripheral circulation, then the pH and pCO_2 will be worse than the actual arterial value. The venous and capillary pO_2 is of negligible value in accessing oxygenation. Lung disease will be associated with a raised pCO_2 and decreased pH. A discussion of blood gases is beyond the scope of this book, but the principles should be known by medical and nursing professionals.

Antenatal screening

Congenital abnormalities of the lung are rare. They may be picked up on antenatal ultrasound. The incidence of congenital diaphragmatic hernia is 1 in 4,000 live births (Spina et al., 2003). The severity of this condition depends on when and how much of the abdominal organs go through the defect into the chest cavity. If this occurs early, then the lungs cannot grow normally and the baby will be born with hypoplastic lungs. The degree of hypoplasticity of the lungs dictates the chances of survival. Other abnormalities include congenital cystic adenomatous malformations, bronchogenic cysts, congenital lobar emphysema, pulmonary agenesis and aplasia, pulmonary hypoplasia, pulmonary sequestration and the scimitar syndrome (Wallis, 2000; Shanmugam et al., 2005).

Conclusion

Most respiratory problems will manifest themselves at or soon after birth. Respiratory distress syndrome will be anticipated in premature infants and transient tachypnoea of the newborn after elective caesarean sections. Congenital diaphragmatic hernia is now often picked up antenatally and delivery should occur at a tertiary neonatal surgical centre. Problems likely to develop after birth include group B streptococcal pneumonia. The astute carer will pick up on the deteriorating or poor feeding pattern, the increased work of breathing and the subtle change in colour. A few simple measurements of temperature, heart and respiratory rate and pulse oximetry will help pick up infants that need further examination.

Cardiac abnormality – a case study

Baby John was born at 39 weeks by spontaneous vaginal delivery; his birth weight was 3.4 kg. His mother Sarah was a primigravida who had an uneventful pregnancy.

He was put to the breast soon after birth and fed well. His first-day examination was done the next morning by the midwife. Upon asking Sarah about family history, the midwife noted that there was no family history of significant congenital heart disease. John was feeding well and had passed urine and meconium.

On examination, he was pink and looked well. His respiratory rate was 40 breaths a minute, his heart rate 130 a minute. His brachial pulses were easily palpable. However, upon auscultation of the heart, the midwife discovered a 3/6 ejection systolic murmur at the left sternal edge and pulmonary area with radiation to the back and the lung fields. His liver was not enlarged and his femoral pulses were palpable on the second attempt (as he started to cry lustily during the examination and needed to be settled). The oxygen saturations in his right hand and left foot were 97%.

He was reviewed by the paediatric registrar who noted that John was well but he did have an obvious systolic murmur. One of the paediatric consultants was on the neonatal unit and performed an echocardiogram. This showed a ventricular septal defect, an overriding aorta and increased velocity in the pulmonary artery.

An appointment was made at the regional cardiac unit for an outpatient review next day.

How would you deal with this situation and what feedback would you give to the mother?

What does your Trust policy say about management of congenital heart conditions?

Look here for resources on congenital heart defects

(see also webpage for much more information on examining the cardiovascular and respiratory systems)

These links give you a simple overview of ventricular septal defect (VSD):

http://emedicine.medscape.com/article/903271-overview

http://www.cdc.gov/ncbddd/heartdefects/ventricularseptaldefect.html

http://www.pediatricct.surgery.ucsf.edu/conditions–procedures/ventricular-septal-defect.aspx

On these sites, you can hear various heart murmurs:

Easy Auscultation

http://www.easyauscultation.com/heart-sounds.aspx?gclid=CNP11Zry1r0CFWzJtAodKysAZA

Auscultation Assistant

http://www.med.ucla.edu/wilkes/intro.html

This site shows you where to place your stethoscope on the chest to hear different murmurs:

Stanford School of Medicine

http://newborns.stanford.edu/PhotoGallery/HeartNL1.html

Here's where you can find information on various congenital cardiac abnormalities and their treatment:

Cincinnati Children's Hospital

http://www.cincinnatichildrens.org/patients/child/encyclopedia/defects/default/

Find help for mothers and fathers here with a child who has a cardiac abnormality:

Children's Heart Federation

http://www.chfed.org.uk/

Example of a leaflet for mothers and fathers of a baby with a heart murmur

http://www.nnuh.nhs.uk/docs%5Cleaflets%5C543.pdf

References

Alenick DS, Holzman IR, Ritter SB (1992) The neonatal transitional circulation: a combined non-invasive assessment. *Echocardiography* **9**, 29–37.

Alvaro RE, Rigatto H (2005) Cardiorespiratory adjustments at birth. In: Avery GB, MacDonald MG, Sesheia MKM, and Mullett MD (eds) *Avery's Neonatology. Pathology and Management of the Newborn*, 6th edn. London: Lippincott Williams & Wilkins.

Andersson O, Hellström – Westas L, Andersson D, Domellöf M (2011) Effect of delayed versus early umbilical cord clamping on neonatal outcomes and iron status at 4 months: a randomised controlled trial. *British Medical Journal* **343**, d7157, DOI: 10.1136/bmj.d7157

Askin D (2009a) Fetal-to-neonatal transition: what is normal and what is not? Part 1. The physiology of transition. *Neonatal Network* **28**(3), 33–36.

Askin D (2009b) Fetal-to-neonatal Transition: what is normal and what is not? Part 2. Red flags. *Neonatal Network* **28**(3), 37–40.

Avery GB, MacDonald MG, Sesheia MKM, Mullett MD (2005) Avery's neonatology. *Pathology and Management of the Newborn*, 6th edn. London: LWW.

Aylott M (2006) The neonatal energy triangle. Part 2. Thermoregulatory and respiratory adaptation. *Pediatric Nursing* **18**(7), 38–42.

Baker MD, Maisels MJ, Marks KH (1984) Indirect BP monitoring in the newborn: evaluation of a new oscillometer and comparison of upper and lower limb measurements. *American Journal of Diseases in Childhood* **138**, 775–778.

Bhutani VK (1997) Extrauterine adaptation. *Seminars in Neonatology* **7**(2), 1–12.

Blackburn ST (2007) *Maternal, Fetal and Neonatal Physiology: A Clinical Perspective*, 3rd edn. St. Louis, MO: Saunders.

Boxwell G (ed) (2010) *Neonatal Intensive Care Nursing*. London: Routledge.

Bricker L, Garcia J, Henderson J, Mugford M, Neilson J, Roberts T, Martin M-A (2000) Ultrasound screening in pregnancy: a systematic review of the clinical effectiveness, cost-effectiveness and women's views. *Health Technology Assessment* **4**(16), 1–193.

Clur SA, Mathijssen IB, Pajkrt E, Cook A, Laurini RN, Ottenkamp J, Bilardo CM (2008) Structural heart defects associated with an increased nuchal translucency: 9 years experience in a referral centre. *Prenatal Diagnosis* **28**, 347–354.

Coggins M, and Mercer JS (2009) Delayed cord clamping. Advantages for infants. *Nursing for Women's Health* **13**(2), 133–139.

Cross KW (1949) The respiratory rate and ventilation in the newborn baby. *Journal of Physiology* **109**, 459–474.

Crossland DS, Furness JC, Abu-Harb M, Sadagopan SN, Wren C (2004) Variability of four limb blood pressure in normal neonates. *Archives of Disease in Childhood Fetal and Neonatal Edition* **89**, 325–327.

Dannevig I, Dale HC, Liestøl K, Lindemann R (2005) Blood pressure in the neonate: three non-invasive oscillometric pressure monitors compared with invasively measured blood pressure. *Acta Paediatrica* **94**, 138–140.

Davies L, McDonald S (eds) (2008) *Examination of the Newborn and Neonatal Health: A Multidimensional Approach*. Edinburgh: Churchill Livingstone.

Dellagrammaticas HD, Wilson AJ (1981) Clinical evaluation of the Dinamap noninvasive blood pressure monitor in pre-term neonates. *Clinical and Physiological Measurement* **2**, 271–276.

Ewer AK, Middleton LJ, Furmston AT, Bhoyar A, Daniels JP, Thangaratinam S, Deeks JJ, Khan KS (2011) Pulse oximetry screening for congenital heart defects in newborn infants (PulseOx): a test accuracy study. *Lancet* **378**, 785–794.

Gnanalingham MG, Mehta BM, Siverajan M, Wild NJ, Bedford CD (2001) Pulse oximetry as a screening test in neonates. *Archives of Disease in Childhood* **84**(Suppl. 1), A35.

Gossett DR, Lantz ME, Chisholm CA (2002) Antenatal diagnosis of a single umbilical artery: is fetal echocardiography warranted? *Obstetric Gynecology* **100**, 903–908.

Granelli A, Wennergren M, Sandberg K, Mellander M, Bejlum C, Inganäs L, Eriksson M, et al. (2009) Impact of pulse oximetry screening on the detection of duct dependent congenital heart disease: a Swedish prospective screening study in 39,821 newborns. *British Medical Journal* **338**, 145–149.

Greenwood RD, Somer A, Rosenthal A, Craenen J, Nadas AS (1977) Cardiovascular abnormalities in the Beckwith–Wiedemann syndrome. *American Journal of Disease in Childhood* **131**, 293–294.

Griebsch I, Knowles RL, Brown J, Bull C, Wren C, Dezateux CA (2007) Comparing the clinical and economic effects of clinical examination, pulse oximetry, and echocardiography in newborn screening for congenital heart defects: a probabilistic cost-effectiveness model and value of information analysis. *International Journal of Technology Assessment in Health Care* **23**, 192–204.

Hill E, Stoneham MD (2000) Practical applications of pulse oximetry. Update in anaesthesia. (11), Article 4. Available from: http://e-safe-anaesthesia.org/e_library/04/Pulse_oximetry_-_practical_applications_Update_2008.pdf (accessed February 2015).

Hoffman JI, Kaplan S (2002) The incidence of congenital heart disease. *Journal of the American College of Cardiology* **39**, 1890–1900.

Katzman GH (1995) The newborn's SpO$_2$: a routine vital sign whose time has come? *Pediatrics* **95**, 161–162.

Kenner C, Wright Lott J (2007) *Comprehensive Neonatal Care: An Interdisciplinary Approach*, 4th edn. London: Saunders.

Kiserud T (2005) The fetal circulation. *Seminars in Fetal and Neonatal Medicine* **10**, 493–503.

Knowles R, Griebsch I, Dezateux C, Brown J, Bull C, Wren C (2005) Newborn screening for congenital heart defects: a systematic review and cost-effectiveness analysis. *Health Technology Assessment* **9**(44), 1–152, iii–iv.

Koppel RI, Druschel CM, Carter T, Goldberg BE, Mehta PN, Talwar R, Bierman FZ (2003) Effectiveness of pulse oximetry screening for congenital heart disease in asymptomatic newborns. *Pediatrics* **111**, 451–455.

Liske MR, Greeley CS, Law DJ, Reich JD, Morrow WR, Baldwin HS, Graham TP, Strauss AW, Kavanaugh-McHugh AL, Walsh WF (2006) Report of the Tennessee Task Force on screening newborn infants for critical congenital heart disease. *Pediatrics* **118**, 1250–1256.

Lundell BPW (1983) Pulse wave patterns in patent ductus arteriosus. *Archives of Disease in Childhood* **58**, 682–685.

Lurie IW, Lazjuk GI, Ussova YI, Presman EB, Gurevich DB (1980) The Wolf–Hirschhorn syndrome. I. Genetics. *Clinical Genetics* **17**(6), 375–384.

Maas NM, Van Buggenhout G, Hannes F, et al. (2008) Genotype-phenotype correlation in 21 patients with Wolf–Hirschhorn syndrome using high resolution array comparative genome hybridisation (CGH). *Journal of Medical Genetics* **45**(2), 71–80.

Mahle WT, Newburger JW, Matherne GP, Smith FC, Hoke TR, Koppel R, Gidding SS, Beekman RH 3rd, Grosse SD (2009) Role of pulse oximetry in examining newborns for congenital heart disease: a scientific statement from the American Heart Association and American Academy of Pediatrics. *Circulation* **120**, 447–458.

Mariani G, Dik PB, Ezquer A, Aguirre A, Esteban ML, Perez C, Jonusas SF, Fustiñana C (2007) Pre-ductal and post-ductal O2 saturation in healthy term neonates after birth. *Journal of Pediatrics* **150**, 418–421.

McDonald SJ, Middleton P, Dowswell T, Morris PS (2013) Effect of timing of umbilical cord clamping of term infants on maternal and neonatal outcomes. *Cochrane Database of Systematic Reviews* (7). Available at: http://onlinelibrary.wiley.com/doi/10.1002/14651858.CD004074.pub3/pdf (accessed February 2015).

Mellander M, Sunnegårdh J (2006) Failure to diagnose critical heart malformations in newborns before discharge: an increasing problem? *Acta Paediatrica* **95**, 407–413.

Mercer JS and Erickson-Owens DA (2012) Rethinking placental transfusion and cord clamping issues. *Journal of Perinatal and Neonatal Nursing.* **6**(3) 202–217.

Mercer J, Skovgaard R (2002) Neonatal transitional physiology: a new paradigm. *Journal of Perinatal and Neonatal Nursing* **15**(4), 56–75.

Milcic TL (2008) Neonatal glucose homeostasis. *Neonatal Network* **27**(3), 203–207.

NIPE (2008) *Newborn and Infant Physical Examination Standards and Competencies.* Available from: http://newbornphysical.screening.nhs.uk/publications (accessed July 2010).

Palethorpe RJ, Farrar D, Duley L (2010) Alternative positions for the baby at birth before clamping the umbilical cord. *Cochrane Database of Systematic Reviews* **2010**(10).

Perrson B (2009) Neonatal glucose metabolism in off spring of mothers with varying degrees of hyperglycaemia during pregnancy. *Seminars in Fetal and Neonatal Medicine* **14**, 106–111.

Persutte WH, Hobbins J (1995) Single umbilical artery: a clinical enigma in modern prenatal diagnosis. *Ultrasound Obstetrics and Gynecology* **6**, 216–229.

Pilz D (2003) Miller–Dieker syndrome. Available from: www.orpha.net/data/patho/GB/uk-MDS.pdf (accessed July 2010).

Rabi Y, Yee W, Chen SY, Singhal N (2006) Oxygen saturation trends immediately after birth. *Journal of Pediatrics* **148**, 590–594.

Reich JD, Miller S, Brogdon B, Casatelli J, Gompf TC, Huhta JC, Sullivan K (2003) The use of pulse oximetry to detect congenital heart disease. *Journal of Pediatrics* **142**, 268–272.

Resuscitation Council Guidelines. (UK) (2010) Newborn Life Support. http://www.resus.org.uk/pages/nls.pdf (accessed May 2014).

Richmond S, Reay G, Abu Harb M (2002) Routine pulse oximetry in the asymptomatic newborn. *Archives of Disease in Childhood. Fetal and Neonatal Edition* **87**, F83–F88.

Riede FT, Wörner C, Dähnert I, Möckel A, Kostelka M, Schneider P (2010) Effectiveness of neonatal pulse oximetry screening for detection of critical congenital heart disease in daily clinical routine-results from a prospective multicenter study. *European Journal of Pediatrics* **169**(8), 975–981.

Roberts D, Kitchiner D (2004) Antenatal diagnosis of fetal heart disease. *Hospital Medicine* **65**, 396–399.

Royal College Obstetricians and Gynaecologists (2015) Clamping of the Umbilical Cord and Placental Transfusion. Scientific Impact Paper No 14, February 2015.

Rudolph AM (2009) Congenital malformations and the fetal circulation. *Archives of Disease in Childhood. Fetal and Neonatal Edition* **95**, F132–F136. Published Online First 25 March 2009. doi: 10.1136/adc.2007.126777.

Rudolph CD, Rudolph AM, Hostetter MK, Lister G, Siegel NJ (eds) (2003) *Rudolph's Pediatrics*. New York: McGraw-Hill, Medical Publication Division.

Sands A, Craig B, Mulholland C, Patterson C, Dornan J, Casey F (2002) Echocardiographic screening for congenital heart disease: a randomized study. *Journal of Perinatal Medicine* **30**(4), 307–312.

Schultz AH, Localio AR, Clark BJ, Ravishankar C, Videon N, Kimmel SE (2008) Epidemiologic features of the presentation of critical congenital heart disease: implications for screening. *Pediatrics* **121**, 751–757.

Shanmugam G, MacArthur K, Pollock JC (2005) Congenital lung malformations: antenatal and postnatal evaluation and management. *European Journal of Cardiothoracic Surgery* **27**, 45–52.

Singh A, Ewer AK (2014) Pulse oximetry screening: do we have enough evidence now? *Journal of Paediatrics and Child Health* **50**(10): 841–842, DOI: 10.1111/jpc.12722.

Spina V, Bagolan P, Nahom A, Trucchi A, Aleandri V, Fabiani C, Giorlandino C (2003) Prenatal diagnosis of congenital diaphragmatic hernia: an update. *Minerva Ginecologica* **55**, 253–257.

Srinivasan R, Arora RS (2004) Do well infants born with an isolated single umbilical artery need investigation? *Archives of Disease in Childhood* **90**, 100–101.

Thangaratina S, Daniels J, Ewer AK, Zamora J, Khan KS (2007) Accuracy of pulse oximetry in screening for congenital heart disease in asymptomatic newborns: a systematic review. *Archives of Disease in Childhood. Fetal and Neonatal Edition* **92**, F176–F180.

Thureen PJ, Deacon J, O'Neill P, Hernandez J (2004) *Assessment and Care of the Well Newborn*. Philadelphia, PA: Saunders.

Tortora GJ, Derrickson BH (2009) *Principles of Anatomy and Physiology*, 12th edn, Hoboken, NJ: John Wiley & Sons.

Toth B, Becker A, Seelbach-Göbel B (2002) Oxygen saturation in healthy newborn infants immediately after birth measured by pulse oximetry. *Archives of Gynecology and Obstetrics* **266**, 105–107.

Tubman TRJ, Shields MD, Craig BG, Mulholland HC, Nevin NC (1991) Congenital heart disease in Down's syndrome: two year prospective early screening study. *British Medical Journal* **302**, 1425–1427.

Valmari P (2007) Should pulse oximetry be used to screen for congenital heart disease?. *Archives of Disease in Childhood. Fetal and Neonatal Edition* **92**, F219–F224.

Van den Hof MC, Wilson RD (2005) Fetal soft markers in obstetric ultrasound. *Journal Obstetrics and Gynaecology Canada* **27**, 592–612.

Wallis C (2000) Clinical outcomes of congenital lung abnormalities. *Pediatric Respiratory Reviews* **1**, 328–335.

Ward-Platt M, Deshpande S (2005) Metabolic adaptation at birth. *Seminars in Fetal and Neonatal Medicine* **10**, 341–350.

Wilson DG (1999) Antenatal detection of congenital heart disease. *Current Paediatrics* **9**, 123–127.

Wren C, Richmond S, Donaldson L (1999) Presentation of congenital heart disease in infancy: implications for routine examination. *Archives of Disease in Childhood. Fetal and Neonatal Edition* **80**, F49–F53.

Zanardo V, Vedovato S, Chiozza L, Faggian D, Favaro F, Trevisanuto D (2008) Pharmacological closure of patent ductus arteriosus: effects on pulse pressure and on endothelin-1 and vasopressin excretion. *American Journal of Perinatology* **25**, 353–358.

Zhao Q-m, Ma X-j, Ge X-I, Liu F, Wu L, Ye M, Liang X-c, Zhang J, Gao Y, Jia B, Huang G-y. (2014) Pulse oximetry with clinical assessment to screen for congenital heart disease in neonates in China: a prospective study. *Lancet* published on line April 23. http://dx.doi.org/10.1016/S0140-6736(14)60198-7 (accessed June 2014).

Zollino M, Murdolo M, Marangi G, Pecile V, Galasso C, Mazzanti L, Neri G (2008) On the nosology and pathogenesis of Wolf–Hirschhorn syndrome: genotype-phenotype correlation analysis of 80 patients and literature review. *American Journal of Medical Genetics, Part C Seminars in Medical Genetics* **148C**(4), 257–269.

CHAPTER 3

The neonatal skin: examination of the jaundiced newborn and gestational age assessment

Morris Gordon[1] and Anne Lomax[2]

[1] Department of Paediatric Gastroenterology, Royal Manchester Children's Hospital, Manchester, UK
[2] Department of Midwifery, University of Central Lancashire, Preston, UK

KEY POINTS

- There should be a consistent approach to skin care in the newborn on both regional and national levels.

- There are different terms used to categorise newborn jaundice. It is important to understand their significance.

- Physiological newborn jaundice can present a challenge to the practitioner with regard to the different investigation and management options.

- Utilising evidence-based consensus guideline documents relating to jaundiced newborns is crucial in supporting best practice options of care.

- By knowing gestational age and growth patterns, the practitioner can identify infants at risk for complications in the postnatal period and amend care plans accordingly.

Introduction

The neonatal skin is the largest organ of the body providing many vital functions as the baby adapts to extra-uterine life. The skin begins its development early on in pregnancy and continues to mature after birth (Jackson, 2008). The roles and functions of the skin are many and varied providing first and foremost a natural barrier against infection if the skin remains intact. This delicate organ plays major part in thermoregulation, the subcutaneous layer of fat insulates the neonate from cold. Skin permeability and water loss further regulate heat exchange and electrolyte balance.

As a sensory organ, the dermal layer of the skin is richly enervated and the neonate can obtain much information about its environment through

---

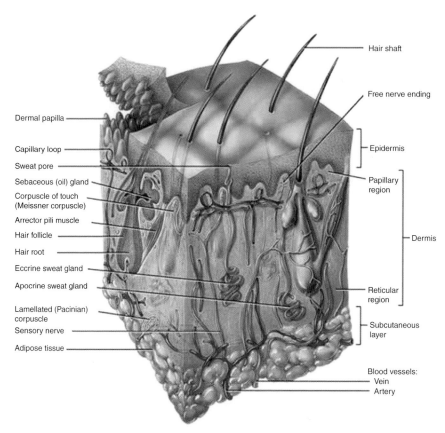

Hair shaft

Free nerve ending

Dermal papilla

Capillary loop

Sweat pore

Sebaceous (oil) gland

Corpuscle of touch
(Meissner corpuscle)

Arrector pili muscle

Hair follicle

Hair root

Eccrine sweat gland

Apocrine sweat gland

Lamellated (Pacinian)
corpuscle

Sensory nerve

Adipose tissue

Epidermis

Papillary
region

Dermis

Reticular
region

Subcutaneous
layer

Blood vessels:
Vein
Artery

Figure 3.1 Components of the epidermis, dermis and subcutaneous tissue. Source: Tortora
and Derrickson (2009). Reproduced with permission of John Wiley & Sons.

perception of changes in temperature, pressure, pain levels and tactile stimulation. Skin-to-skin contact with its mother soon after birth can facilitate
the neonate's normal neurological adaptation and behavioural state. It can
stabilise thermoregulation and help establish a closer maternal–infant bond,
laying down the foundations for future physiological well-being (Kenner and
Wright-Lott, 2007).

   The three main layers of the skin consist of an outermost layer called the epidermis, a middle layer called the dermis and an underlying layer of subcutaneous
fat or hypodermis (Figure 3.1).

   The layers of the skin will now be examined in more detail, *starting with the
innermost layer first.*

   This underlying layer of subcutaneous white adipose tissue (hypodermis)
consists mainly of fat deposits and connective tissue and has a lobular structure. White adipose tissue is deposited in most significant amounts in the last
trimester of pregnancy and forms an insulatory layer and calorie store for

postnatal life. This white fat differs from brown fat or brown adipose tissue. The latter has a more abundant blood, glucose and nerve supply and is responsible for non-shivering thermoregulation in the newborn (see also Chapter 2).

Above the subcutaneous fat layer lies the dermis. This layer is made up of connective tissue, nerves blood and lymphatic vessels. Around 90% of the connective tissue component is collagen with elastic and rectangular fibres. Fibroblasts within the dermis produce elastin, collagen and mucopolysaccharides giving the dermis a characteristic strength and elasticity. Development of this fibrous complex begins around 8–12 weeks of pregnancy and continues to mature after birth. Hair follicles and sebaceous glands are also contained within the dermis. Above the dermis lies the epidermis, which is made up of the following layers:
- Stratum germinativum/basalis (innermost layer)
- Stratum spinosum
- Stratum granulosum
- Stratum corneum (outermost layer).

At the dermal/epidermal junction is the innermost layer of the epidermis: the stratum basalis or basal cell layer. This layer is important for the integrity of the skin and new cells called keratinocytes are being continually produced here. Keratinocytes are the major cells of the epidermis containing intracellular lipid. As new cells appear at the basal layer, they move up through the stratum granulosum and towards the outer layers of the skin. In doing so, they lose the majority of lipid content which then surrounds the dry flatted cells and causes them to stick to each other to form a tough outer layer of skin called the stratum corneum. There are 10–20 layers of the stratum corneum in full-term infants (Jackson, 2008). As the cells continue to move towards the skin surface, the cohesive forces lessen and desquamation (shedding) occurs. The outermost stratum corneum protects the neonate from dehydration and the entry of bacteria or chemical substances that may be applied topically. In fetal life, as the skin matures, the basal cell layer of the epidermis develops down-growths which penetrate into the dermis and form ridges. This genetically controlled process produces groves on the surface of the hands and soles of the feet. The epidermal ridges found on the fingers eventually develop into fingerprints. If chromosomal makeup is abnormal as in Down's syndrome, the extent to which the epidermal rides develop will be affected. This can result in the diagnostic appearance of a distinct palmer and/or plantar crease pattern after birth (Blackburn, 2007).

The topmost layer of skin is continually being shed and, *in utero*, dead cells from the stratum corneum mix with secretions from sebaceous glands to form the thick white greasy substance called vernix caseosa. This starts around 20 weeks' gestation and increases in amount until approximately 36 weeks. It then begins to disappear. At term, it is mainly found in the creases of the newborn (Lund et al., 1999). Melanocytes are also found within the lower layers of the epidermis, production of melanin and thus pigmentation start before birth. In babies of African origin or Asian babies, clusters of melanocytes can

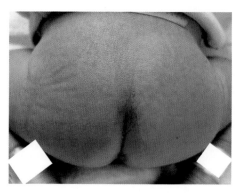

Figure 3.2 Mongolian blue spot. Reproduced with kind permission of Dr Malcolm Battin, Auckland City Hospital.

form in the dermis. These can be recognised clinically as Mongolian blue spots (Figure 3.2), which cover the buttocks, back and sometimes shoulders of the newborn. As pigmentation of the skin develops, the Mongolian spots disappear (Kenner and Wright-Lott, 2007).

The neonatal skin continues to mature within the first few days by a process of water loss, desquamation and drying out of the stratum corneum. At birth, newborn skin looks pale and fairly transparent, sometimes with localised oedema. Vernix caseosa acts as a natural moisturiser and protects the outer layers of the skin to allow normal adaptation to the new aerobic environment (Trotter, 2008). In the first week, superficial skin peeling often occurs on the hands and feet with normal underlying skin; this is thought to be part of the natural maturation process. The skin then becomes comparable to that of an adult in thickness, providing a vital barrier to the environment. Despite this, the neonatal skin is more permeable to substances applied topically, substances such as drugs or chemicals can be absorbed rapidly.

The pH of the neonatal skin is naturally alkaline and virtually sterile at birth. In response to its new aerobic environment, the neonatal skin quickly changes to a more acid state known as the 'acid mantle'. The acid mantle is thought to influence both the colonisation of skin and the normal adaptation of the stratum corneum. This usually happens within the first week (Jackson, 2008).

Assessment of the neonatal skin

Colour

The full-term newborn baby from white ethnic groups will exhibit a generally pale skin colour. In the first 24–48 hours, the hands, feet and circumoral areas may be slightly cyanosed until normal circulatory and respiratory adaptation has taken place. Acrocyanosis (hands and feet) is a common finding after birth and will usually resolve within a few days. Assessment of cyanosis in the neonate may

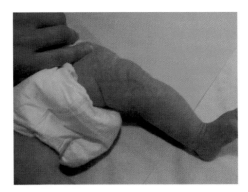

Figure 3.3 Cutis marmorata. Reproduced with kind permission of Dr Malcolm Battin, Auckland City Hospital.

present problems for some practitioners and the use of pulse oximetry during this assessment merits further consideration (O'Donnell et al., 2007). This has been discussed in greater depth in Chapter 2.

Evidence of pallor in the neonate may indicate anaemia, hypoxia or shock arising from poor peripheral perfusion. Pallor may also indicate the presence of infection (Kenner and Wright-Lott, 2007). Cutis marmorata (Figure 3.3) may be seen as a response to chilling and can be identified by a bluish mottling effect appearing on the trunk and limbs. It usually disappears when the infant is warmed. A midline demarcation in colour may be observed in the newborn period known as Harlequin sign; this is due to a temporary vasomotor disturbance in newborns and is not thought to be harmful in the healthy newborn.

In the first few hours after birth, the neonate may develop an intense red colour (plethora) and is common in infants with an excess of red blood cells (polycythaemia). In an effort to break down the extra-red blood cells, a physiological hyperbilirubinaemia may occur leading to a yellow discolouration of the skin known as jaundice. This can take up to 48 hours to develop and appears to some degree in 60–70% of full-term infants. The condition is usually self-limiting but can be prolonged for a few weeks in breastfed infants (Deken, 2008). Jaundice that appears immediately after birth or is present within the first 24 hours must be regarded as pathological in nature and warrants immediate referral to a paediatrician. Jaundice will be discussed in greater depth later on in this chapter.

Care of the neonatal skin: a consistent approach to practice

Health-care professionals who perform examination of the newborn are in an ideal position to influence choices made by women and their families to help ensure good maternal health. Moreover, the examination can provide a valuable opportunity to advise women on health promotion issues such as nutrition, baby bathing and cord care practices

National guidance on the standards necessary to define 'good practice' within maternity services is crucial. Development of practice guidelines help guarantee a high level of quality and consistency but they must be informed and under-pinned by current research-based evidence and they must be applied using an individualised approach. Mothers and babies should have access to a practitioner who provides a flexible but informed attitude to care designed to meet their individual needs.

Despite this, there is currently no recognised national guidance outlining best skin care practice for the full-term infant in any detail. Paucity of well-designed research studies on this topic has been identified by several authors (Atherton and Mills, 2004; Walker et al., 2005; Hale, 2007; Jackson, 2008; Trotter, 2008; Atherton, 2009).

Both the World Health Organisation (WHO, 2003) and the National Institute for Clinical Excellence (NICE, 2014) have made reference to neonatal skincare in their publications but without entering into any great depth.

Research has been undertaken in the United States (US) by the Association of Women's Health Obstetrics and Neonatal Nurses/National Association of Neona-tal Nurses (AWHONN/NNAN); however, this study was primarily concerned with the preterm baby (Lund et al., 1999). More recently, this organization has pub-lished an evidence-based clinical practice guideline (AWHONN, 2007) available from their website https://www.awhonn.org/awhonn/.

Midwife Sharon Trotter provided us with an in-depth evidence-based view of neonatal skin care practices in the United Kingdom. This has been achieved through extensive work on the effects of manufactured skin care products on the neonatal skin (Trotter, 2002, 2004, 2006a, 2006b, 2008).

The aims of essential skin care in the newborn immediately following deliv-ery are to preserve the natural lipid barrier, allow normal bacterial colonisation to take place, allow the acid mantle to develop undisturbed and facilitate nat-ural separation of the umbilical cord. The use of synthetic detergents would disturb these vital processes and so plain water is advocated for the first bath immediately following delivery. This practice should continue for at least the first month following birth, and then soaps, etc. should be introduced only grad-ually. Under no circumstances must products be used on unbroken skin (Trotter, 2008). Trotter goes on to advocate that vernix caseosa is left on the skin as added protection in the first few days – this guideline is also upheld by the WHO in its publication on *Pregnancy, Childbirth, Postpartum and Newborn Care* (2003). If a moisturiser is needed after a few weeks, an emollient-based moisturiser should only be used. To protect against nappy rash, a thin layer of petroleum jelly is recommended.

Similarly, the cord should be left undisturbed and bathing avoided until sep-aration has occurred. The nappy should be folded down to expose the cord at each change. If an umbilical flare or any obvious signs of infection should develop, a swab may need to be taken for culture and sensitivity (Trotter, 2008).

More recently, Lavender et al (2013) conducted a study into comparison of water versus wash product on newborn skin over a 14-day period. They found that the wash product did not appear to significantly cause changes in skin structure, hydration or pH of the skin. The rate of transepidermal water loss was also thought to be unaffected. In addition, Ness et al. (2013) reviewed current evidence regarding neonatal skin care practices and concluded that mild pH neutral skin care products were safe to use on the full-term newborn skin. They went on to suggest that use of emollients has little benefit in preventing skin infections but may have a role in skin barrier maturation and repair. NICE (2014) remain consistent with their 2006 advice on neonatal skin care, recommending that plain water only should be used together and a 'non perfumed soap' only if necessary.

Common skin lesions in neonate

The skin of the neonate may exhibit a variety of dermatological conditions. Some of these may be present at the time of the initial examination and will more than likely cause anxiety to the mother and father. Practitioners who undertake examination of the newborn should be familiar with common skin disorders. Careful assessment of skin integrity together with knowledge of normal variations and appropriate referral will contribute to accurate diagnosis and timely intervention. Integrity of the skin may have been affected at delivery with damage to skin and underlying tissue. During delivery, the presenting part may have been subjected to pressure trauma resulting in oedema and haematoma formation. Instrumental delivery with forceps or vacuum extraction can cause additional damage and breaks in the skin can occur from the use of fetal scalp electrodes used in fetal monitoring or from fetal scalp blood sampling (Blackburn, 2007). Ecchymosis or bruising may also be present and if extensive may contribute to the degree of physiological jaundice that is likely to develop. Petechiae are pinpoint haemorrhagic spots on the skin distributed over the trunk and face and are caused by pressure of delivery and rotation through the birth canal. Evidence of petechiae on the face may also be associated with delivery of infants where the umbilical cord is wrapped tightly around the neck. They will usually fade within a few days; however, a petechial rash that becomes more extensive may be indicative of infection or a bleeding disorder and may warrant further investigation (Lund and Kuller, 2007).

Non-infectious skin disorders
Erythema toxicum neonatorum
This is a harmless self-limiting condition, which can develop within 72 hours of birth. It is characterised by erythematous pustules, which contain eosinophils usually involving the face and trunk but may develop anywhere on the body (Figure 3.4). It will resolve spontaneously over several days.

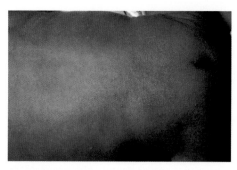

Figure 3.4 Erythema toxicum neonatorum. Reproduced with kind permission of Dr Malcolm Battin, Auckland City Hospital.

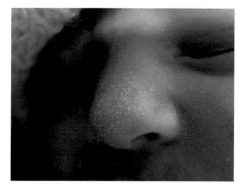

Figure 3.5 Milia. Reproduced with kind permission of Dr Malcolm Battin, Auckland City Hospital.

Milia

These are small white follicular cysts commonly known as milk spots (Figure 3.5). They normally appear in clusters on the cheeks, forehead, nose and nasolabial folds and clear within the first 4 weeks of life. They are believed to be the result of retention of keratin and sebaceous material.

Miliaria

This is commonly known as prickly heat and presents as superficial clear vesicles or deep, grouped red papules on forehead and skin folds in the first weeks of life. It is caused by obstruction of eccrine or sweat glands due to oedema of the stratum corneum and is associated with overheating in the neonate. The lesions will resolve in a few hours if the infant is kept cool and dry.

Neonatal acne

These are small red papules and pustules on the face and can be observed in approximately 20% of neonates (Figure 3.6). It is otherwise known as cephalic

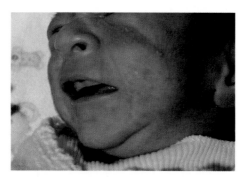

Figure 3.6 Neonatal acne. Reproduced with kind permission of Dr Malcolm Battin, Auckland City Hospital.

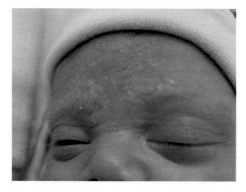

Figure 3.7 Cradle cap. Reproduced with kind permission of Dr Malcolm Battin, Auckland City Hospital.

pustulosis and is believed to be caused by the influence of maternal hormones on the infant's sebaceous glands. It will usually resolve around 3 months of age.

Seborrhoeic dermatitis (cradle cap)
Commonly seen on the scalp of the newborn but can also occur in the axillae, groins and napkin areas (Figure 3.7). It is characterised by scaling lesions with a greasy feeling and is thought to be a reactive response to irritants. However, bacterial infection can exacerbate this condition.

Sucking blisters
These are a common finding and can be recognised as clear blisters, which appear on the skin – usually the hands and fingers (Figure 3.8). They are present at birth and develop as a result of *in utero* sucking.

Transient neonatal pustulosis
This disorder is present at birth and mainly seen in black neonates. Small vesicles and pustules appear over the face, limbs and back, but there is no associated

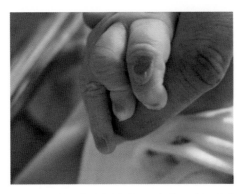

Figure 3.8 Sucking blister. Reproduced with kind permission of Dr Malcolm Battin, Auckland City Hospital.

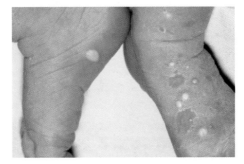

Figure 3.9 Transient neonatal pustulosis. Reproduced with kind permission of Dr Malcolm Battin, Auckland City Hospital.

erythema (Figure 3.9). Neonates can be isolated unnecessarily as infection is often wrongly suspected. The pustules may continue to appear for weeks but eventually subside leaving brown scaly macules. There is no treatment required (Verbov, 2000; Tappero and Honeyfield, 2010; Thureen et al., 2005; Lund and Kuller, 2007; Sethuraman and Mancini, 2008).

Infectious skin disorders
Impetigo

This is the most common skin infection and can be caused by *Staphylococcus aureus* or *Streptococcus pyogenes*. There are two types, the less common bullous impetigo appears as superficial pus-filled blisters in the napkin area around the umbilicus and over the trunk (Figure 3.10). It can be treated with appropriate antibiotic treatment. The more common non-bullous (or 'crusted' impetigo) presents with erythematous papules and vesicles.

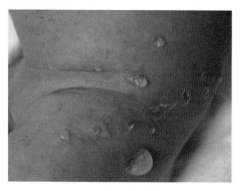

Figure 3.10 Bulbous impetigo. Reproduced with kind permission of Dr Malcolm Battin, Auckland City Hospital.

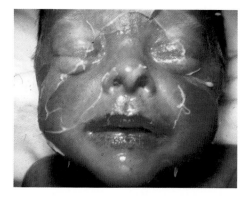

Figure 3.11 Scalded skin syndrome. Reproduced with kind permission of Dr David Clark.

Staphylococcal scalded skin syndrome

This is a fairly uncommon disorder caused by *Staphylococcus aureus*, sometimes seen in full-term infants. It can begin with localised infection characterised by an erythematous rash that forms clusters of fluid-filled blisters within 12–14 hours of initial symptoms. The skin visibly separates leaving raw areas (Figure 3.11). There is an accompanying hyperpyrexia and evidence of poor feeding and handling. Sites for colonisation of *Staphylococcus aureus* are around the mouth, nose and umbilicus. Lesions can also be found on the perineum. The severity of peeling will depend on the effects of the toxin to the skin but scarring should not be expected to occur. Treatment is with an antistaphylococcal agent.

Neonatal herpes

This condition is usually acquired through the infected genital tract during vaginal delivery although vertical transmission from an infected mother can also occur. The condition has the potential to develop incrementally into a severe infection carrying a high mortality rate. Skin lesions are evident in the first stages and appear as raised vesicles with accompanying erythema. These may develop into pustules within a few days. The lesions most commonly occur around the eyes, scalp, mouth and umbilical regions with involvement of the presenting part in many cases. The condition may progress to involve the central nervous system and go on to be disseminated more widely in the later stages. It should be noted that absence of skin involvement does not rule out the presence of the disease. Prompt referral and treatment is vital.

Candida infection

The condition can be either transmitted *in utero* from ascending vaginal infection or acquired after birth. Lesions will manifest around 1 week of age. If the infection has been transmitted *in utero*, the lesions will be more widespread over the neonate's skin and appear in great numbers as erythematous papules and pustules. Upon rupture, the outer layers of the skin become red and excoriated. In localised infection acquired after birth, neonates are most commonly infected in the mouth and napkin areas. In oral candidiasis, the infection typically presents as white plaques on the tongue and cheeks. In the napkin area, the rash is moist with small yellow or white pustules accompanied in some cases with skin erosion. Antifungal treatment is necessary. Failure to respond to treatment should alert the practitioner to the possibility of a compromised immune system (Verbov, 2000; Rudolph et al., 2002; Atherton and Mills, 2004; Lund and Kuller, 2007; Sethuraman and Mancini, 2008; Atherton, 2009).

Common lesions involving pigment

Skin pigment develops in stages in the normal neonate. In fetal life, melanocytes gradually increase in number as pregnancy progresses and transport melanin from the dermis to the basal cells of the epidermis. Melanin is responsible for skin colour and production in newborns is relatively low and some lesions if not present at birth may take time to develop. We have already reviewed the presence of benign Mongolian blue spots at birth produced by clusters of melanocytes in the dermis. These areas of hyperpigmentation are more common in babies of African origin and will tend to fade over the first 2–3 years of life.

Café-au-lait spots

These are brown, well-defined patches less than 3 cm diameter, which will become darker and more apparent with time. They represent areas of increased melanin and keratinocytes and can occur anywhere in the body. Café-au-lait spots are not generally associated with a syndrome; however, large or multiple patches may be indicative of neurofibromatosis.

Pigmented naevi

Around 3% of neonates will manifest this type of lesion at birth. It can appear as a dark brown patch on the lower back or buttocks with possible prominent

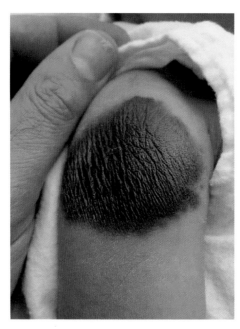

Figure 3.12 Pigmented naevus. Reproduced with kind permission of Dr Malcolm Battin, Auckland City Hospital.

speckling around the periphery of the lesion (Figure 3.12). They are due to a benign proliferation of melanocytes in the dermis and/or epidermis and usually present as a solitary patch. The major clinical concern with these lesions is the development of malignancy and must be monitored closely for changes in size or shape (Batt, 2000; Moss, 2000; Verbov, 2000; Rudolph et al., 2002; Tappero and Honeyfield, 2010; Lund and Kuller, 2007; Sethuraman and Mancini, 2008).

Common vascular birthmarks

Vascular lesions can be explained in two ways. The first category of birthmarks can be described as haemangiomas, which signify proliferation of the vasculature up to approximately 12 months of age. Growth then stabilises up to approximately 18 months of age when they involute spontaneously over the following 5–10 years.

The second category can be described as vascular malformations, which signify developmental abnormalities of the capillary, lymphatic, venous or arterial blood vessels. These are congenital malformations that grow but do not involute spontaneously.

Salmon patch haemangioma (naevus simplex) or 'stork marks'

These appear most commonly on the nape of the neck, eyelids and glabella in around 50% of neonates. Stork marks can be recognised as dull red patches

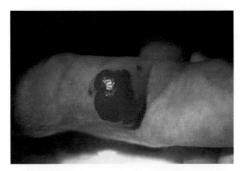

Figure 3.13 Strawberry haemangioma. Reproduced with kind permission of Dr David Clark.

containing superficial capillaries which blanch on pressure. They will resolve spontaneously; no treatment is necessary.

Strawberry haemangioma
This is a raised lobular capillary haemangioma that occurs in approximately 10% of neonates by the age of 1 year and is not always present at birth. It has a bright red colour and may be single or multiple and can frequently have both superficial and deep tissue properties (Figure 3.13). The tumours are mostly benign but can cause problems in the proliferative phase depending on location. Once involuted, the deeper haemangiomas may leave fibrous tissue.

Cavernous haemangioma
This is similar to the strawberry haemangioma but penetrates deeper into the underlying tissue and occur less commonly. It will increase in size after birth but, as with other haemangiomas, will resolve spontaneously.

Port wine stain (naevus flammeus)
These birthmarks fall into the category of vascular abnormalities and so do not follow the pattern of haemangiomas. They present as pink or bright red vascular patches, which consist of mature capillaries in the dermis (Figure 3.14). They are present in approximately 0.3% of neonates. Most port wine stains occur as an isolated lesion whose size remains static without spontaneous resolution over time. These birthmarks commonly appear over the face and can thicken and darken with time. Most port wine stain birthmarks are isolated; however, they can also be associated with various syndromes depending on location. Sturge–Weber syndrome is characterised by a port wine stain that involves the skin served by the trigeminal nerve and so facial birthmarks are a common association. Children with this syndrome may also present with seizures and glaucoma and/or orbital vascular abnormalities. In Klippel–Trénaunay syndrome, the extremities are usually involved, and as the child grows, venous varicosities and bony overgrowth become evident. In Cobb syndrome, the port wine stain is usually seen along with spinal cord vascular malformation.

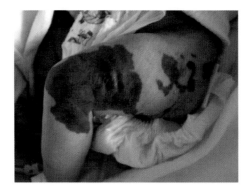

Figure 3.14 Port wine stain. Reproduced with kind permission of Dr Malcolm Battin, Auckland City Hospital.

Examination of the jaundiced newborn

Introduction

Jaundice describes yellow staining of the skin and eyes. It is caused by excessive levels of the bile pigment bilirubin. It is the most common problem encountered in newborns, occurring in 50% of full-term infants and 85% of preterm infants (Levene et al., 2008). Usually, this finding is not of any danger to newborns and is merely a reflection of normal adaptive processes at birth. It is important for the newborn examiner to be aware of the more sinister origins of jaundice and when they may present. It is also important to understand the direct dangers of high levels of bilirubin to a newborn and ways this can be managed. In this chapter, we discuss the mechanisms that lead to jaundice in a way that helps the reader understand physiological and pathological causes of jaundice. We also discuss the evidence base for investigation and management of jaundice in newborns and direct the reader to some useful up-to-date resources to direct care.

Physiology of neonatal jaundice

The red blood cells in our body are constantly being broken down by macrophages to be replaced with new cells. When this happens, the red pigment in our blood cells (haemoglobin) is also broken down. The 'haem' portion creates the bile pigment biliverdin as a by-product. This is converted to bilirubin; the yellow pigment that causes jaundice. This is an entirely normal process and is continuous. The bilirubin will travel to the liver in the blood, usually attached to albumin, which renders it non-toxic, and then a key process takes place within the liver. The bilirubin is conjugated, a reaction that converts the bilirubin, so it is water soluble. From the liver, this water-soluble conjugated bilirubin finishes its journey by being excreted in bile and travelling into the gut. It can be passed into the stool after further breakdown by gut bacteria, giving the characteristic colour to stools. It can also be converted by the gut bacteria

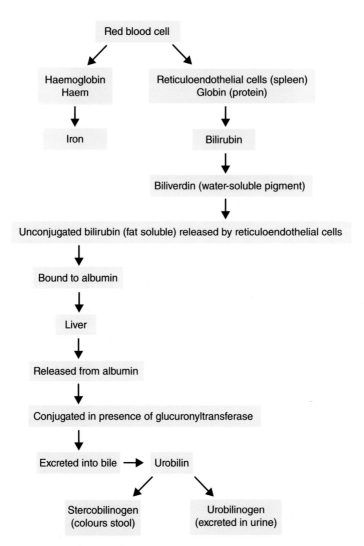

Figure 3.15 Physiology of neonatal jaundice.

to urobilinogen and reabsorbed from the gut and passed by the kidneys giving colour to urine (Figure 3.15).

This normal process should keep levels of bilirubin in the blood low at all times, so normally one would never appear jaundiced in day-to-day life. If we contrast that situation with the situation at birth, there are a number of factors that affect the status quo. When a neonate is born, for the first time their liver is asked to take the load of the bilirubin conjugation that up till now the mother has been dealing with through the placenta. The newborn's liver takes a while to perform its function as an adult's would and so is less able to process the bilirubin load. In addition, a newborn breaks down blood cells twice as fast as an adult because of shortened blood cell life and a proportionately higher amount of cells in the blood (Maisels, 2007). At the final stage of bilirubin excretion, because of a lower bacterial load in the gut, much of the conjugated water-soluble bilirubin cannot be converted into urobilinogen. Consequently, it ends up being broken down back into unconjugated bilirubin, further increasing unconjugated bilirubin levels. All these mechanisms together cause the so-called physiological jaundice.

Dangers of newborn jaundice

As previously mentioned, bilirubin will travel in the blood temporarily bound to albumin. This removes the toxic effects of bilirubin by specifically reducing its ability to leave the intravascular space and cross the blood–brain barrier. Despite the extremely large bilirubin load a newborn has to deal with, they are still able to bind very large amounts of this free unconjugated bilirubin to albumin. There are times when the amount of bilirubin produced is so high that it simply overwhelms the newborn's binding capacity, or alternatively due to sickness or prematurity, their binding capacity is reduced. In either of these scenarios, there may be an excess of unconjugated bilirubin that, because it is unbound and lipid soluble, is able to cross the blood–brain barrier. Kernicterus was a term initially used as a pathological diagnosis when bilirubin staining was found in the brain, but the term is generally used now to describe bilirubin encephalopathy; the clinical nervous system findings of bilirubin toxicity. The classic signs of severe bilirubin encephalopathy are hypertonia, drowsiness, poor feeding, hypotonia and alternating tone (Johnson et al., 1999). Recently, a grading scheme was described (Volpe, 2001) that allows an accurate documentation of the severity of acute bilirubin encephalopathy. Death can occur from kernicterus, usually due to respiratory failure and coma, or intractable seizures.

With the current trend of early postnatal discharges, a kinder, gentler approach to the management of full-term newborns with jaundice has developed (Dodd, 1993). This may explain why the incidence of kernicterus appears to have increased in the 1990s, and a recent UK study (Manning et al., 2007) reported a surprising number of cases of kernicterus in recent years, in line with similar trends in US figures (Newman and Maisels, 2000). There have been such concerns with this worrying finding that in 2001, the Joint Committee on Accreditation of Healthcare Organizations (JCAHO) in the United States issued a sentinel event alert for kernicterus and suggested units worldwide adopt strategies of more aggressive screening and management (Anonymous, 2001).

Categorising newborn jaundice

When discussing newborn jaundice, a number of different terms and methods are used that may cause confusion. Before progressing, these need clarification. The first form of categorisation has already been discussed, i.e. jaundice is unconjugated or conjugated. Unconjugated jaundice is the most common form of jaundice encountered and is dangerous in its own right, as this bilirubin can cross the blood–brain barrier and cause kernicterus. Conjugated jaundice is generally described when more than 10% of the total bilirubin is conjugated. This cannot cause kernicterus and in itself is not dangerous. It does, however, point to potentially serious and even life-threatening illnesses and so still demands urgent investigation. Knowing which form of jaundice a baby is suffering from will direct investigations appropriately.

The next categories are early jaundice and prolonged or late jaundice. Early jaundice usually refers to jaundice in the first 24 hours of life. This is of concern because all the mechanisms described in the previous sections that cause physiological jaundice are not likely to take place in these early hours of life. This raises the concern of a pathological cause, which will be discussed in detail next. Prolonged or late onset jaundice varies in specific definitions. Generally, 2 weeks of age in a term baby and 3 weeks in a preterm baby are taken as the boundaries for reconsidering a diagnosis of physiological jaundice. This prolonged jaundice can be conjugated or unconjugated and depending on this, investigations may be planned accordingly.

Finally, jaundice may be categorised as physiological or pathological. This simply describes whether the jaundice is as a result of the normal processes previously discussed or whether an underlying reason is at play. It may not be clear which is the case in a newborn, but investigations must be planned in a logical, evidence-based and safe manner so as not to risk missing a potentially unwell newborn. Physiological jaundice most commonly occurs at between 2 and 5 days of age, although this does not mean it cannot occur earlier or persist later into the newborn period.

Assessing newborn jaundice

Traditionally, practitioners tend to use a visual assessment of clinical jaundice as a method of classifying severity of hyperbilirubinaemia. We would strongly discourage this practice, as it is very hard to distinguish the level of bilirubin in this way. For example, perceiving a difference of 60 mg/dL of bilirubin clinically is not possible, but in a 24-hour-old newborn, this is the difference between the 50th and 95th percentiles (Maisels, 2007) and would have massive clinical implications if confused. Therefore, particularly in the early hours of a newborn's life, serum blood levels should be checked if jaundice is seen clinically. In older term newborns that are clinically well and have no risk factors for underlying disorders, judgement must be used when deciding whether to send a blood sample. Certainly, it could be strongly argued that if you are questioning whether or not to send a sample if you have concerns about a newborn's jaundice, sending a sample is probably the correct action. Up until recently, treatment thresholds for jaundice were set based on experience from the first half of the last century (Rennie, 2005). The campaign by Newman and Maisels (2000) for a kinder and gentler approach to jaundice and the backlash from this have led to much more evidence-based ways of charting risk in newborn's with jaundice by the creation of clear nomograms (Bhutani et al., 1999). Most units have adapted versions for use locally and these must be used as the basis for treatment decisions, given the previously mentioned rise in severe hyperbilirubinaemia.

Early jaundice

Generally, if a newborn becomes jaundiced in the first 24 hours of life, it is deemed to be early jaundice. Although we have discussed many physiological reasons for jaundice, in early jaundice, it is more likely that there is an alternative pathological cause. In particular, a bilirubin level rising at a rate of greater than 10 μmol/L per hour in the first 24 hours of life is highly suggestive of an increased red cell breakdown (haemolysis) (Johnston et al., 2003a, 2003b). It should be assumed that haemolysis is the cause of early jaundice until proven otherwise, so, in this context, investigations must be instigated (Levene et al., 2008). Consideration of the risk factors, symptoms and signs of sepsis must also be made, and in light of these concerns, a paediatric review is recommended for all cases of jaundice within the first 24 hours of life.

Haemolytic disease of the newborn

Haemolysis may result from blood group incompatibility, congenital abnormalities of red cell shape or structure or inherited deficiencies of red cell enzymes. Sepsis can also exaggerate the normal haemolytic process. A haemolytic process will lead to an unconjugated jaundice. The most common and urgent cause to identify has traditionally been rhesus incompatibility between the mother and the newborn. This is an alloimmune condition that develops in a fetus when IgG antibodies that have been produced by a rhesus-negative blood group mother pass through the placenta causing fetal red cell breakdown and resulting jaundice. In 1966, two groups from the United Kingdom and the United States demonstrated that anti-D IgG prophylaxis soon after delivery prevented sensitisation in Rh-negative women. The WHO in 1971 recommended that a dose of 25 μg (125 IU) of anti-D immunoglobulin should be given intramuscularly for every 1 mL of feto–maternal haemorrhage of Rh-positive packed RBCs or 2 mL of whole blood. This effective strategy was followed up in 1998 with advice from the American College of Obstetrics and Gynaecology suggesting routine maternal anti-D prophylaxis of rhesus-negative women at 28 weeks' gestation. This is now widely adopted in the United Kingdom with the aim of reducing the frequency and severity of rhesus haemolytic disease of newborns. Guidance for screening of infants born to at-risk mothers currently varies across the United Kingdom, as the impact of the new prophylactic programme is recognised. Current evidence (Gordon and Bhadoria, 2008) would point to a strategy of routinely screening cord blood samples of at-risk babies. Tests should include a blood group, full blood count and particularly a bilirubin level, as this is an accurate indicator of the need for immediate treatment escalation. The Direct Coombs test is less useful in pregnancies where prophylaxis was administered, as a weak positive result is possible and this may not be significant. Consultation of up-to-date local guidelines is suggested.

Physiological jaundice

Resulting from the mechanisms discussed earlier, this is an extremely common newborn problem that rarely needs active intervention. Presence of certain risk factors can increase the frequency and severity of physiological jaundice, such as low birth weight, prematurity or male gender. Use of nomograms and other tools already discussed will guide therapy, as there are still circumstances when a physiological jaundice can require active management.

Prolonged/late onset jaundice

Jaundice that begins or persists past 14 days of age in a full-term newborn must prompt further consideration of specific history, risk factors and the need for a series of investigations. There are a number of conditions that will be excluded in initial screening tests and most units will have clear guidance on this process. These policies will usually involve community midwifery services liaising with inpatient paediatrics to organise a review and basic blood tests, although many midwives will begin by performing a split bilirubin level within the community setting. The key question that this addresses is whether the jaundice is conjugated or unconjugated. There are huge numbers of possible causes in both situations, but this differentiation is key, as early recognition of an obstructive jaundice is paramount. This is so named as it is due to obstruction of bile flow and results in a conjugated jaundice. The uncommon presentation of a baby with conjugated persistent jaundice, pale stools and dark urine suggests this obstructive picture and urgent referral for investigation at a national paediatric liver centre is indicated. The most common findings in this case are biliary atresia and neonatal hepatitis (Andres, 1996). In the case of biliary atresia, prompt surgical intervention can significantly reduce morbidity and so time is of the essence. The British Society of Gastroenterology Hepatology and Nutrition published guidelines on the investigation of such newborns in 2007 (Anonymous, 2007), which are available for reference at https://bspghan.org.uk/documents/Investigation%20of%20Conjugated%20hyperbilirubinaemia%202012.pdf.

Management of newborn jaundice

A majority of newborns will not require active medical intervention for jaundice, as it will be physiological and not of a significantly high level to be of danger. Monitoring of the newborn's progress can be done within the community, with escalation and involvement of other services only if there are concerns with the child's clinical state or if a biochemically alarming picture develops. There are cases where the level of hyperbilirubinaemia will be such that, as well as treatment of a possible underlying cause, management will be needed to prevent possible kernicterus. Options include phototherapy, exchange transfusion or medication. Phototherapy works by infusing light energy which is absorbed by bilirubin and changes it into forms that can be excreted directly or can bypass the liver altogether for excretion. Easily and safely administered, this is a common therapy found on all postnatal wards. By contrast, exchange transfusion is now a much less common therapy. It involves a large blood transfusion with simultaneous removal of the newborn's blood. This is a complex procedure which rapidly reduces bilirubin levels and slows the haemolytic process. With the reduction in rhesus haemolytic disease, it is now much less commonly indicated and tends to be performed at specialist centres, where possible, due to the loss of expertise at local level. Finally, there are drugs that can improve bile flow and lower bilirubin levels, but these are not the mainstay of treatment, with one exception. In the case of a haemolytic jaundice, administration of intravenous immunoglobulin may be used to prevent an exchange transfusion. As this is a pooled blood product, its use must be considered carefully. A new guideline published by the National Institute for Health and Clinical Excellence (NICE, 2014) recommends alterations to current NHS practice, particularly regarding recognition and management of neonatal jaundice. This can be found at https://www.nice.org.uk/guidance/qs57.

Assessment of gestational age

A gestational age assessment evaluating physical and neuromuscular charac-teristics can be performed as part of the initial examination of the newborn. Estimation of gestational age is possible because there is a predictable pattern of physical changes that occur throughout gestation. Although some hospitals make gestational age assessment a routine practice, other establishments have devel-oped criteria for performing the assessment based on birth weight, suspected intrauterine growth restriction, post-maturity or suspected prematurity.

Even in infants who weigh 3–3.5 kg, a careful and accurate assessment of gestational age needs to be undertaken to verify term status. This helps identify potential feeding and respiratory problems that are more common with selected gestational ages and increases the likelihood of timely referral and early intervention during the immediate newborn period. By knowing gestational age and growth patterns, the practitioner can identify infants at risk for complications in the postnatal period and amend care plans accordingly (Simpson and Creehan, 2008).

Originally, the most popular assessment tool was the Dubowitz scoring system based on assessment of neurological and external criteria (Dubowitz et al., 1970). Later on, Ballard et al. (1979) revised the scoring system by reducing the number of criteria assessed. The assessment became more accurate and quicker to perform.

A further modification by Ballard in 1991 called the New Ballard Score (Ballard et al., 1991) provided an instrument that could also include the assessment of extremely premature babies in various ethnic groups infants. The examination is separated into two parts: firstly, an assessment of maturity of neuromuscular function and secondly, assessment of physical characteristics. The special features of this measurement tool can be seen in Figures 3.16a–c. Scores from both parts are added together to determine gestational age. The New Ballard Score can give an accurate assessment of gestational age until at least 7 days of life and is now the most widely used tool (Sasidharan et al., 2009). More information on the New Ballard Score can be found at www.ballardscore.com.

Accurate assessment of gestational age depends on experience of the practitioner and knowledge of the neonate's medical history (see also Chapter 1).The recall of the last menstrual period, information gained from early ultrasound scan dating and physical assessment using the New Ballard assessment score are the three basic methods of accurate assessment of gestational age (Thilo and Rosenburg, 2003).

An infant whose gestational age can be calculated as between 37 and 42 weeks is considered *term*. An infant whose gestational age is calculated as less than 37 completed weeks is classified as *preterm* and the infant whose gestational age can be calculated as greater than 42 weeks is classed as *post-term* (Sola et al., 2003).

Valuable information about maturity and neurological state can also be obtained by quiet observation of the infant and discussion with the mother about her perception of the baby's behaviour (for more information on neonatal behavioural states, see Chapter 8). Information can be obtained from the mother with regard to the baby's general handling, alertness, feeding and sleeping patterns. Observation of the baby feeding can give information on rooting, sucking and swallowing reflexes. General handling of the infant can give an indication of the infant's responses to external stimuli. The fetus's neurologic development will follow a predictable pattern and continues at a constant rate during maturation. The interpretation of neurologic assessment will, therefore, depend on gestational age of the infant, also on experience of the practitioner. The more mature infant will respond very differently to the preterm baby and so accurate assessment of gestational age is important. Primitive reflexes present at birth represent only lower level motor function and will disappear with development and increasing gestational age (Blackburn, 2007). Primitive reflexes start at around 32 weeks' gestation and disappear completely between 6 and 12 weeks of age in the term neonate. Observation of these reflexes beyond

PHYSICAL MATURITY

SIGN	SCORE							SIGN SCORE
	-1	0	1	2	3	4	5	
Skin	Sticky, friable, transparent	gelatinous, red, translucent	smooth pink, visible veins	superficial peeling &/or rash, few veins	cracking, pale areas, rare veins	parchment, deep cracking, no vessels	leathery, cracked, wrinkled	
Lanugo	none	sparse	abundant	thinning	bald areas	mostly bald		
Plantar Surface	heel-toe 40-50mm: -1 <40mm: -2	>50 mm no crease	faint red marks	anterior transverse crease only	creases ant. 2/3	creases over entire sole		
Breast	imperceptible	barely perceptible	flat areola no bud	stippled areola 1-2 mm bud	raised areola 3-4 mm bud	full areola 5-10 mm bud		
Eye / Ear	lids fused loosely: -1 tightly: -2	lids open pinna flat stays folded	sl. curved pinna; soft; slow recoil	well-curved pinna; soft but ready recoil	formed & firm instant recoil	thick cartilage ear stiff		
Genitals (Male)	scrotum flat, smooth	scrotum empty, faint rugae	testes in upper canal, rare rugae	testes descending, few rugae	testes down, good rugae	testes pendulous, deep rugae		
Genitals (Female)	clitoris prominent & labia flat	prominent clitoris & small labia minora	prominent clitoris & enlarging minora	majora & minora equally prominent	majora large, minora small	majora cover clitoris & minora		
						TOTAL PHYSICAL MATURITY SCORE		

(a)

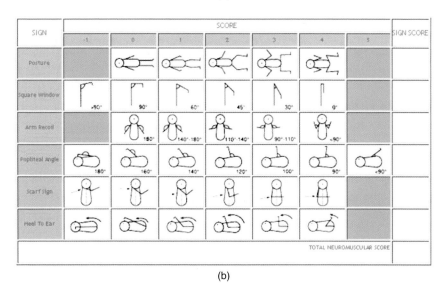

(b)

Figure 3.16 (a) New Ballard Score: physical maturity. (b) New Ballard Score: neuromuscular maturity. (c) New Ballard Score: total score (neuromuscular and physical). Source: Ballard et al. (1991). Reproduced wtih permission of Elsevier.

MATURITY RATING TABLE

TOTAL SCORE (NEUROMUSCULAR + PHYSICAL)	WEEKS
-10	20
-5	22
0	24
5	26
10	28
15	30
20	32
25	34
30	36
35	38
40	40
45	42
50	44

(c)

Figure 3.16 (*continued*)

this time may be indicative of abnormal neurological development (Levene et al., 2008).

The baby should be examined within a thermal neutral environment approximately 2 hours after a feed and the baby should be observed lying quietly in the supine position. Symmetry of reflexes is best assessed with the infant in a neutral midline position.

Newborn reflexes

The following details some of the more common reflexes that can easily be elicited at the time of the newborn examination giving the practitioner information about lower level motor function, neurological state and general muscle tone.

Moro reflex

This reflex can demonstrate symmetry of movement when the baby is held in the supine position. The baby's head is allowed to drop back a few centimetres in a sudden movement. The response involves abduction of the arms with the hands and fingers open and legs extended (Figure 3.17). A startled look and, sometimes, a cry will accompany this response. The Moro reflex can stabilise position and prevent rolling. Asymmetry of movement may indicate brachial plexus injury or clavicular fracture. Complete absence of response indicates more severe central nervous system damage.

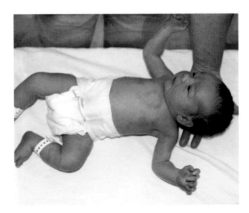

Figure 3.17 Moro reflex.

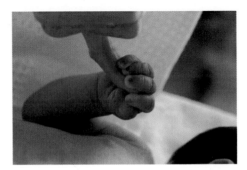

Figure 3.18 Grasp reflex.

Grasp responses

The palmer grasp response is elicited by stimulating the palm of the infant's hand with the practitioner's finger. The response is tight flexion of the fingers into the palm (see Figure 3.18). Care should be taken not to stimulate the back of the hand at the same time to avoid conflicting responses. Both hands are assessed. Sucking may also produce a palmer grasp response. If absent or weak, central nervous system depression will be suspected. A similar assessment can be undertaken on the soles of the infant's feet to elicit the plantar grasp reflex.

Babinski reflex

This is demonstrated by stimulating the sole of the foot producing plantar flexion. This reflex disappears with development. Absence of this reflex may indicate spinal nerve damage (see Figure 3.19).

Rooting, sucking reflexes

The rooting reflex should be easily assessed by stroking the cheek of the infant causing the head to turn in that same direction and the mouth to open. Placing a

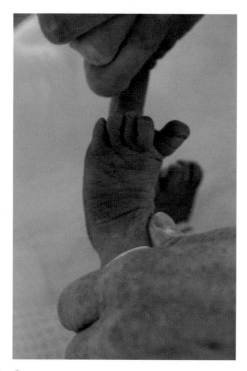

Figure 3.19 Babinski reflex.

clean finger in the baby's mouth should elicit the sucking reflex. An assessment can then be made regarding the rate rhythm and strength of suck.

Tonic neck reflex

Turning the head on to one side should cause the arm and leg on that side to extend. The limbs on the opposite side should flex and the baby should be able to break the posture after a short time under normal circumstances. This reflex is not fully developed until approximately 1 month of age. Again, this response can prevent rolling.

Stepping reflex

This response is present by 34 weeks but is another of the primitive reflexes that will disappear with development. The infant is placed in the standing position on a firm surface with the weight applied to the foot in contact with the surface. That leg extends while the other leg makes a stepping movement. The head and body straighten (Figure 3.20).

Neurological assessment can sometimes be unpredictable as only lower motor function capabilities can be assessed at this early stage. Some babies who appear normal may go on to develop handicap later. Caution should be exercised when giving feedback to the mother and father regarding neurological

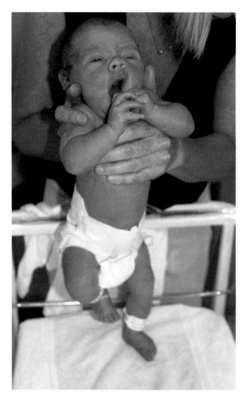

Figure 3.20 Stepping reflex.

assessment (giving feedback to the mother and father will be discussed in detail in Chapter 7).

Growth charts

In the 1960s, growth standards were measured using the Tanner Whitehouse charts (Royal College of Paediatrics and Child Health (RCPCH), 2000). The information gathered was based on children born in the 1950s who were almost exclusively artificially fed. Over time, the validity of the charts came into question as it was recognised that factors such as method of feeding, gender and race affected growth patterns in a way that could not be accurately represented on the Tanner charts.

In 1990, the growth charts were updated to better reflect growth patterns from a larger cross section of infants (RCPCH, 2009). In 1997, WHO initiated the *Multicentre Growth Reference Study* (WHO, 2004) in order to develop even better standards for measuring and assessing healthy growth. The new charts were developed based on breastfeeding babies with 'optimal' growth projections rather than 'average' projections. Those included had to be healthy term infants who were breastfed exclusively for at least 4 months. Mothers had to be non-smoking

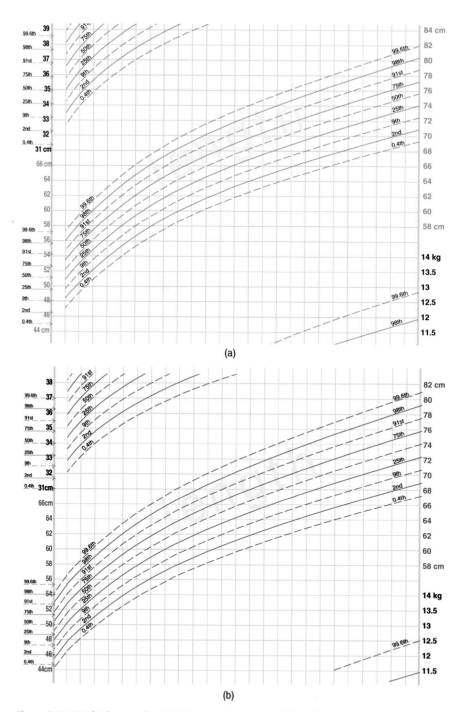

(a)

(b)

Figure 3.21 Weight-for-age chart: (a) Boys: 0–6 months and (b) Girls: 0–6 months. Source: www.who.org. Reproduced with kind permission of WHO.

and living in comfortable economic circumstances. Data were collected from six countries – the United States, Norway, India, Ghana, Brazil and Oman.

The new WHO *Child Growth Standards* were published in 2006 (WHO, 2006) and have several following key characteristics:
- Exclusively breastfed infants are recognised as the 'norm'.
- They provide an international standard for growth representing infants from six participating countries.
- They allow measurement of the body mass index against an agreed standard for infants to 5 years of age.
- They provide a link between physical growth and motor development depicting six key motor development milestones.

In 2007, the Scientific Advisory Committee on Nutrition (SACN) recommended that the charts be adopted in the United Kingdom (RCPCH, 2009). Figures 3.21a and b provide an example of weight-for-age charts for 0–6 months in boys and girls. The full range of new charts can be found at www.who.int/childgrowth or at the Royal College of Paediatrics and Child Health webpage http://www.rcpch.ac.uk/.

Conclusion

Newborn jaundice is the most common abnormality encountered when examining a newborn. Key areas we have highlighted include the importance of monitoring serum bilirubin levels, rather than relying on visual assessment to assess jaundiced infants. We have also reviewed the changes in management of women at risk from rhesus sensitisation over recent years and the impact this has had on practice. Finally, we have highlighted the recent guidance published by NICE for the care of the jaundiced neonate and the guidance from BSPGHAN for the management of the infant with prolonged jaundice and we would urge readers to review these documents.

A careful and accurate assessment of gestational age needs to be undertaken to verify term status even in babies in the 3 kg range. This helps identify potential feeding and respiratory problems. The likelihood of timely referral and early intervention is, therefore, increased in the immediate newborn period. By knowing gestational age and growth patterns, the practitioner can identify infants at risk for complications in the postnatal period and amend care plans accordingly.

Physiological jaundice and umbilical infection – a case study

Susan is a 32-year-old woman (gravida 2 para 1). She also has a 4-year-old daughter who is well. She gave birth 2 days ago at home to baby Paul, who was in good condition at birth and weighed 3.7 kg. Susan has breastfed Paul but has found that he does not settle well after feeds and always seems to be hungry.

On day 3, the community midwife visited and undertook a full examination of the newborn and found the following:

Weight 3.3 kg

Respiration rate 46 breaths per minute

Heart rate 115 beats per minute

Temperature 36.6 °C

Mum reported that Paul was breastfeeding frequently but did not stay long on the breast before appearing tired. He has been sleeping for only short periods of time.

The midwife noticed that Paul was slightly jaundiced and the skin around the umbilicus was red. The rest of the assessment was normal.

The midwife documented that Paul had lost more than 10% of his birth weight, was mildly jaundiced and had an umbilical flare. She then arranged for Susan to take Paul to her general practitioner the following day.

The midwife observed Paul at the breast and gave advice regarding correct attachment. She also contacted the local breastfeeding support midwife and arranged a visit. The midwife planned to return to visit Susan the following day also to weigh Paul again on day 6 and to monitor the redness around the umbilicus.

The midwife also advised Susan regarding care of her baby's cord.

What support is available in your Trust to help you deal with a situation like this?

Acknowledgements

The author Morris Gordon thanks Gabrielle Mew and Cassandra Gordon for their assistance in editing the text for the section on neonatal jaundice.

Look here for resources on neonatal infection and management of jaundice

Antibiotics for Early Onset Neonatal Infection NICE Guidelines 2012 http://www.nice.org.uk/Guidance/cg149

An interactive learning tool to help you recognise the sick baby https://www.spottingthe-sickchild.com/

Topical Umbilical Cord Care for Prevention of Infection and Neonatal Mortality http://www.ncbi.nlm.nih.gov/pmc/articles/PMC3785148/pdf/emss-53628.pdf

Trends in Umbilical Cord Care: Scientific Evidence for Practice http://www.sciencedirect.com/science/article/pii/S1527336904000972#

Neonatal Jaundice NICE Guidelines 2014 https://www.nice.org.uk/guidance/qs57

Post-natal care: routine post-natal care for women and their babies. NICE Guidelines 2014 http://www.nice.org.uk/guidance/CG37

Neonatal Jaundice: evidence Update March 2012. http://www.evidence.nhs.uk/documents/neonatal-jaundice-evidence-update-2012-final-version.pdf

Early recognition of neonatal hyperbilirubinaemia and its emergent treatment. http://www.sciencedirect.com/science/article/pii/S1744165X06000199

References

Andres JM (1996) Neonatal hepatobiliary disorders. *Clinical Perinatology* **23**(2), 321–352.

Anonymous (2001) Kernicterus Threatens Healthy Newborns. Sentinel Event Alert. Issue 18. USA: JCAHO. Available from: http://www.jointcommission.org/assets/1/18/SEA_18.pdf (accessed February 2010).

Anonymous (2007) *British society of Gastroenterology, Hepatology and Nutrition Guidelines. Investigation of Neonatal Conjugated Hyperbilirubinaemia.* Edinburgh: SIGN. Available from: http://bspghan.org.uk/document/liver/InvestigationofNeonatal Conjugatedhyperbilirubinaemia. pdf (accessed February 2010).

Association of Women's Health Obstetric and Neonatal Nurses (2007) *Neonatal Skin Care: Evidence-based Clinical Practice Guideline.* 3rd edn. AWHONN. https://www.awhonn.org/awhonn/store/productDetail.do?productCode=ENSC-3-13 (accessed February 2015).

Atherton D, Mills K (2004) What can be done to keep babies skin healthy? *RCM Midwives Journal* **7**(7), 288–290.

Atherton DJ (2009) Managing healthy skin for babies. *Infant* **5**(4), 130–132.

Ballard JL, Novak KK, Driver M (1979) A simplified score for assessment of fetal maturation of newly born infants. *Journal of Pediatrics* **95**, 769–774.

Ballard JL, Khoury C, Wedig K, Wang L, Eilers-Walsman BL, Lipp R (1991) New Ballard Score expanded to include extremely premature infants. *Journal of Pediatrics* **119**, 417–423.

Batt K (2000) Management of large birthmarks. *Seminars in Neonatology* **5**(4), 325–332.

Bhutani VK, Johnson L, Sivieri EM (1999) Predictive ability of a predischarge hour-specific serum bilirubin for subsequent significant hyperbilirubinaemia in healthy term and near term newborns. *Pediatrics* **103**, 6–14.

Blackburn ST (2007) *Maternal, Fetal and Neonatal Physiology: A Clinical Perspective*, 3rd edn. St. Louis, MO: Saunders.

Deken (2008) Neonatal jaundice: implications for newborn health. In: L Davis and S McDonald (eds) *Examination of the Newborn and Neonatal Health-A Multidimensional Approach*. Edinburgh: Churchill Livingstone.

Dodd KL (1993) Neonatal jaundice: a lighter touch. *Archives of Disease in Childhood* **68**: 529–533.

Dubowitz LMS, Dubowitz V, Goldberg C (1970) Clinical assessment of gestational age in the newborn infant. *Journal of Pediatrics* **77**, 1–10.

Gordon M, Bhadoria R (2008) Neonatal Haemolytic Disease and the Use of the Direct Coombs Test. Paper presented at Regional Neonatal Scientific Meeting (MANPEG/NORPEG), Royal Preston Hospital Preston, UK, 13th November 2008. Wigan, UK: Royal Albert Edward Infirmary.

Hale R (2007) Protecting neonates' delicate skin. *British Journal of Midwifery* **15**(4), 231–235.

Jackson A (2008) Time to review newborn skin. *Infant* **4**(5), 186–171.

Johnson L, Brown AK, Bhutani VK (1999) BIND: a clinical score for bilirubin induced neurologic dysfunction in newborns. *Pediatrics* **104**(Suppl), 746.

Johnston P, Flood K, Spinks K (2003a) Haematological problems and jaundice. *The Newborn Child*, 9th edn. Chapter 12. London: Churchill Livingston, pp. 183–200.

Johnston PGB, Flood K, Spinks K (2003b) Clinical assessment of the newborn baby. *The Newborn Child*. Chapter 5. London: Churchill Livingstone, pp. 59–77.

Kenner C, Wright-Lott J (2007) *Comprehensive Neonatal Care: An Interdisciplinary Approach*, 4th edn. London: Saunders.

Lavender T, Bedwell C, Roberts SA, Turner M A, Cater LA, Cork MJ (2013) Randomised controlled trail evaluating a baby wash product on skin barrier function in healthy term neonates. *Journal of Obsteric, Gynecologic, and Neonatal Nursing* **42**(2),203–214.

Levene M, Tudehope D, Sinha S (2008) *Essential Neonatal Medicine*, 4th edn. Oxford: Blackwell Publishing.

Lund CH, Kuller JM (2007) The integumentary system. In: C Kenner and J Wright-Lott (eds) *Comprehensive Neonatal Care: An Interdisciplinary Approach*, 4th edn. London: Saunders.

Lund C, Kuller J, Lane A, Wright-Lott J, Raines DA (1999) Neonatal skin care: the scientific basis for practice. *Journal of Obstetrics and Gynaecology and Neonatal Nursing* **28**(3), 241–254.

Maisels MJ (2007) Neonatal hyperbilirubinaemia. In: R Polin and M Yoder (eds) *Workbook in Practical Neonatology*, 4th edn. Chapter 5. Philadelphia, PA: Saunders, Elsevier.

Manning D, Todd P, Maxwell M, Platt MJ (2007) Prospective surveillance study of severe hyperbilirubinaemia in the newborn in the UK and Ireland. *Archives of Disease in Childhood. Fetal and Neonatal Edition* **92**, F342–F346.

Moss C (2000) Genetic skin disorders. *Seminars in Neonatology* **5**(4), 311–320.

Ness MJ, Davis DMR, Carey WA (2013) Neonatal skin care: a concise review. *International Journal of Dermatology.* **52**:14–22.

Newman TB, Maisels MJ (2000) Less aggressive treatment of neonatal jaundice and reports of kernicterus: lessons about practice guidelines. *Pediatrics* **105**, 242–245.

NICE (2014) Routine Postnatal Care of Women and Their Babies. NICE Clinical Guide no 37. https://www.nice.org.uk/guidance/cg37 (accessed April 2015).

O'Donnell CPF, Kamlin COF, Davis PG, Carlin JB, Morely CJ (2007) Clinical assessment of infant colour at delivery. *Archives of Disease in Childhood. Fetal and Neonatal Edition* **92**, 465–467.

RCPCH (2000) Growth Reference Charts for Use in the United Kingdom. Available from: www.rcpch.ac.uk (accessed June 2010).

RCPCH (2009) UK-WHO Growth Charts: Fact Sheet 2. What is the difference? Available from http://www.rcpch.ac.uk/child-health/research-projects/uk-who-growth-charts/uk-who-growth-chart-resources-0-4-years/uk-who-0#0-4 (accessed February 2015).

Rennie J (2005) *Roberton's Textbook of Neonatology*, 4th edn. Chapter 29. Oxford: Elsevier, Churchill Livingston.

Rudolph AM, Kamei RK, Overby KJ (eds) (2002) *Rudolph's Fundamentals of Pediatrics*. New York: McGraw-Hill, Medical Publication Division.

Sasidharan K, Dutta S, Narang A (2009) Validity of New Ballard Score until 7th day of postnatal life in moderately preterm neonates. *Archives of Disease in Childhood. Fetal and Neonatal Edition* **94**, 39–44.

Sethuraman G, Mancini AJ (2008) Neonatal skin disorders and the emergency medicine physician. *Clinical Pediatric Emergency Medicine* **9**(3), 200–209.

Simpson K, Creehan PA (2008) *Association of women's health, obstetric, and neonatal nurses. Perinatal Nursing*, 3rd edn. Philadelphia, PA: Lippincott Williams & Wilkins.

Sola A, Rogido MR, Partridge JC (2003) The perinatal period. In: CD Rudolph, AM Rudolph, MK Hosetter, G Lister, NJ Siegel (eds) *Rudolph's Rudolphs Pediatrics*. Chapter 4. New York: McGraw-Hill, Medical Publication Division.

Thilo EH, Rosenburg AA (2003) The newborn infant. In: AR Hayward, MJ Levin, JM Sondheimer, WW Hay (eds) *Current Pediatric Diagnosis and Treatment*, 16th edn. Chapter 1. New York: McGraw-Hill.

Tappero EP, Honeyfield ME (2010) *Physical Assessment of the Newborn*, 4th edn. Santa Rosa, CA: NICU Ink.

Thureen PJ, Deacon J, O'Neill P, Hernandez J (2005) *Evaluation and Care of the Newborn Infant.* Missouri, USA: Elsevier, Saunders.

Tortora GJ and Derrickson BH (2009) *Principles of Anatomy and Physiology*, 12th edn. John Wiley & Sons.

Trotter S (2002) Skincare for the newborn: exploring the potential harm of manufactured products. *RCM Midwives Journal* **5**(11), 576–578.

Trotter S (2004) Care of the newborn: proposed new guidelines. *British Journal of Midwifery* **12**(3), 152–157.

Trotter S (2006a) Neonatal Skincare: why change is vital. *RCM Midwives Journal* **9**(4), 134–138.

Trotter S (2006b) *Baby Care: Back to Basics*. Troon, Scotland, UK: TIPS Limited.

Trotter S (2008) Neonatal Skincare and cord care: implications for practice. In: L Davis and S McDonald (eds) *Examination of the Newborn and Neonatal Health A Multidimensional Approach*. London: Elsevier.

Verbov J (2000) Common skin conditions in the newborn. *Seminars in Neonatology* **5**, 303–310.

Volpe JJ (2001) *Neurology of the Newborn*. 4th edn. Philadelphia, PA: WB Saunders.

Walker L, Downe S, Gomez L (2005) Skin care in the well term newborn: two systemic reviews. *Birth* **32**(3), 224–228.

WHO (2003) *Pregnancy*, Childbirth, Postpartum and Newborn Care. Available from: http://whqlibdoc.who.int/publications/2006/924159084X_eng.pdf?ua=1 (accessed February 2015).

WHO (2006) Child Growth Standards. Available from: http://www.who.int/childgrowth/1_what.pdf (accessed September 2009).

WHO (2004) The Multicentre Growth Reference Study. Available from: http://archive.unu.edu/unupress/food/fnb25-1s-WHO.pdf (accessed September 2009).

CHAPTER 4

Examination of the head, neck and eyes

Carmel Noonan[1], Fiona J. Rowe[2] and Anne Lomax[3]

[1] Aintree University Trust, Liverpool, UK
[2] Directorate of Orthoptics and Vision Science, University of Liverpool, Liverpool, UK
[3] Department of Midwifery, University of Central Lancashire, Preston, UK

KEY POINTS

- Ocular structures in the brain are well organised by 6 weeks' gestation; therefore, exposure to teratogenic agents in the first trimester may result in ocular defects.

- There is a critical period of development of visual acuity in early childhood such that pathology during this time will result in significantly impaired development.

- For babies with unilateral cataracts, treatment must take place urgently where the therapeutic 'window of opportunity' may be as little as 6 weeks.

- Early detection of any abnormality that may crucially interfere with visual impairment permits effective treatment.

Examination of the head and neck

Introduction

During the examination, the shape, size and symmetry of the head in relation to the face and rest of the body should be noted. Knowledge of delivery details will indicate presentation and allow an assessment of the degree of expected moulding (see Chapter 1). The skull of a newborn is still in the process of being calcified and the soft bones readily alter in shape with passage through the birth canal as a result of external pressure. A cephalic delivery will give rise to a narrowed biparietal diameter and a more prominent vertex, whilst a breech delivery may result in an after-coming head which exhibits an increased anterior/posterior diameter and appears flatter on top. The mother and father can be reassured that normal moulding will resolve within a few days.

A measurement of the occipitofrontal diameter should always be taken and this should be within the range of 32–36 cm for a full-term infant. Apart from

---

Examination of the Newborn: An Evidence-Based Guide, Second Edition. Edited by Anne Lomax.
© 2015 John Wiley & Sons, Ltd. Published 2015 by John Wiley & Sons, Ltd.
Companion Website: www.wiley.com/go/lomax/newborn

Table 4.1 Common malformations of the skull at birth.

Caput succedaneum. This condition usually arises following prolonged labour and results in subcutaneous swelling which crosses the suture lines. It usually resolves within a few days.

Cephalhaematoma. This type of birth injury can occur following instrumental delivery, and in some cases an underlying skull fracture may be present. The bleed occurs between the skull bone and the periosteum and is caused by friction during birthing. The swelling, therefore, does not cross the suture lines and may take up to 24 hours to accumulate following birth and may be unilateral or bilateral. In infants with large haematomas, jaundice may become a problem. The swelling usually resolves within 6–12 weeks.

Craniotabes. Sometimes referred to as 'a ping-pong ball skull' (Levene et al., 2008). Areas of the skull bone are soft and spring back into place once depressed. The parietal bones are the most commonly affected areas and the condition is usually confined to the suture borders. It can be linked to more serious disorders such as rickets or osteogenesis imperfecta.

Craniosynostosis. This is a somewhat rarer finding in which the suture bones have become prematurely fused, resulting in a palpable ridge. This sometimes affects the size of the anterior fontanelle, making it look smaller than usual.

Plagiocephaly. In this condition, the occipital region appears flat on one side and is believed to be due to the baby's posture *in utero*. This condition can be exacerbated after birth if the baby is placed on its back in the cot. There is a tendency to rotate the head slightly to one side. There is no associated pathology and the condition usually resolves by itself.

normal moulding of the head, the most common forms of variations in newborns, which can affect shape, size, symmetry and occipitofrontal circumference, are summarised in Table 4.1.

The bones, sutures and fontanelles of the skull can be identified on examination. The fontanelles and sutures give the skull flexibility and accommodate the rapidly growing brain in infancy. In healthy full-term infants, the anterior fontanelle appears as a diamond shape at the point where the frontal and parietal bones meet. It is usually slightly concave but can look bulging if the baby is crying or if there is a condition of raised intracranial pressure. The anterior fontanelle usually closes around 18 months of age. The posterior fontanelle is triangular in shape and found at the junction of the sagittal and lambdoidal sutures. It can be closed at birth or takes approximately 3 months to close after birth.

The scalp of newborns may have been bruised or lacerated during delivery or by the application of a fetal scalp electrode. A condition which may easily be mistaken for a scalp wound is cutis aplasia (Figure 4.1). This is a localised congenital absence of skin which can occur anywhere on the body but is most commonly seen on the scalp. The lesions may be solitary or multiple and may be a normal variation; however, they can have an association with trisomy 13, Patau syndrome (Tappero and Honeyfield, 2009) (see also Chapter 7).

The face may give an indication of dysmorphic features which may be distinctive of a particular syndrome (see Chapter 7). The location and relationship of eyes, ears, nose and mouth should be noted. Evidence of birth trauma may be recognised as facial paralysis where the facial muscles on one side appear

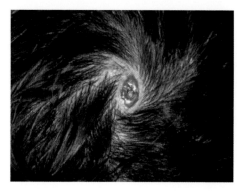

Figure 4.1 Cutis aplasia. Reproduced with kind permission of Dr Malcolm Battin, Auckland City Hospital.

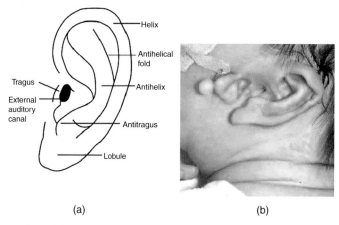

(a)   (b)

Figure 4.2 (a) Physical features of the external ear. (b) Periauricular skin tags. Reproduced with kind permission of Dr Malcolm Battin, Auckland City Hospital.

to droop. This affects the overall symmetry of the face, particularly when the baby cries. The condition can be caused by nerve damage from the application of forceps or from compression of the facial nerve against the sacral promontory during birth (Fuloria and Kreiter, 2002).

The ear position should be similar on both sides. The anatomy of the normal ear can be seen in Figure 4.2a. The upper margin should be at the same level as the eyes and low set ears may be associated with chromosomal abnormalities or urogenital malformations. However, a finding of low set ears on their own may be a normal variation. Periauricular pits may be present and are a common finding; these are an inherited autosomal dominant feature (Rudolph et al., 2003). Other minor craniofacial anomalies such as skin tags may be seen anterior to the ear (Figure 4.2b). Evidence suggests that the presence of ear pits and periauricular skin tags may indicate significant risk of hearing impairment and that these infants should be routinely screened soon after birth (Roth et al., 2008). Some practitioners may choose to examine the inner ear for evidence of the tympanic membrane; however, this is not necessary unless alerted by the history or evidence of other findings (Thureen et al., 2005).

The baby will normally undergo a hearing test shortly after birth. Despite the fact that it is important to obtain a detailed family history, some babies with hearing loss have no relevant family history of note. The incidence of significant permanent congenital hearing impairment (PCHI) is about 1 in 1,000 live births in most developed countries although this may be 3–4 times higher in certain communities or parts of the United Kingdom (UK NSC, 2008). Universal screening for hearing problems is offered to all newborns in England, Northern Ireland and Scotland in the first week of life (UK NSC, 2008). Commonly, hearing impairment is caused by loss of hair cells in the inner ear. In addition, a malformation may occur that affects the small bones that transmit vibrations in the eardrum. The aim of the NHS Newborn Hearing Screening programme is to achieve early detection of such problems and to provide high-quality care and support for babies and their families. The programme also aims at offering all newborn babies a hearing test within the first 2 weeks of birth (UK NSC, 2008; DH, 2009).

The nose shape may vary depending on familial traits. The two nares should be centrally placed and patent, any positional deformities could be as a result of delivery. Most newborns are obligatory nose breathers, and patency can be observed when the baby is breathing normally at rest. Choanal atresia is a congenital defect where the back of the nasal passages can be blocked by an abnormal bony or soft tissue development in fetal life. The baby with choanal atresia may present as cyanotic at rest, but this improves upon crying as the oral airway is used. Nasal flaring may be indicative of respiratory distress, particularly if the baby is cold (Johnston et al., 2003).

The mouth should open symmetrically and, as mentioned earlier, facial palsy can be noted upon crying. The newborn may be noted to have a receding mandible, resulting in micrognathia; this is most commonly associated with Pierre Robin's syndrome (Tappero and Honeyfield, 2009). On examination of the mouth, Epstein's pearls may be seen and appear as small white cysts on the gums or commonly at the junction of the hard and soft palates. Sublingual cysts called 'ranula' may be seen. These are harmless and are a common normal finding but may need to be removed if they interfere with feeding.

Examination of the soft and hard palates
Cleft lip and palate

The incidence of cleft lip and palate in the United Kingdom is approximately 1:700 live births (Cleft Lip and Palate Association (CLAPA), 2009). This means that around 1000 babies are born in this country with some variation in this craniofacial anomaly.

Early diagnosis and referral to a specialist team are essential to successful care, treatment and positive health outcome. An essential component of any approach to the care of a baby who is born with an oral cleft is the provision of a responsive and evidence-based service. By 2008, UK cleft care had been organised into nine Regional Specialist Managed Networks with established links to maternity units. In addition, national standards for care had been agreed by the Nurse Special Interest Group, Cleft Lip & Palate (Bannister, 2008; CLAPA, 2007).

There is some evidence to suggest, however, that current procedures for examining the lip and palate are inadequate and, as a result, delay can occur in identification and referral of some forms of oral clefts (Habel et al., 2006). Following a survey of mothers and fathers, CLAPA reported that there was a delay in detection of around 10% of clefts (CLAPA, 2009). This can result in adverse effects on growth, development and timely referral for medical or surgical procedures.

Practitioners should be aware of the correct procedure when undertaking the examination of the mouth and palate. A recent cleft lip and palate survey of midwives in Scotland demonstrated that knowledge of the incidence, associated problems and treatment of cleft lip and palate was low. The authors went on to suggest that there was a need for increased training amongst professionals who are undertaking this examination. Additional training would boost midwives' confidence and lead to a better detection and referral rate (Chalmers, 2012).

The hard and soft palates, gums and lips should be checked for clefts. The uvula may be visualised to rule out bifid uvula, which is classified as a mild form of cleft palate. The examination should involve full inspection with a torch and use of a wooden spatula to depress the tongue so that direct vision of the posterior palate and uvula can be achieved. Examination by digital palpation alone is no longer thought to be sufficient to aid detection (Habel et al., 2006). To view an informative video about cleft lip and palate called 'Easing the First Few Hours', go to http://www.clapa.com/pros/article/1123/.

Also see the website that accompanies this book for more links and information.

At the time of writing, the Royal College of Paediatricians and Child Heath (RCPCH) in collaboration with key partners was in the process of developing a best practice guideline to improve the timely detection of cleft palates in neonates. Publication of the guideline was published in September 2014 (RCPCH, 2014).

Erupted teeth may be observed in the mouth and are common in approximately 1 in 2,000 newborns (Fuloria and Kreiter, 2002). These will require removal particularly if loose. A large protruding tongue (macroglossia) may be associated with syndromes such as Beckwith–Wiedemann, Down's or hypothyroidism (see also Chapter 7).

Tongue-tie

Tongue-tie may be noted where the frenulum on the underside of the tongue prevents complete protrusion and restricts mobility of the tongue. In a mild form of the condition, only a thin mucous membrane attaches the tongue to the floor of the mouth. In severe cases, the tongue is actually fused in place. The condition affects between 3–7% of births and has a greater incidence in boys (Finigan, 2014a). Tongue-tie can create problems when breastfeeding as the restriction interferes with correct attachment to the breast. In the interests of encouraging mothers to breastfeed for as long as possible, early diagnosis of tongue-tie is essential. In some cases, tongue-tie can go on to affect speech as the child gets older. Where appropriate, surgical division can be undertaken soon after birth, a procedure currently supported by the National Institute for Health and Clinical Excellence (NIHCE, 2005).

A clinical audit of a frenulotomy service in the North West of England was undertaken between 2007 and 2012. Surgical division of the frenulum was performed on 2,509 babies in all. Results from the audit revealed that 96% of mothers and fathers reported an immediate improvement in breastfeeding with better attachment, leading to a more comfortable experience. Mothers and fathers who bottle-fed their babies also reported an improvement (Finigan, 2014b). Finigan goes on to highlight that today, this kind of service provision is lacking and more research is needed to calculate the short- and long-term benefits of developing this service more widely in the United Kingdom. More information about the extent of the provision of tongue-tie services in the United Kingdom can be found at The Association of Tongue Tie Practitioners (ATP) website http://www.tongue-tie.org.uk/index.html. The ATP was formed in 2012 by a group of tongue-tie specialists whose aims are to raise awareness of the condition and provide support for mothers and fathers to help them access safe and effective care. The group also provides information and education for professionals who wish to refer babies with tongue-tie. The site identifies regions in the United Kingdom where ATP members who provide this service can be accessed. See the website which accompanies this book for more links and information on tongue-tie.

Moving on, the neck may appear as rather short but should have full movement. The head should be able to turn as far as the shoulder in both directions. The neck should be examined for any masses, the most common being the sternomastoid tumour. This is a small painless swelling in the sternomastoid muscle associated with undue traction on the neck during delivery. The swelling will resolve in a few weeks and physiotherapy may be recommended in some cases. Fracture of the clavicles may also be a feature, particularly if there is a history of a difficult delivery. These are the most common broken bones in newborns and movement of the arm on the affected side may be limited and cause pain. On examination, the practitioner may notice some irregularity along the clavicle with possible discolouration of the skin at the site (Fuloria and Kreiter,

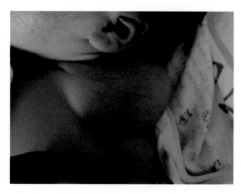

Figure 4.3 Cystic hygroma. Reproduced with kind permission of Dr Malcolm Battin, Auckland City Hospital.

2002). Cystic hygroma is the most common cyst seen in the neck and can be described as a multiloculated lymphatic lesion (Figure 4.3). The cyst can vary in size and may cause airway obstruction or feeding difficulties. Webbing of the neck may alert the practitioner to the possibility of Turner syndrome (see Chapter 7).

Examination of the eye

Introduction

Examination of the eye in newborns is principally aimed at detecting any abnormality that may crucially interfere with visual development in a baby. It is estimated that prenatal events may contribute to abnormal ocular development in up to 61% of the paediatric population in the United Kingdom, with further aetiological factors in the neonatal and childhood period contributing to additional pathology (Rahi and Cable, 2003). Perinatal and neonatal events include prematurity, complications of labour and neonatal infections. Significant improvements in the management of labour over the past 30 years and progress in the treatment of retinopathy of prematurity (ROP) have notably reduced these once leading causes of visual impairment in newborns (Bodeau-Livinec et al., 2007). In a recent national audit examining visual impairment in children in the United Kingdom, at least 75% of cases were found to have pathological disorders that were neither potentially preventable nor indeed treatable. In the United States, the leading three causes of visual impairment in the paediatric population were cortical visual impairment, ROP and optic nerve hypoplasia (Steinkuller et al., 1999). The early and prompt recognition of potentially treatable causes of visual impairment in children permits effective therapies. Disturbances of visual impairment have serious lifelong implications for social adaptation and early development including impaired mobility, restricted hand–eye coordination with long-term handicap

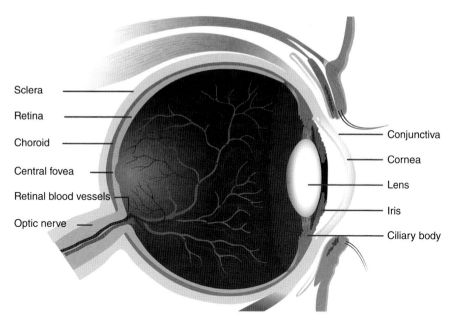

Sclera

Retina

Choroid

Central fovea

Retinal blood vessels

Optic nerve

Conjunctiva

Cornea

Lens

Iris

Ciliary body

Figure 4.4 Anatomy of the eye.

affecting mainstream education and independence (O'Connor et al., 2007). For vulnerable children who have an untreatable disorder, early detection allows for timely provision of professional advice, genetic counselling of heritable disorders and formulation of developmental priorities including an educational programme.

Embryology

Development of the eye occurs relatively early in comparison to other organ systems. Ocular structures and the brain are well organised by 6 weeks. If the mother is exposed to teratogenic agents in the first trimester, ocular defects may occur. At birth, the anteroposterior diameter of the eye is almost 70% that of an adult. The anterior structures constitute the cornea, ocular lens and pigmented iris. As the eye grows in the first few months, the central nervous system is also developing. Myelination of the visual pathways is not complete until at least 2 years of age. The anatomy of the eye is shown in Figure 4.4.

Physiology

At birth, visual acuity is approximately at the 1/60 Snellen level (3.3/200 or 1.5 logMAR equivalent). This accelerates dramatically in the first year of life – reaching adult levels at around 3 years of age. There is a critical period of visual development in the early years, such that pathology during this time will result in significantly impaired visual development. This is well known from seminal studies of children born with congenital cataracts undergoing surgery in their early childhood years. Despite lens replacement, optimal optical correction vision is significantly impaired. Clearing of the media should take place by the first few months of life in order to allow a relatively normal visual life (Jain et al., 2010). For babies with unilateral cataract, treatment must take place urgently where the therapeutic 'window of opportunity' may be as little as 6 weeks following birth. In the United Kingdom, robust visual screening programmes for congenital cataracts and other media opacities occur as part of a routine physical examination of newborn babies and a further assessment takes place at 6 weeks after birth (http://www.screening.nhs.uk/congenitalcataracts).

History taking and examination of the newborn

The clinician will take into account the detailed information provided in the obstetrical and paediatric case notes (see also Chapter 1). Family history, maternal health and previous pregnancies should be noted including prenatal loss. Details of the pregnancy are required including illnesses during pregnancy and a maternal drug history. The mother should be asked specifically if there is any history of hereditary eye problems, for example, congenital cataracts. If the baby is premature or has a very low birth weight, this may indicate the need for a more formal structured ophthalmic assessment. In neonatal practice, the leading three conditions include ocular leukocoria, retinoblastoma and ophthalmia neonatorum. The most common eye problem encountered by midwives in newborns is 'sticky watery eyes' (discussed later in this chapter).

Clinical examination

Preliminary observations

Whilst taking a history from the mother, the baby's general appearance should be observed. Orbital asymmetry, abnormal lid position/structure and strabismus may be apparent.

Observations to consider include the following: Do the eyes look symmetrical? Is the cornea clear? Are the eyes larger or smaller than you would expect? Is the pupil symmetrically round?

If the baby is asleep whilst scheduling the examination visit, one should undress the baby or remove a layer of clothing, to reduce the body temperature. This may be sufficient to arouse the baby. Likewise, if the baby is distressed, the clinician may need to return at a later time when the infant is less agitated and settled. It should be noted that when babies cry, they squeeze their eyelids shut and examination is virtually impossible.

As practice does vary, examination and management of eye problems should be conducted in line with local trust policy. The relevant NIPE process map (UK NSC, 2008) should also be considered within this context and can be viewed in Figure 4.5.

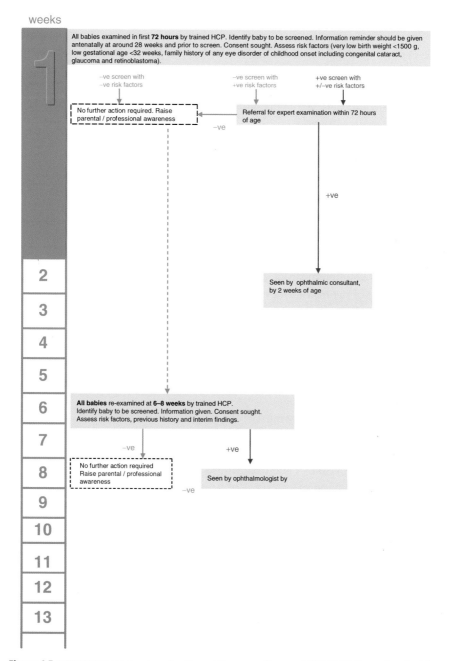

weeks

1

All babies examined in first **72 hours** by trained HCP. Identify baby to be screened. Information reminder should be given antenatally at around 28 weeks and prior to screen. Consent sought. Assess risk factors (very low birth weight <1500 g, low gestational age <32 weeks, family history of any eye disorder of childhood onset including congenital cataract, glaucoma and retinoblastoma).

–ve screen with –ve risk factors

–ve screen with +ve risk factors

+ve screen with +/–ve risk factors

No further action required. Raise parental / professional awareness

Referral for expert examination within 72 hours of age

–ve

+ve

Seen by ophthalmic consultant, by 2 weeks of age

2

3

4

5

6

All babies re-examined at **6–8 weeks** by trained HCP. Identify baby to be screened. Information given. Consent sought. Assess risk factors, previous history and interim findings.

7

–ve

+ve

8

No further action required Raise parental / professional awareness

Seen by ophthalmologist by

–ve

9

10

11

12

13

Figure 4.5 NIPE Process map: examination of the eyes. Source: NIPE 2008. Reproduced with kind permission of HMSO.

Direct ophthalmoscopy

The handheld direct ophthalmoscope is the instrument often utilised to examine the eyes. Ensure the room is adequately darkened. Face the baby away from light sources such as the window or overhead fluorescent lighting. Difficulties in visualising the ocular 'red reflex' can occur if the light source of ophthalmoscope is poor, the room is inadequately darkened, the pupil is too small or there is too much light scatter from the cornea.

  Steps in how to use the direct ophthalmoscope
- The examining room should be either semi-dark or completely dark.
- Select '0' on the illuminated lens.
- Start with a small aperture.
- Take the ophthalmoscope in the examiner's right hand.
- Hold the ophthalmoscope vertically in front of the examiner's right eye.
- Direct the light beam towards the baby.
- Place your right index finger on the edge of the lens dial.
- Position the ophthalmoscope approximately 6 in (15 cm) in front and slightly to the right of the newborn's eye.
- Direct the light beam into the pupil. A 'red reflex' should appear.

'Sight-threatening' eye problems

Leukocoria

A white-coloured pupillary reflex seen when an ophthalmoscope is shone at the pupil (Figure 4.6).

  Causes include the following:
- Congenital cataracts
- Retinoblastoma
- Infection: Toxoplasmosis and toxocariasis
- Developmental abnormalities: For example, persistent hyperplastic primary vitreous (PHPV)
- ROP

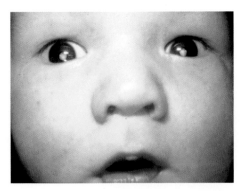

Figure 4.6 Leukocoria.

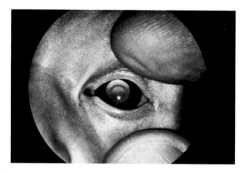

Figure 4.7 Congenital cataracts. Reproduced with kind permission of Dr David Clark.

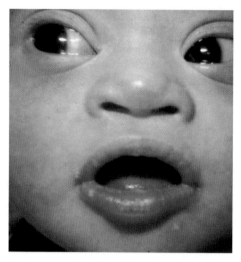

Figure 4.8 Down's syndrome. Reproduced with kind permission of Dr David Clark.

Congenital cataracts

Congenital cataracts present classically as leukocoria, i.e. a white pupil, or present with a dull red reflex. They occur in up to 2–3 per 10,000 births. Most children born with cataracts are otherwise healthy and many will have other family members born with cataracts (see Figure 4.7). In some cases, cataracts may be associated with syndromes such as Down's syndrome (Figure 4.8). The eye may also be smaller than its fellow eye.

Causes include the following:

- Idiopathic (most common)
- Familial autosomal dominant disorders
- Galactosaemia
- Rubella or 'measles' – also causes microcephaly, congenital heart defects, corneal clouding and viral induced retinopathy.

Urgent referral is required to the paediatric service for a full metabolic workup and babies must be referred to the ophthalmologist (within days). The ophthalmologist will assess if emergency surgery is indicated. A few congenital cataracts are small and only require monitoring or may require aggressive therapy for amblyopia ('lazy eye').

Retinoblastoma

This is a malignant tumour of the retina and represents the most common intraocular tumour of childhood. The incidence is 44 per million births in Europe (MacCarthy et al., 2006). One-third of tumours may be bilateral. If the tumour is bilateral, the baby will almost certainly have a heritable form of the tumour. Up to 85% of unilateral retinoblastoma tumours are not inherited. The lesion often appears as a 'white mass' growing into the vitreous and can cause a 'white pupil'. Urgent referral and assessment is essential by a paediatric ophthalmologist and medical oncologist in a specialist centre. Five-year UK survival rates are excellent (>95%). If tumours are bilateral, there is a 48% risk that infants will over time develop another soft tissue tumour. Less than 5% of babies develop a secondary soft tissue tumour if the retinoblastoma is unilateral (MacCarthy et al., 2006).

Infections (TORCH)

While most maternal infections during pregnancy do not damage the developing fetus, there are several notable exceptions including the TORCH infections (i.e. toxoplasmosis, syphilis, rubella, cytomegalovirus (CMV) and *Herpes simplex*). A number of these have decreased in prevalence due to the introduction of vaccinations, antivirals and antibiotics, e.g. rubella, syphilis and *Herpes simplex*. Only primary toxoplasmosis can cause infection in a fetus, whereas CMV can cause infections in successive pregnancies (Villena et al., 2010).

Toxoplasmosis

Toxoplasmosis is the most common cause of posterior uveitis in older children. It is caused by the protozoa *Toxoplasma gondii*. Domestic cats are the definitive host and humans may also acquire the infection by ingestion of parasitic cysts in contaminated meat. Eighty to ninety per cent of humans infected are entirely asymptomatic. In 2007, France recommended that a national laboratory-based surveillance system should be established to accurately monitor the disease. A total of 272 congenital cases were identified, the majority of cases infected being asymptomatic. The incidence rates for symptomatic congenital toxoplasmosis are found to be 0.34 per 10,000 live births (Abdel-Fattah et al., 2005).

Toxocara

Toxocara canis is the common intestinal parasite worm found in dogs. Infection is acquired in humans when the ova of the nematode are inadvertently ingested.

It is estimated that 4% of healthy people in Britain are infected with *Toxocara canis* (Barriga, 1988). Congenital disseminated toxoplasmosis may manifest itself with extraocular findings such as intrauterine growth retardation, microcephaly, microphthalmia, congenital cataracts, uveitis, hearing defects, osteomyelitis, hepatosplenomegaly, lymphadenopathy, dermal erythropoiesis, carditis and congenital heart disease.

Cytomegalovirus (CMV)

Congenital CMV infection only rarely gives rise to ophthalmological abnormalities (Kenneson and Cannon, 2007). When they do occur, they include cataract, optic atrophy and chorioretinitis. A number of asymptomatic newborns infected with congenital CMV will present with permanent childhood hearing impairment during early childhood (Korver et al., 2009).

Ophthalmia neonatorum

This is a notifiable disease, which presents with unilateral or bilateral purulent conjunctivitis within a few days of birth. The baby must be assessed by an ophthalmologist and swabs taken for bacteria, *Chlamydia* and viral cultures. Always suspect *Neisseria gonorrhoea* – 'Gonorrhoea' or *Chlamydia* until proven otherwise (Quirke and Cullinane, 2008). Of interest, 20% of neonatal conjunctivitis admitted to Cork University Hospital, Ireland, between July 2002 and December 2006, was secondary to *Gonorrhoea*. The most common identifiable infection, however, was *Chlamydia*. Systemic and topical antibiotic therapy is essential in the management of this debilitating condition. The mother and father should also be referred to a sexually transmitted disease clinic for treatment.

Developmental abnormalities
Persistent hyperplastic primary vitreous (PHPV)

The space at the back of the eye, behind the ocular lens, is normally filled with a clear jelly-like material referred to as the vitreous. Children with PHPV are born with a hazy, scarred vitreous. The vitreous may often be adherent to the back of the lens and areas of the retina. This may significantly damage parts of the eye and lead to other eye conditions such as the following:
- The lens may become hazy (cataracts).
- The retina may peel from the back of the eye (retinal detachment).
- Pressure in the eye can rise (glaucoma).
- The eye can be smaller than usual (microphthalmia).

It is unclear why the vitreous does not develop correctly. Most cases of PHPV occur sporadically although some may run in families. Usually, the condition affects only one eye. The most common manner in which PHPV presents may be a scenario in which the normally dark pupil in a child's eye looks pale or whiter than expected. In a study from Pakistan, the incidence of PHPV in neonates with leukocoria was found to be 4% (Haider et al., 2008).

Retinopathy of prematurity (ROP)

ROP is an eye disease that affects babies born prematurely. It is caused by disorganised growth of retinal blood vessels, which may result in scarring and retinal detachment. ROP can be mild and may resolve spontaneously, but may lead to blindness in serious cases. As such, all preterm babies born less than 32 weeks' gestation or weighing less than 1,500 g are at risk for ROP and are screened by an ophthalmologist. The incidence of ROP has decreased dramatically over the past 20 years. This is despite the increasing survival of very low birth weight babies due to improved intensive care of newborns (Dhaliwal et al., 2008). Early treatment with laser is the key to management. Advanced/untreated ROP also presents with leukocoria. In severe ROP with associated retinal detachment, vitreoretinal surgery may only achieve palliative success.

Non-accidental injury

A newborn with leukocoria or ocular trauma may be a victim of non-accidental injury (NAI) (Kivlin, 2001) (see also the website that accompanies this book). Retinal haemorrhages are the most common finding on fundal examination in 'shaken baby' syndrome. In any child younger than 3 years of age, the presence of extensive bilateral retinal haemorrhages raises a very strong possibility of abuse, which must be thoroughly investigated. Poor visual function following NAI is most likely due to traumatic brain injury (Kivlin et al., 2000). Injuries may also result in subluxed or dislocated lenses, glaucoma, cataracts, retinal detachment or optic atrophy (Green et al., 1996).

Congenital glaucoma buphthalmos ('ox eye')

This is a very rare congenital disorder affecting less than 0.05% of newborns (Papadopoulos et al., 2007; Aponte et al., 2010). The baby may present with signs and symptoms of raised intraocular pressure. The mother and father or health-care workers may notice watery eyes and/or extreme sensitivity of the newborn to bright light. The condition is usually bilateral but may also present asymmetrically. Clinical features include large eyes ('ox eyes') with a wider corneal diameter than usual. This may be the only obvious sign. Cloudy corneas and extreme irritability may also occur. A baby will go blind if the condition is not detected and treated early (Figure 4.9).

The differential diagnosis of newborns presenting with congenital glaucoma include the following:

- *Corneal oedema:* Birth trauma, metabolic conditions, rubella and infections such as *Herpes simplex*
- *Enlarged cornea:* Axial myopia, megalocornea and osteogenesis imperfecta
- *Watery eyes:* Conjunctivitis, nasolacrimal duct obstruction, corneal abrasion and ocular inflammation

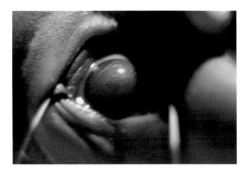

Figure 4.9 Congenital glaucoma. Reproduced with kind permission of Dr David Clark.

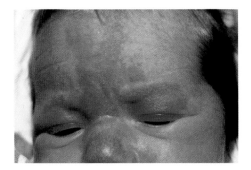

Figure 4.10 Capillary haemangioma. Reproduced with kind permission of Dr David Clark.

Capillary haemangioma (strawberry naevus)

These swellings appear at birth or shortly afterwards (see Figure 4.10) (see also Chapter 3). Lesions may increase in size over the next few months and may threaten vision development if the haemangioma progression occludes the margins of the eye and obscures the visual axis. They most commonly occur in the supra nasal orbit regions and eyelids. They may be treated with local injection of steroids or laser treatment, and more recently propranolol has been shown as an effective treatment. If left untreated, they usually cease growing by 1 year of age. Complete spontaneous regression by 5 years of age is the common outcome (in 80–90%).

Ptosis

A neonate with an upper lid drooping ('ptosis') across the visual axis should be referred urgently to the ophthalmologist. This is a similar clinical priority to congenital cataracts in that lesions blocking the visual axis during the critical period of visual development will result in stimulus deprivation and amblyopia. Ptosis in children occurs for a variety of reasons. Despite a long list of potential causes, simple or congenital ptosis is the common form. For the clinician examining an infant, a third nerve palsy, capillary haemangioma or lid birth trauma need to be out ruled.

Strabismus and eye movements

It is unusual for one eye to be misaligned in a neonate. Strabismus ('squint') more commonly develops as an early-onset condition from 2 to 3 months of age with more common types of strabismus occurring from the age of 2 years and onwards. Where strabismus is seen in the newborn period, it may indicate injury sustained during birth with coexistent abnormal eye movements relating to damage to the cranial nerves that supply the extraocular muscles. The lateral rectus muscle enervated by the VI cranial nerve is particularly susceptible as it is the outermost extraocular muscle.

'Non-sight-threatening' eye problems
'Watery eyes' due to nasolacrimal duct obstruction

Nasolacrimal duct obstruction commonly presents with watery eyes. It occurs because the opening at the lower end of the nasolacrimal duct is often partially obstructed for several months following birth. The mother and father can be reassured that this nuisance condition will resolve in over 90% of babies by 1 year of age. Cleaning with sterile water and daily gentle finger massage over the lacrimal sac at the medial canthus may help open the drainage system. Antibiotics are only rarely required. For persistent watering after the age of 1 year, referral to the ophthalmologist is recommended so that treatment to dilate the nasolacrimal duct can be undertaken.

Conclusion

The sequence of the examination of the head, neck and eyes by the practitioner will, like the rest of the examination, depend on the cooperation of the newborn. This may necessitate an opportunistic approach. Examination of the head, neck and eyes requires careful attention as many malformations or variations from the normal can be visible in this region. Early recognition and referral of ocular abnormalities are crucial in order to prevent permanent visual damage.

Tongue-Tie (Ankyloglossia) – a case study

Carol was a 25-year-old primigravida who after an uneventful pregnancy gave birth to full-term healthy baby boy called Simon.

Simon's condition at birth was good (Apgars were 8 at 1 minute and 9 at 5 minutes), and he had skin-to-skin contact immediately. Carol attempted a breastfeed straight away.

At 12 hours old, Simon was examined by the midwife and on examination of the mouth he was found to have a tongue-tie. The midwife referred the baby to the duty paediatrician. He told Carol that the abnormality would not cause a problem and so no action was taken. Carol and her baby were discharged home shortly after.

Initially, the baby fed well; however, when the community midwife visited Carol on day 4, she found that Carol was upset and frustrated, her nipples were becoming very sore and she was finding it difficult to satisfy Simon with breastfeeds. Carol talked about changing to bottle feeds as she was convinced this would be easier for Simon.

The midwife encouraged Carol to continue to breastfeed and arranged for her to see her general practitioner (GP).

Her GP referred Simon to their nearest tongue-tie clinic for frenulotomy. In the meantime, the midwife arranged for Carol to have extra help with feeding from the breastfeeding support midwife. The breastfeeding support midwife suggested Carol to express her milk and bottle-feed Simon until he could be seen at the tongue-tie clinic.

Simon was treated 2 weeks later and was able to attach to the breast and feed successfully immediately after treatment.

Think about how you would address this problem within your Trust.

What information do you have available to give to the mother and father of a baby with tongue-tie?

See the accompanying website for photos of tongue-tie before and after surgery.

Look at these resources for more information on tongue-tie:

Information on tongue-tie from Southampton Children's Hospital. http://www.uhs.nhs.uk/OurServices/Childhealth/Tonguetie/Tonguetie.aspx

Listen to the radio 4 programme: A mother talks about her experience of having a baby with tongue-tie: http://www.bbc.co.uk/programmes/b03vdx7t

Exploding the Myths on Tongue Tie http://www.infantgrapevine.co.uk/pdf/inf_009_exm.pdf

Finigan V (2014a) Tongue Tied. *Midwives* (2), 54.

Finigan V (2014b) Overcoming Tongue Tie. *Midwives* (3), 48–49.

NHS Institute for Innovation and Improvement http://www.institute.nhs.uk/case_studies/nhs_live/frenulotomy_clinic_for_tongue_tied_babies.html

Association of Tongue Tie Practitioners http://www.tongue-tie.org.uk/index.html

Baby friendly initiative –Locations where tongue-tie can be divided. http://www.unicef.org.uk/BabyFriendly/Parents/Problems/Tongue-Tie/Locations-where-tongue-tie-can-be-divided/

Help for mothers and fathers:

NHS Choices http://www.nhs.uk/conditions/tongue-tie/Pages/Introduction.aspx

Babycentre http://www.babycentre.co.uk/a552046/tongue-tie

In the news: Desperate families need better help with tongue-tie http://www.bbc.co.uk/news/health-26199591

Voices: Mothers and fathers of tongue-tie babies http://www.bbc.co.uk/news/health-26241665

NICE (2005) has approved the division of tongue tie: https://www.nice.org.uk/guidance/ipg149

http://www.nursinginpractice.com/article/tongue-tie-assessment-referral-and-outcomes

References

Abdel-Fattah SA, Bhat A, Illanes S, Bartha JL, Carrington D (2005) TORCH test for fetal medicine indications: only CMV is necessary in the United Kingdom. *Prenatal Diagnosis* **25**(11), 1028–1031.

Aponte EP, Diehl N, Mohney BG (2010) Incidence and clinical characteristics of childhood glaucoma: a population-based study. *Archives in Ophthalmology* **128**(4), 478–482.

Bannister P (2008) Management of infants born with a cleft lip and palate. Part 1. *Infant* **4**(1), 5–8.

Barriga OO (1988) A critical look at the importance, prevalence and control of toxocariasis and the possibilities of immunological control. *Veterinary Parasitology* **29**(2–3), 195–234.

Bodeau-Livinec F, Surman G, Kaminski M, Wilkinson AR, Ancel PY, Kurinczuk JJ (2007) Recent trends in visual impairment and blindness in the UK. *Archives of Disease in Childhood* **92**(12), 1099–1104.

Chalmers E (2012) Cleft lip and Palate in Scotland: a survey. *The Practising Midwife*, **15**, 10–15.

CLAPA (2009) Understanding cleft lip and palate. Available from http://www.clapa.com/medical/cleft_lip_article/107/ (accessed May 2014).

CLAPA (2007) Regionalisation of Cleft lip and Palate services: has it worked? Available from http://www.clapa.com/documents/Full%20report%20final.pdf (accessed May 2014).

Dhaliwal C, Fleck B, Wright E, Graham C, McIntosh N (2008) Incidence of retinopathy of prematurity in Lothian, Scotland, from 1990 to 2004. *Archives of Disease in Childhood. Fetal and Neonatal Edition* **93**(6), F422–F426.

DH (2009) The Healthy Child Programme. Pregnancy and the First Five Years of Life. Department for Children, Schools and Families.

Finigan V (2014a) Tongue tied. *Midwives* (2), 54.

Finigan V (2014b) Overcoming tongue tie. *Midwives* (3), 48–49.

Fuloria M, Kreiter S (2002) The newborn examination. Part 1. Emergencies and common abnormalities involving the skin, head, neck, chest and respiratory and cardiovascular systems. *American Family Physician* **65**(1), 61–68.

Green MA, Lieberman G, Milroy CM, Parsons MA (1996) Ocular and cerebral trauma in non-accidental injury in infancy: underlying mechanisms and implications for paediatric practice. *British Journal Ophthalmology* **80**(4), 282–287.

Habel A, Elhadi N, Sommerlad B, Powell J (2006) Delayed detection of cleft palate: an audit of newborn examination. *Archive of Disease in Childhood Fetal and Neonatal Edition* **91**, 238–240.

Haider S, Qureshi W, Ali A (2008) Leukocoria in children. *Journal of Pediatric Ophthalmology and Strabismus* **45**(3), 179–180.

Jain S, Ashworth J, Biswas S, Lloyd IC (2010) Duration of form deprivation and visual outcome in infants with bilateral congenital cataracts. *Journal of American Association Pediatric Ophthalmology and Strabismus* **14**(1), 31–34.

Johnston PGB, Flood K, Spinks K (2003) *The Newborn Child*. Churchill: Livingstone.

Kenneson A, Cannon MJ (2007) Review and meta-analysis of the epidemiology of congenital cytomegalovirus (CMV) infection. *Reviews in Medical Virolology* **17**(4), 253–276.

Kivlin JD (2001) Manifestations of the shaken baby syndrome. *Current Opinions in Ophthalmology* **12**(3), 158–163.

Kivlin JD, Simons KB, Lazoritz S, Ruttum MS (2000) Shaken baby syndrome. *Ophthalmology* **107**(7), 1246–1254.

Korver AM, de Vries JJ, Konings S, de Jong JW, Dekker FW, Vossen AC, Frijns JH, Oudesluys-Murphy AM (2009) DECIBEL collaborative study group. DECIBEL study: Congenital cytomegalovirus infection in young children with permanent bilateral hearing impairment in the Netherlands. *Journal of Clinical Virology* **46**(Suppl 4), S27–S31.

Levene MI, Tudenhope DI, Thearle MJ (2008) *Essentials of Neonatal Medicine*, 3rd edn. Oxford: Blackwell Science.

MacCarthy A, Draper GJ, Steliarova-Foucher E, Kingston JE (2006) Retinoblastoma incidence and survival in European children (1978–1997). Report from the Automated Childhood Cancer Information System project. *European Journal of Cancer* **42**(13), 2092–2102.

NIHCE (2005) *Division of Ankyloglossia (tongue tie) for Breastfeeding*. London: National Institute for Clinical Excellence.

UK NSC (2008) UK NSC Policy Database. Hearing (newborn) Online. Available from: http://www.screening.nhs.uk/hearing-newborn (accessed 12 August 2009).

O'Connor AR, Wilson CM, Fielder AR (2007) Ophthalmological problems associated with preterm birth. *Eye (Lond)* **21**(10), 1254–1260.

Papadopoulos M, Cable N, Rahi J, Khaw PT (2007) The British infantile and childhood glaucoma (BIG) eye study. *Investigative Ophthalmology of Visual Science* **48**(9), 4100–4106.

Quirke M, Cullinane A (2008) Recent trends in chlamydial and gonococcal conjunctivitis among neonates and adults in an Irish hospital. *International Journal of Infectious Diseases* **12**(4), 371–373. Epub 21 February 2008.

Rahi JS, Cable N (2003) British Childhood Visual Impairment Study Group. Severe visual impairment and blindness in children in the UK. *Lancet* **362**(9393), 1359–1365.

Roth DA, Hildesheimer M, Bardenstein S, Goidel D, Reichman B, Myaan-Metzger A, Kuint J (2008) Periauricular skin tags and ear pits are associated with permanent hearing impairment in newborns. *Pediatrics* **122**, 884–890.

Royal College of Paediatricians and Child Health (2014) Best practice guidelines to the examination of the neonatal palate scope. Available from: http://www.rcpch.ac.uk/rcpch-guidelines-and-standards-clinical-practice#in-development (accessed May 2014).

Rudolph CD, Rudolph AM, Hostetter MK, Lister G, Siegel NJ (eds) (2003) *Rudolphs Pediatrics*. New York: McGraw-Hill, Medical Pub.

Steinkuller P, Du L, Gilbert C, Allen Foster A, Collins ML, Coats DK (1999) Childhood blindness. *Journal of American Association Pediatric Ophthalmology and Strabismus* **3**(1), 26–32.

Tappero EP, Honeyfield ME (2009) *Physical Assessment of the Newborn*, 4th edn. Petaluma, CA: NICU Ink.

Thureen PJ, Deacon J, O'Neill P, Hernandez J (2005) *Assessment and Care of the Well Newborn*. Philadelphia, PA: Saunders.

Villena I, Ancelle T, Delmas C, Garcia P, Brezin AP, Thulliez P, Wallon M, King L, Goulet V (2010) Congenital toxoplasmosis in France in 2007: first results from a national surveillance system. *European Surveillance* **15**(25), 19600.

CHAPTER 5

Examination of the newborn abdomen and genitalia

Morris Gordon

Paediatric Gastroenterology, Royal Manchester Children's Hospital, Manchester, UK

KEY POINTS

- A clear and evidence-based algorithm for abdominal and genital examination is helpful when assessing the neonate.

- There appears to be lack of clarity surrounding the term 'bilious vomiting' amongst mother and fathers and professionals. It is important to understand the significance of this finding in the context of abdominal examination.

- An appreciation of the literature pertaining to the incidence and management of undescended testes is necessary to provide best practice.

- Did you know there is a difference between undescended testicles and normal retractile testicles?

Examination of the newborn abdomen

The abdominal examination is an area in which neonatal abnormalities are rare. Those often read about are gross abnormalities that are quite obvious on initial inspection. This should not detract from the examiner giving this portion of the examination the same attention as any other, as the early findings in neonates with abdominal problems may be subtle.

An approach to abdominal examination

Key to this portion of the examination, more than any other, is a good history from the mother and father. Ask them whether the baby has passed meconium and record this clearly in the documentation. Ask about feeding and particularly about any vomiting. If vomiting is present, ask the mother and father to describe the colour. It is advised that you do not use the term bilious while asking the mother and father about vomiting as there tends to be a misunderstanding

---

Examination of the Newborn: An Evidence-Based Guide, Second Edition. Edited by Anne Lomax.
© 2015 John Wiley & Sons, Ltd. Published 2015 by John Wiley & Sons, Ltd.
Companion Website: www.wiley.com/go/lomax/newborn

between the perceived meaning and the medical use of this term. A recent piece of work (Roy et al. 2007) highlighted professional confusion with the issue, showing that while doctors, midwives and neonatal nurses were very confident labelling clearly dark green aspirates or vomits as bile, there was much more uncertainty with yellow non-bilious aspirates. If there has been vomiting that you feel may have been bilious, ask the mother and father if they have any clothes they can give you to examine yourself. Although non-bilious vomiting does not exclude bowel obstruction, all bilious vomiting in a neonate demands further investigation and, if present, an immediate paediatric review is recommended.

Before proceeding further with the examination, expose the abdomen completely and make sure your hands are warm:

- *Inspect the abdomen.* Observe its shape. A scaphoid (sunken) abdomen suggests congenital diaphragmatic hernia and needs more detailed examination. Mild and variable abdominal distension is normal, but a persistent distension could suggest bowel obstruction or intra-abdominal fluid (ascites) and, therefore, needs further evaluation.
- *Palpate for abdominal organs or masses.* A liver can be felt in normal infants at a size of up to 2 cm below the costal margins. A splenic tip may also be felt in normal newborns. Kidneys may also be palpated. If any masses or organ enlargement is palpated, further investigation is required.
- *Palpate and percuss for a bladder.* This should not usually be palpable above the umbilicus and, if felt, ask the mother and father whether the baby has urinated and again arrange further investigation.
- *Listen for bowel sounds.* These should be easily heard throughout the abdomen.
- Examine the umbilical stump and confirm the presence of two arteries and a vein. A single artery increases the chances of other congenital anomalies. Local policies for further investigation should be consulted. Check for signs of infection on the abdomen.
- Inspect for the presence of the anus and confirm it is not ectopically placed. The presence of faeces does not exclude a problem, so make sure to see the anus itself.

Deviations from the norm

There are a number of possible abnormalities that you may encounter, many touched upon in the suggested method of examination. As the vast majority of these abnormalities are rare and will require specialist attention, a detailed discussion is outside the scope of this chapter. Instead, the focus of this section is on the recognition of the most clinically important abdominal presentations and their causes.

Bowel obstruction

Although this is not a common finding, bowel obstruction is an extremely important abdominal condition as the consequences to an infant can be devastating
and prompt treatment can lead to improved outcomes. It is best to consider bowel
obstruction anatomically, divided into upper and lower gastrointestinal (GI) tract
causes, as there are symptomatic differences in presentation.

Upper GI obstruction

- Early vomiting (bilious or non-bilious)
- Possible respiratory symptoms with feeds

Tracheo–oesophageal fistula describes a spectrum of disorders which are characterised by abnormal anatomy that leads to an aberrant connection between the
trachea and oesophagus. The frequency of this condition is estimated to be 1 in
3,000 births (Goyal et al. 2006), making it one of the more common paediatric
surgical problems. When an affected neonate feeds, depending on the specific
anatomy, varying amounts of feed may enter the trachea and the neonate will
display respiratory symptoms. Investigation is with plain X-ray, contrast studies
or computer tomography and management by surgery.

Duodenal atresia is the third most common atresia of the GI tract. The estimated incidence is 1 in 20,000 live births, about 30% of infants with duodenal
atresia having Down's syndrome (Beers and Berkow 1999). Vomiting usually
starts within hours after birth and again, depending on the specific anatomy of
the blockage, may or may not be bilious. An x-ray of the abdomen may show
large air-filled spaces – the so-called double bubble sign. Management of dehydration is required, followed by surgery.

Lower GI obstruction

- Failure to pass meconium
- Abdominal distension
- Vomiting (late sign)

Intestinal malrotation is a congenital anomaly of the developmental process of rotation of the midgut. It can be asymptomatic, but obstruction may
occur due to compression of the duodenum by the abnormal anatomy (Beattie
et al. 2009). Volvulus is complete obstruction caused by abnormal twisting of the
bowel, which may also cause ischaemia of the bowel. Presentation will be poor
feeding, bilious vomiting and occasionally rectal bleeding. A range of imaging
modalities may be used to aid diagnosis, with intervention being surgical.

The meconium sometimes becomes thickened and congested in the ileum,
a condition known as meconium ileus. Below this level, the bowel is narrow
and there is an empty micro-colon. Above the level of the obstruction, there
are several loops of hypertrophied bowel distended with fluid. No meconium is

passed, and abdominal distension and vomiting appear soon after birth. Approximately 90% of meconium ileus cases are in patients with cystic fibrosis, although in contrast only 20% of children with cystic fibrosis suffer with the condition (Stephenson et al. 2000). Again, a range of imaging modalities may be used for diagnosis, with intervention being surgical. Investigations for cystic fibrosis are essential in these cases.

Hirschsprung's disease involves an enlargement of the colon caused by bowel obstruction, resulting from an aganglionic section of bowel that starts at the anus and progresses upwards (Skinner 1996). The incidence cited is 1 in 15,000 births. Suspect the condition in any child who does not pass meconium in the first 48 hours after birth. Other symptoms include abdominal distension and constipation. Diagnosis is by rectal suction biopsy of a narrowed section. Treatment is by surgical removal of the affected gut.

Necrotising enterocolitis

Necrotising enterocolitis (NEC) is a condition in which areas of gut undergo tissue death. The condition is typically one associated with prematurity, but 10% of cases occur in term infants (Raboei 2009). Despite being identified 150 years ago, the cause of the condition remains unclear (Obladen 2009). Historically, it was believed that NEC arose predominantly from ischaemic injury to the immature GI tract, yet current thinking is that many factors are likely to be involved. These may include issues related to the introduction and increase in feeds and alterations in the normal bacteria of the GI tract (Thompson and Bizzarro 2008).

The condition may present with variable signs, with obstruction being only one element. Symptoms include vomiting, abdominal distension and per rectum bleeding. Progression to a discoloured abdomen will follow with rapid deterioration of the baby's condition resulting in the baby needing intensive support. This will be associated with peritonitis and bowel perforations. Diagnosis is largely clinical, but a plain X-ray may uncover several possible signs of the extensive bowel disease.

Treatment may be medical, including keeping the child nil by mouth and giving parenteral nutrition, antibiotics, general cardiovascular support and gut decompression by nasogastric tube. If the disease is more severe and not responding to medical therapy or when there is evidence of bowel perforations, surgical management may be needed, allowing the dead portions of bowel to be resected. As disease may be extensive, infants can be left with very small lengths of viable bowel and can suffer in the long term with short gut syndrome – essentially the inability for the gut to absorb adequate nutrition to sustain the infant. Despite advances in neonatal care, the outcomes from this condition have not improved in the last 30 years (Mshvildadze and Neu 2009). This has led to a focus on prevention, with current methods being investigated, including the speed of introduction of feeds and the use of probiotic agents.

Although rare, early recognition of the disease will allow management to be instigated and so the diagnosis should be considered in any child with evidence of bowel obstruction that is also systemically unwell.

Examination of the newborn genitalia

The genital examination in a newborn is often a problematic area and despite progress in newborn examination as a whole, the genital element has not been well researched. In the vast majority of newborns, a rather quick and cursory examination of the genitalia takes place that may not pay sufficient attention to a number of pertinent details. This section of the chapter will highlight relevant development issues and introduce and discuss common and important deviations from the norm, based on the most up-to-date evidence. This will be accompanied by a practical guide to the genitalia examination which will discuss this evidence and give useful tips on common abnormalities; 'red flag' findings that need immediate action and consideration of how to talk to the mother and father when specific genital anomalies are discovered.

Development of genitalia and determinants of sex

It is important when discussing genital examination to have an understanding of the developmental basis for the sex organs, making it easier to appreciate deviations from the norm.

There are a number of ways in which we may consider the determination of sex. The external genitalia are the most obvious. One may also consider chromosomes and specifically the presence or absence of the male Y chromosome. Finally, recognition of whether gonads are testes or ovaries may also be considered. It might seem rather pointless to discuss these three aspects as they all describe the same state, namely, an infant's gender. The importance of these other aspects of gender will become apparent as we discuss the rare circumstance of genital abnormalities.

At the start of development, a fetus will be without gender. The first stage of differentiation is controlled by the chromosomes. If the fetus is male, there will be a gene on the Y chromosome known as the SRY (referring to the sex determining region of Y chromosome). This produces a protein known as testis determining factor (TDF), as well as several other sex determining factors. It is the presence of these proteins and factors that initiates the process of male sex determination, by causing the gonads to develop into testes. At this point, a fetus will have two small embryological ducts known as the Wolffian and the Mullerian ducts. If TDF influences the primitive gonads to become testes and these produce the male sex hormone testosterone, the Wolffian ducts are stimulated to form the rest of the male internal sex organs, while the Mullerian structures are simply left as undeveloped remnants. In a female fetus, the lack of TDF leaves gonads to

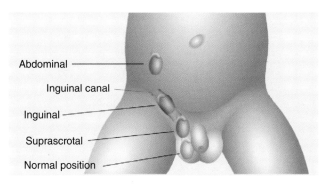

Abdominal

Inguinal canal

Inguinal

Suprascrotal

Normal position

Figure 5.1 Descent of the testes.

become ovaries, and in that case, the Wolffian structures are not stimulated and simply remain as remnants and, in their absence, the Mullerian system develops into the female sex organs. This process highlights how the chromosomes and gonads are both key to the determination of the gender of a neonate.

In the normal development of a male fetus, the testes develop in the abdominal cavity, just as the ovaries do. At about 28 weeks of fetal life, they start their descent through the internal inguinal ring into the inguinal canal and then to the external inguinal ring and finally into the scrotum (Figure 5.1). This process is usually completed by birth, so if an infant is born premature, they are much more likely to have an undescended testicle. In between 2 and 4% of males, the testes may be undescended (Jackson et al. 1986), with 7 out of 10 of these continuing to descend normally by 12 months of age (Acerini et al. 2009).

The neonatal period is well recognised as the most appropriate time for testes examination. This is because a child is quite immobile, which aids the process. More importantly, the cremaster reflex, which allows the testes to be lifted from the scrotum and can lead to the appearance of undescended testicle, is not well developed at birth.

An approach to genitalia examination

The following is a structured approach to newborn genital examination, which draws on a number of texts (Thilo and Rosenberg 2003, Sniderman and Taeusch 2004, Rennie 2005, Thureen et al. 2005). At this point in your newborn examination, you may wish to ask the mother and father if the baby has passed urine and if so, if they have noticed a normal stream in a boy. Make sure the baby is clean and your genital view is not obstructed before beginning. It is especially important to warm your hands.

Male examination

Table 5.1 offers a perspective as to the relevant actions for each of the findings mentioned. As practice does vary, local policy should be consulted. The relevant

Table 5.1 Examination of the genitalia: deviations from the norm.

Male		Female	
Abnormality	Action (red flag findings in italics)	Abnormality	Action (red flag findings in italics)
Unilateral palpable undescended testes	Routine paediatric urology referral or follow-up in the community	Ambiguous genitalia	*Urgent paediatric and paediatric urology referral*
Unilateral impalpable undescended testes	Routine paediatric urology referral	Inguinal hernia, reducible	Routine paediatric urology referral. Warn mother and father of signs of incarceration
Bilateral palpable undescended testes	Routine paediatric urology referral	Inguinal hernia, not reducible	*Emergency, paediatric surgical referral*
Bilateral impalpable undescended testes with normal penis	*Paediatric review within 24 hours*	Prominent clitoris/labial swelling	*Urgent paediatric review*
Bilateral impalpable undescended testes with abnormal penis	*Urgent paediatric and paediatric urology referral*		
Hypospadias	Routine paediatric urology referral. Advise against circumcision (prepuce is important for reconstruction)		
Epispadias	Routine paediatric urology referral		
Ambiguous genitalia	*Urgent paediatric and paediatric urology review*		
Hydrocele	Routine paediatric urology referral		
Inguinal hernia, reducible	Routine paediatric urology referral. Warn the mother and father of signs of incarceration		
Inguinal hernia, not reducible	*Emergency paediatric surgical referral*		

NIPE process map (UK National Screening Committee 2008) (Figure 5.2) should also be considered within this context.
- Inspect the penis and confirm that it is an appropriate size (normally around 3 cm, less than 2.5 cm being abnormal), noting that in some children, suprapubic fat can make the penis appear shorter.
- Confirm that the overall appearance of the scrotum is normal. Examine the scrotum and confirm that the scrotal skin is wrinkled (normal rugosity). The

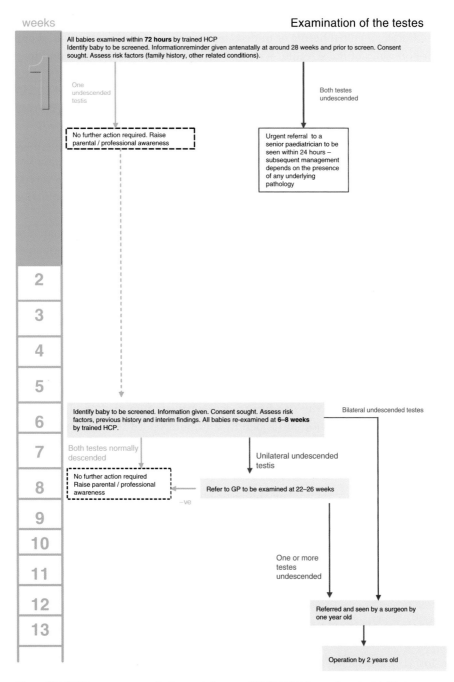

weeks   Examination of the testes

All babies examined within **72 hours** by trained HCP
Identify baby to be screened. Informationreminder given antenatally at around 28 weeks and prior to screen. Consent
sought. Assess risk factors (family history, other related conditions).

One
undescended
testis

Both testes
undescended

No further action required. Raise
parental / professional awareness

Urgent referral to a
senior paediatrician to be
seen within 24 hours –
subsequent management
depends on the presence
of any underlying
pathology

2

3

4

5

6   Identify baby to be screened. Information given. Consent sought. Assess risk
factors, previous history and interim findings. All babies re-examined at **6–8 weeks**
by trained HCP.

Bilateral undescended testes

7   Both testes normally
descended

Unilateral undescended
testis

8   No further action required
Raise parental / professional
awareness

Refer to GP to be examined at 22–26 weeks

–ve

9

10

11   One or more
testes
undescended

12

13   Referred and seen by a surgeon by
one year old

Operation by 2 years old

Figure 5.2 NIPE process map. Undescended testes. (NIPE 2008. Reproduced with kind permission of HMSO.)

scrotum should be symmetrical, as asymmetry may indicate the presence of a hydrocele, inguinal hernia or undescended testis. A dark discoloration of one or both sides of the scrotum, with or without swelling, is abnormal and may indicate torsion and requires immediate surgical review (see below).

- Do not attempt to withdraw the foreskin, as it is entirely normal for the foreskin to be adherent to the glans of the penis in infants. There is no need to see the urethral meatus as long as the prepuce is normally formed, there is not chordee (bending of the penis) and the infant has passed urine. If the prepuce is abnormal (i.e. opened on the ventral/bottom side), it is likely the infant has got hypospadias (see the section Hypospadias) and the urethral meatus should be identified to classify the abnormality. It is particularly important to describe if the penis is straight or if there is chordee.
- Observe for any groin swelling that may indicate an inguinal hernia. If a swelling can be reduced with gentle pressure in the direction of the inguinal canal, it is likely to be an inguinal hernia. A painful swelling in the groin needs urgent surgical review as this may be an incarcerated hernia. Remember, if no testes are in the scrotum, they may be what you can feel in the groin.
- With a thumb and finger at the topside of the scrotum, palpate down to confirm the presence of a testis of normal size (1–1.5 cm approximately). If this is successful, your examination is complete. If you do not feel a testicle, continue to the next step.
- This step should allow you to differentiate between palpable and impalpable undescended testis. With two fingers gently palpate from the top of the groin down towards the scrotum to identify an undescended testis. If you do not palpate the testis at all, this may be because of your examination skills, because the testis is in the abdomen or it is atrophic (and thus too small to feel or not there at all).
- If you are able to manipulate the testis into the scrotum, remove your fingers and observe. A testis that remains in the scrotum for some time without any further support is a normal retractile testis. If it 'snaps back' into its initial position, this is a true undescended testis (this explains why in your past experience you may have encountered disagreement amongst practitioners as to whether an undescended testicle is present in a neonate).

Female examination

- Inspect the genitalia to confirm that the general anatomy appears correct. You may notice a normal mucoid discharge that occurs in response to maternal oestrogens.
- Confirm the presence of normal labia majora, without fusion, with normal skin (this should not contain rugae, like a scrotum) and this should cover the labia minora in a term infant.

- Part the labia majora to view the labia minora. The clitoris will be at the upper border of the labia minora at the 12 o'clock position and should be of normal size.
- At this point, the urethral opening will be visible below the clitoris and then below that the hymen will be visible in the vagina.
- Note the presence of any mucoid cysts or skin tags around the vagina. There may be some swelling to the labia minora in response to maternal hormones. This is normal, but abnormalities in the skin texture or colour and a large clitoris are not.
- Observe for any groin swelling that may be inguinal hernia. If a swelling can be reduced with gentle pressure in the direction of the inguinal canal, it is likely to be an inguinal hernia. A painful swelling in the groin needs urgent surgical review as this may be an incarcerated hernia (bowel and/or ovary stuck in the inguinal canal with potential for ischaemia).

Undescended testicles

Undescended testicles are also referred to as cryptorchidism (Figure 5.3). Quoted incidence rates vary, but are generally accepted at birth to be 2–4% in full-term male infants and 1% at 1 year of age (Jackson et al. 1986, Acerini et al. 2009).

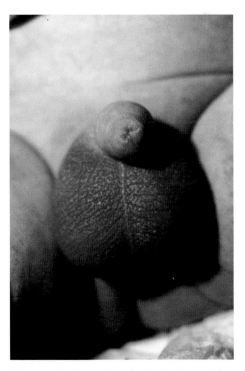

Figure 5.3 Undescended left testicle. (Reproduced with kind permission of Dr David Clark.)

In preterm infants, these figures are much higher, as normal testicular descent is not completed until late into pregnancy. The majority of undescended testicles are palpable, either in a normal route of descent in the groin, or in an ectopic position, most commonly in the perineum lateral to the scrotum.

There are several reasons why recognising undescended testicles is important. There are increased rates of fertility problems in later life if no intervention is made, thought to be related to the increased temperatures the testicles are exposed to. There is an increased risk of malignancy, which could again be related to temperature or possibly could be a spurious link due to the later age at diagnosis, given the difficulties in palpating an undescended testicle. Finally, there are the cosmetic and psychosocial concerns associated with the problem. Considering the anaesthetic risk and the low chance of any testis that is undescended at 1 year of age proceeding to descend naturally, advice from the American Academy of Pediatrics states intervention should take place optimally at around 1 year of age (Anonymous 1996) and global consensus is definitely to intervene before the age of 2 years (Khatwa and Menon 2000).

Management has been tried by medical hormonal methods, with reported success ranging from 6% to 65% (Rajfer et al. 1986), but many of these studies were uncontrolled and are thought to have included many retractile testes initially, thereby skewing the results. Double-blind placebo-controlled trials have shown these methods to be ineffective (Madden 2008).

The common treatment for this condition is surgery. The procedure is known as an orchidopexy and is a fairly simple operation in the majority of cases. It involves making an incision in the groin, exposing the testicle, removing the tissue that is keeping it stuck in the groin and then making a further incision in the scrotum to allow it to be placed there. A newer method (Bianchi and Squire 1989) has been used over the last 20 years and a long-term study (Gordon et al. 2010) has shown that it achieves the same result through a single scrotal incision, thus causing less pain, quicker wound healing and a better cosmetic result. The largest published literature review to date on orchidopexy (Docimo 1995) reports an overall success rate of 95.9% for this procedure. This procedure should be performed by paediatric urologists with an expertise in dealing with this condition and its possible long-term complications, highlighted previously.

Testicular torsion

Testicular torsion can be a cause of a discoloured scrotum in the newborn (Figure 5.4). This condition involves twisting of the testicle on itself and limited blood supply through the twisted vessels, which is very harmful and can rapidly lead to the death of a testicle. It can occur at any age, but if it occurs during delivery, as the baby will not be able to show symptoms, the testicle may simply die and this causes the discoloration. If this is seen, you must arrange an urgent paediatric urological review.

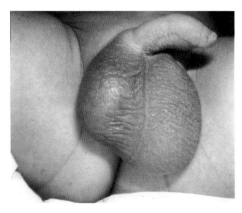

Figure 5.4 Right testicular torsion. (Reproduced with kind permission of Dr David Clark.)

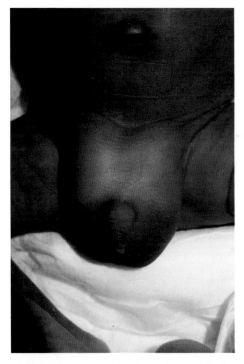

Figure 5.5 Inguinal hernia. (Reproduced with kind permission of Dr David Clark.)

Inguinal hernia

This is caused by the persistence of a connection between the scrotum and abdominal cavity and so abdominal fluid (hydrocele) or loops of bowel may pass into the inguinal canal and be felt as a lump (Figure 5.5). It is important to note because it is possible that loops of bowel may become incarcerated and thus irreducible. This is a surgical emergency as the bowel loops will have poor blood supply and will become ischaemic and then necrotic, with disastrous results for the infant. This concern is the reason why the operation is performed so early in life, despite the slight increase in anaesthetic risk. If the lump is reducible, a routine referral is made to a paediatric urologist. Clear advice must be given to the mother and father that if the lump seems to get stuck, is tender or red, or the child becomes irritable or has symptoms of bowel obstruction, they must attend their nearest A&E department.

Hydrocele

This describes the passage of fluid into the scrotum so it appears large and fluctuant. Light from a torch will pass through the fluid-filled scrotum. It is painless and harmless to the child and on examination gentle pressure on the scrotum will reduce the size of the scrotum by draining the fluid back into the abdomen. It occurs in 2–5% of boys, but the vast majority resolve spontaneously by 1 year of age, so no action is needed (Madden 2008). It is related to inguinal hernia, the difference being that the opening into the abdominal cavity is not large enough to allow anything other than fluid through. If it is still present after 2 years of age, the mother and father should see their general practitioner (GP) to request a paediatric urological review.

Hypospadias

This is a problem with the development of the penis's tissues on its lower aspect that leads to an abnormal opening of the urethra, as well as possibly problems with the foreskin and a downward curvature to the head of the penis (Figure 5.6). Like many conditions, it can vary in severity along a spectrum, but overall occurs in 1 in 300 males (Khatwa and Menon 2000). When a case is

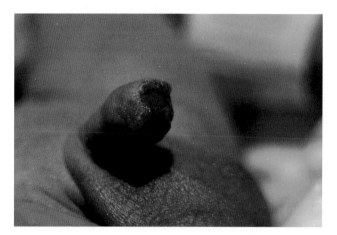

Figure 5.6 Hypospadias.

identified and both testes are in the scrotum, routine paediatric urology referral should be made. Repairs usually take place around 12 months of age.

Epispadias

Epispadias is the most severe congenital penile abnormality. It is extremely rare (1:117,000 males) (Gearhart et al. 1998). The majority of infants are incontinent of urine until major urological reconstruction is performed. Do not confuse a normal penis with a slightly dorsally opened prepuce with epispadias. In classic epispadisa, there are severe dorsal chordees and the urethra is opened on the dorsum of the penis. In the United Kingdom, epispadias and the other condition within the bladder exstrophy spectrum (bladder exstrophy and cloacal exstrophy) are treated only in two centres of excellence: Royal Manchester Children's Hospital and Great Ormond Street in London. Epispadias requires a routine paediatric urological referral, but it is advisable to order an urgent ultrasound of the renal tract to rule out associated urological abnormalities.

Ambiguous genitalia

The occurrence of genital ambiguity and intersex disorders is rare, but given the implications it has both from a medical and a familial psychosocial perspective, it is of great importance for the newborn examiner to have some familiarity with the topic. Understanding the basis of the problem is essentially simple when the developmental pathway of the genitalia, as discussed previously, is considered. There are many causes, possibly two of the most important being androgen insensitivity syndrome and congenital adrenal hyperplasia (Figure 5.7a and b).

Congenital adrenal hyperplasia (CAH)

This is the most common cause of ambiguous genitalia, occurring in 1 in 15,000 newborns and although the term covers a large number of conditions, generally it causes XX females to be overvirilised and therefore have masculinised external genitalia. This is an autosomal recessive condition which leads to impaired

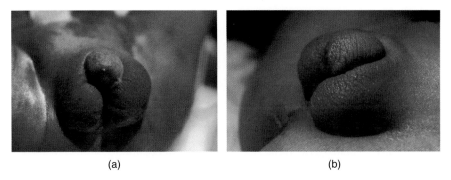

(a)   (b)

Figure 5.7 (a) Androgen insensitivity syndrome. (b) Congenital adrenal hyperplasia.

production of glucocorticoids (which are the body's natural steroids) and mineralocorticoids (such as aldosterone, involved in saving salt). The precursors for these are the sex hormones and therefore, as the body desperately tries to produce the missing hormones, it produces much higher amounts of testosterone as a side effect. This is what can lead to an overvirilised female with ambiguous genitalia, despite having normal internal female genitalia. This condition can present in a severe salt wasting form due to aldosterone insufficiency and those neonates can become very dehydrated within a few days and this may be life-threatening. It is this diagnosis that is the main medical reason for urgent investigation in ambiguous genitalia. Treatment is with replacement of salt and hormones followed by lifelong medication. Surgical reconstruction of the external genitalia is performed in the first few months of life by a dedicated paediatric urology team.

Androgen insensitivity syndrome

This occurs in XY males and leads to an abnormal testosterone receptor so the body cannot respond to testosterone and develops phenotypically as a female. As already discussed, developmentally what makes an XY fetus become masculinised is testosterone and if the body cannot respond to this, you get a female neonate with a blind-ending vagina and intra-abdominal testis.

The routine neonatal clinical examination cannot spot this abnormality; however, if there is a family history for this disorder, further investigation needs to be recommended. Usually, the diagnosis happens at the time of an inguinal herniotomy where the surgeon finds the testis within the inguinal sac!

Although the two conditions discussed are relatively simple to understand, the wider issues of gender assignment, anxieties of the mother and father and associated cultural issues are much more complicated. The first question all mothers and fathers ask is the gender of the neonate. If you have any doubt when you first see a baby, you must ask for an expert opinion and avoid guessing. A severe undervirilised male with severe hypospadias and bilateral undescended testicles may look like a female, and on the other hand, congenital adrenal hyperplasia can easily look like a male with undescended testicles. Figure 5.7a and b shows two images of infants with ambiguous genitalia. Can you tell just by looking which is XX and which is XY and would you feel happy to assign gender to this child? Cooperation between the experienced paediatric and paediatric urology teams can resolve the enigma, as often the clinical examination is not sufficient.

Referring to the baby without gender is difficult and mothers and fathers will have numerous detailed questions and concerns. Explaining the intricacies of gender assignment, particularly balancing chromosomal sex against the best gender assignment in terms of the child's future function, is very difficult. If you do see a case, explain to the mother and father that occasionally children do have genitalia that are not as well defined as in other children. Explain that there are many causes and, depending on what is seen on tests and scans and therefore the cause and treatments available, it is best not to assign a gender until they have spoken to the experts.

There is a growing body of research discussing these issues, particularly the interplay of genes and environment on gender in intersex disorders (Diamond 1997, Kuhnle and Krahl 2002), accompanied by a change in practice by professionals, with much more advanced surgical techniques allowing for better cosmetic and functional results. Nevertheless, if you ever encounter a neonate with these problems, much more important to the mother and father will be your ability to listen, to understand and to support them through an extremely difficult time (see Chapter 7 for further information on giving feedback to mothers and fathers).

Conclusion

While it is rare to find abnormalities on abdominal examination of the newborn, when present, such abnormalities can be of great significance. History from mothers and fathers is of paramount importance for this portion of the examination, specifically regarding feeding, vomiting and bowel function. Examination of the genitalia is far more likely to yield an abnormal finding, with undescended testicles commonly encountered. We have offered a table of abnormalities and a suggested course of action for each of these problems when encountered, which can be integrated with the readers' local policies to help guide practice.

Acknowledgements

The author would like to thank Raimondo M. Cervellione, Consultant Paediatric Urologist, for his assistance in the writing of the text. The author would also like to thank Gabrielle Mew and Cassandra Gordon for their assistance in editing the text.

Undescended testes (cryptorchidism) with associated hypospadias – a case study

Baby Steven was born at 38 weeks and weighed 3.2 kg. His mother had an uneventful antenatal period and no problems during labour. At birth, the amniotic fluid was meconium-stained, but Steven cried vigorously and was in good condition (Apgars were 9 at 1 minute and 10 at 5 minutes).

Steven's observations were as follows:

Respiration rate: 40 breaths a minute

Heart rate: 120 beats a minute.

Temperature: 36.8 °C

Colour: centrally pink

Steven was put to the breast and sucked well. At 8 hours old, his mother told the midwife that she thought Steven had difficulty passing urine as it 'just dripped from his penis', also that his penis looked 'an odd shape' and not like how her other child had looked a birth. The midwife performed a full examination, which revealed an abnormally placed urethral meatus, and she also noted that his scrotum was empty. All other aspects of this examination were normal.

The midwife immediately referred Steven to the paediatrician who confirmed a diagnosis of hypospadias with bilateral undescended testes. Because Steven presented with a combination of cryptorchidism and hypospadias, the paediatrician arranged blood tests to rule out female virilisation associated with Congenital Adrenal Hyperplasia. This condition can result in severe salt wasting and dehydration within days of birth and, if suspected, should be treated as an urgent referral. He also referred Steven to the local children's hospital for corrective surgery.

How would you deal with this situation in your Trust?

How would you help the mother and father understand this condition?

Look at these resources for more information on undescended testes and hypospadias:

Hypospadias http://emedicine.medscape.com/article/1015227-overview

An example of information for mothers and fathers http://www.gosh.nhs.uk/medical-information/search-for-medical-conditions/hypospadias/hypospadias-information/

Management of undescended testes http://eje-online.org/content/159/suppl_1/S87.long

Undescended testes and torsion http://adc.bmj.com/content/98/1/77.full.pdf+html

Jorgen T, McLacnlan R, Cortes D, Nation TR, Balic A, Southwell B, Huston JM (2010) What is new in cryptorchidism and hypospadias: a critical review on the dysgenesis hypothesis. *Journal of Pediatric Surgery* **45**, 2074–2086.

Forest MG, Nicolino M, David M, Morel Y (2005) The virilised female: endocrine background. *BJU International* **93**(3), 35–43.

Congenital Adrenal Hyperplasia http://emedicine.medscape.com/article/919218-overview

Congenital adrenal Hyperplasia support group for mothers and fathers http://www.livingwithcah.com/

References

Acerini CL, Miles HL, Dunger DB, et al. (2009) The descriptive epidemiology of congenital and acquired cryptorchidism in a UK infant cohort. *Archives of Disease in Childhood* **94**, 868–872.

Anonymous (1996) Timing of elective surgery on the genitalia of male children with particular reference to the risks, benefits, and psychological effects of surgery and anesthesia. Section on urology. *Pediatrics* **97**, 590–594.

Beattie M, Dhawan A, Puntis J (2009) Paediatric gastroenterology, hepatology and nutrition. *Oxford Specialist Handbooks in Paediatrics*. Chapter 29. Oxford: Oxford University Press.

Beers M, Berkow R (1999) *The Merk Manual*, 17th edn. Chapter 19. Philadelphia: Merk & Co, Inc.

Bianchi A, Squire BR (1989) Transcrotal Orchidopexy: orchidopexy revised. *Pediatric Surgery International* **4**, 189–192.

Diamond M (1997) Sexual identity and sexual orientation in children with traumatized or ambiguous genitalia. Journal of Sex Research **2**. Available from: http://www.thefree library.com/Sexual+identity+and+sexual+orientation+in+children+with+traumatized ... - a019551973 (accessed 12 January 2011).

Docimo SG (1995) The results of surgical therapy for cryptorchidism: a literature review and analysis. *Journal of Urology* **154**, 1148–1152.

Gearhart JP, Mathews R, Taylor S, Jeffs RD (1998) Combined bladder closure and epispadias repair in the reconstruction of bladder exstrophy. *Journal of Urology* **160**, 1182–1185, discussion 1190.

Gordon M, Cervellione RM, Morabito A, Bianchi A (2010) 20 years of transcrotal orchidopexy for undescended testis: results and outcomes. *Journal of Pediatric Urology* **6**(5), 506–512.

Goyal A, Jones MO, Couriel JM, Losty PD (2006) Oesophageal atresia and tracheo-oesophageal fistula. *Archives of Disease in Childhood. Fetal and Neonatal Edition* **91**, F381–F384. DOI:10.1136/adc.2005.086157.

Jackson MB, Chivers C, Pike MC, et al. (1986) Cryptorchidism: an apparent substantial increase since 1960. *British Medical Journal* **293**, 1401–1404.

Khatwa UA, Menon PSN (2000) Management of undescended testis. *Indian Journal of Pediatrics* **67**, 449–454.

Kuhnle U, Krahl W (2002) The impact of culture on sex assignment and gender development in intersex patients. *Perspectives in Biology and Medicine* **45**, 85–103.

Madden N (2008) In: D Thomas, P Duffy, A Rickwood (eds) *Essentials of Paediatric Urology*. Chapter 18. London: Informa Healthcare.

Mshvildadze M, Neu J (2009) Probiotics and prevention of necrotizing enterocolitis. *Early Human Development* **85**(Suppl. 10), S71–S74. Epub 24 September 2009.

Obladen M (2009) Necrotizing enterocolitis: 150 years of fruitless search for the cause. *Neonatology* **96**(4), 203–210. Epub 29 April 2009.

Raboei EH (2009) Necrotizing enterocolitis in full-term neonates: is it aganglionosis? *European Journal of Pediatric Surgery* **19**(2), 101–104. Epub 9 April 2009.

Rajfer J, Handelsman DJ, Swerdloff RS (1986) Hormonal therapy in cryptorchidism. *New England Journal of Medicine* **314**, 466–470.

Rennie JM (2005) *Robertson's Textbook of Neonatology*. New York: Churchill Livingstone.

Roy R, Gordon M, Watson L, Edi-Osagie N (2007) Recognition of bilious aspirates in a tertiary neonatal centre. *Acta Pædiatrica* **96**(Suppl. 456), 67.

Skinner MA (1996) Hirschsprung's disease. *Current Problems in Surgery* **33**(5), 389–460.

Sniderman S, Taeusch W (2004) Evaluation and care of the normal newborn. In: W Taeusch, R Ballard, C Gleason (eds) *Avery's Diseases of the Newborn*. Chapter 7. Philadelphia: Elsevier, Saunders.

Stephenson T, Marlow N, Watkin S, Grant J (2000) *Pocket Neonatology*. Chapter 16. London: Churchill Livingstone, p. 311.

Thilo E, Rosenberg A (2003). In: Hayward AR, Levin MJ, Sondheimer JM (eds) *Current Pediatric Diagnosis & Treatment*. Chapter 1. Stamford, CT: Appleton & Lange.

Thompson AM, Bizzarro MJ (2008) Necrotizing enterocolitis in newborns: pathogenesis, prevention and management. *Drugs* **68**(9), 1227–1238.

Thureen PJ, Deacon J, Hernandez JA (2005) *Evaluation and Care of the Newborn Infant*. Missouri: Elsevier Saunders.

UK National Screening Committee (2008) *Newborn and Infant Physical Examination: Standards and Competencies*. London: NHS.

CHAPTER 6

Developmental dysplasia of the hip and abnormalities of the foot

Robin W. Paton[1,2] and Naomi Davis[3]

[1] Orthopaedic Department, University of Manchester, Manchester, UK
[2] East Lancashire Hospitals NHS Trust, Blackburn, Lancashire, UK
[3] Royal Manchester Children's Hospital, Central Manchester University Hospitals NHS Foundation Trust, Manchester, UK

KEY POINTS

- The definition of developmental dysplasia of the hip (DDH) is vague and can deteriorate or improve. This makes research into treatment methods difficult as there can be false-positive and false-negative cases.

- The successful treatment of DDH by splintage has never been confirmed by comparative or randomised studies.

- Universal or selective ultrasound screening programmes cannot be advocated at present. There is inadequate evidence to support their value in significantly reducing the incidence of irreducible dislocation of the hip in DDH when compared to clinical screening methods alone.

- The majority of foot deformities can be accurately diagnosed on clinical examination alone.

- Treatment of foot deformities is aimed towards function and the ability to wear normal shoes.

Developmental dysplasia of the hip

Definition

DDH was a term coined by Klisic (1989) in the 1980s. DDH is a spectrum of disease ranging from dysplasia of the hip to irreducible dislocation. This wide definition of hip abnormality can be confusing as it ranges from the minor immature hip dysplasia which develops normally by 3 months of age to complex prenatal irreducible hip dislocation which may require multiple or complex hip and pelvic surgery (Figure 6.1). Klisic viewed the condition as a dynamic disorder that may resolve or deteriorate with growth. Bialik et al. (1999), Graf et al. (1999) and

---

Examination of the Newborn: An Evidence-Based Guide, Second Edition. Edited by Anne Lomax.
© 2015 John Wiley & Sons, Ltd. Published 2015 by John Wiley & Sons, Ltd.
Companion Website: www.wiley.com/go/lomax/newborn

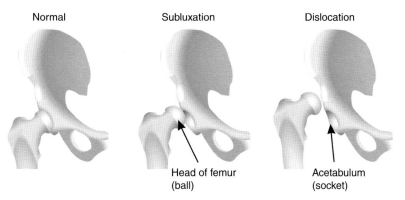

Normal   Subluxation   Dislocation

Head of femur   Acetabulum
(ball)   (socket)

Figure 6.1 Dislocation of the hip.

Rosendahl et al. (1994) attempted to classify DDH sonographically into physiological (most Graf Type II A and Graf Type II B dysplasias) and pathological (some or all Graf Type IIC, Graf Type III, Graf Type IV and irreducible hip dislocation).

Dysplasias or dislocations of the hip secondary to neuromuscular disorders and syndromal conditions are excluded from the definition of DDH as they are secondary to the primary condition not developing de novo (Bialik et al. 1999).

Consequences of DDH

DDH of the hips is a condition that can develop into serious debilitating hip pathology in childhood, adolescent and adult life (Lloyd-Roberts 1955, Engesaeter et al. 2008). An irreducible hip dislocation will result in a short-legged gait, limited hip movement, osteoarthrosis of the hip and back problems secondary to the short leg if not diagnosed and treated in the neonate or infant. Serious debilitating hip pain usually develops within the third decade if the hip is not treated successfully in the neonate or infant (Jones et al. 2000). Avascular necrosis of the femoral head, secondary to open surgical or closed treatment with a splint or hip spica, may accelerate the hip pathology resulting in severe hip symptoms a decade earlier than in the natural history of the condition (Jones et al. 2000). Unsuccessful treatment of the irreducible hip dislocation may, therefore, be more damaging than no treatment at all. Dysplasia of the hip may result in severe osteoarthrosis in adulthood. The Norwegian hip register reported that 29% of hip replacements in patients under the age of 60 years are secondary to hip dysplasia (Engesaeter et al. 2008). Due to the consequences of this potentially serious childhood condition, much effort has been undertaken at national and international levels in order to diagnose and treat the condition in the neonate and infant (Clarke et al. 1985, SMAC guidelines (SMAC 1986,

Graf 1987). These preventative attempts with clinical and ultrasound hip screening can be time-consuming and expensive with mixed results (Macnicol 1990, Clegg et al. 1999, Paton 2005). The effectiveness of such programmes is at best controversial.

DDH: incidence

Due to the imprecise nature of the definition of DDH, pathological DDH is difficult to define accurately. Irreducible dislocation is the most measurable of the pathologies, and the incidence of irreducible dislocation is usually used to compare the effectiveness of clinical and ultrasound screening programmes. Irreducible dislocation is more common in females (6:1) and is more common on the left side (2:1) (Milbrandt and Sucato 2004), and unilateral irreducible dislocation is considerably more common than bilateral irreducible dislocations (>6:1) (personal series). The incidence of irreducible hip dislocation varies between 0.1 per 1,000 in New Zealand (Hadlow 1988) and 0.5–0.8 per 1,000 in the United Kingdom (Macnicol 1990, Paton 2005). In clinically unscreened populations, the incidence may be 1.6 per 1,000 (Catford et al. 1982). The probable reason why in universal clinical and ultrasound screening there is still an irreducible dislocation rate is that not all irreducible hip dislocations are secondary to primary clinical instability occurring at birth. Some of the clinical instabilities may not be identified by neonatal clinical examination, some irreducible hip dislocations may be prenatal and some may be associated with certain dysplasias, which were clinically stable at birth but may progress to irreducible dislocation (Rosendahl et al. 1994).

Dysplasia may be initially diagnosed sonographically in the neonate, and this abnormality may be physiological or pathological. Ninety to hundred per cent of stable sonographic hip dysplasias (Graf Type II) develop normally without treatment by 9–12 weeks of age (Castelein et al. 1992, Marks et al. 1994, Rosendahl et al. 1994, Wood et al. 2000, Holen et al. 2002). In general, Graf Type III and Graf Type IV pathological instabilities are treated as pathological and are splinted, although there are no proper controlled trials to confirm that splintage as a treatment is effective (Jones et al. 2000, Shipman et al. 2006).

Adolescent and adult dysplasia may not be related to sonographic neonatal dysplasia. Theoretically, this dysplasia could be secondary to abnormalities of the acetabular growth plate developing up to the end of growth at skeletal maturity. The incidence of radiological hip dysplasia in the adult population is unknown, but is thought to be in the order of over 1% of the total population (Tönnis 1987). The percentage of hip dysplasia progressing to symptomatic osteoarthrosis is unknown.

Clinical hip joint instability

Subluxable and dislocatable hips diagnosed clinically or by ultrasound imaging may spontaneously resolve. Barlow (1962) in a clinical study in the 1960s noted that 88% of unstable hips stabilised within weeks. Gardiner and Dunn (1991) in a controlled trial confirmed that 71% of unstable hips stabilise within 2 weeks. Two per cent of newborns may have instability at birth, but only 0.1–0.2% develop irreducible dislocation (Toma et al. 2001). Persistent Ortolani positive hips and those with poor acetabular development are found to be at high risk of developing a progressive deterioration of major dysplasia or irreducibility in the future if not treated (Boeree and Clarke 1994, Lerman et al. 2001, Bache et al. 2002, Paton et al. 2004).

Clinical screening

In the United Kingdom, the recommended clinical screening examination for instability of the hip is undertaken in newborns and again at 6–8 weeks (SMAC 1986). There is controversy on the effectiveness of these clinical guidelines (Jones et al. 2000). The last major review of the UK national guidelines prior to 2008 was in 1986.

The National Screening Committee (NSC) has been reviewing these guidelines since 2002 and a change in the national guidelines was published in 2008 (Newborn and Infant Physical Examination (NIPE) guidelines). These guidelines have been endorsed by the UK NSC and National Institute for Clinical Excellence (NICE). The 2008 guidelines are currently being updated, and it is expected that the local primary care trusts will 'roll out' this new set of standards and competencies soon.

In summary, the NIPE guidelines recommend that all babies' hips should ideally be examined by the Ortolani and Barlow hip tests within 24 hours and certainly within 72 hours of birth. If a clinical abnormality is detected, these babies should have an ultrasound imaging of the hip joints within 2 weeks of age. If there is a positive ultrasound, these babies should have an expert consultation (usually a paediatric orthopaedic surgeon) within 3–4 weeks of age. If a baby has the 'risk factors' of breech presentation or a strong family history but a normal clinical examination of the hip joints, these hips should have an ultrasound imaging of the hip joints by 6 weeks of age. If these babies have a positive risk factor, a negative examination and a positive ultrasound imaging, these babies should have an expert consultation by 6–8 weeks of age.

The clinical hip examination should be repeated at between 6 and 8 weeks of age, usually in the primary care scenario.

There is evidence that small well-trained teams of doctor(s), nurses or physio-therapists may be more effective than using inexperienced SHOs/trainee doctors (Hadlow 1988, Macnicol 1990).

The Ortolani hip screening examination test

This is undertaken by elevation and abduction of the femur resulting in a reloca-tion of the dislocated hip (Milbrandt and Sucato 2004). This is usually associated with a palpable clunk in reduction. The sensitivity of this test is 60% and the specificity is 100% (Jones 1998). There are, therefore, some false negatives, but virtually no false positives. Robinson (1998) noted that in two-thirds of irre-ducible cases, the Ortolani test failed to identify the hip pathology.

The Barlow clinical examination test

The action of adduction and depression of the femur dislocates a dislocatable hip (Milbrandt and Sucato 2004). However, the positive predictive value of this test is only 0.22 (Patel 2001). This means that the test is positive in the presence of the disease in only 22% of cases, a poor clinical test.

See the website (Step By Step Guide to the Examination of the Newborn) to access a video about hip examination.

Clinical screening

In an ideal screening test, the sensitivity, specificity and positive predictive val-ues should all be as close to 100% as possible – 100% sensitivity means that the test is 'positive in disease' by the absence of false negatives and 100% speci-ficity means that the test is 'negative in health' by the absence of false positives. Positive predictive value indicates that the test is positive if the patient has the disease. The clinical screening manoeuvres of Ortolani and Barlow clearly do not reach the clinical screening ideal. In view of this, Jones (1998) stated that the clinical assessment of instability of the hip should be considered as a hip 'surveillance' test rather than a true screening test. Medico–legally, if a clinical screening test is undertaken by an individual who has been properly trained and assessed as competent in the clinical test and a late irreducible dislocation occurs, this should not be considered negligent due to the poor sensitivity and positive predictive value of the tests. Clinical tests of instability, however, are still of value as a positive test should not be ignored as treatment of a persistently unstable hip may prevent deterioration to major dysplasia or irreducible dislo-cation, although the numbers of irreducible dislocation prevented by treatment may be low (Bache et al. 2002, Paton et al. 2004). Clinical screening programmes identify more cases of hip instability than in the absence of clinical screening, although due to the spontaneous resolution rate, the numbers of irreducible hip dislocations prevented may be low. This increases the risk of over-treatment. The general view is that clinically unstable hips should be treated (Jones et al. 2000).

Other clinical signs

After 3 months of age, unilateral limitation of hip abduction may be a useful clinical test with a sensitivity of 70% and a specificity of over 90% (Jari et al. 2002). Asymmetrical skin creases in the absence of limitation of hip abduction is not associated with DDH (Lehmann et al. 2000, Shipman et al. 2006). Clicks can be associated with hip pathology although the majority of cases with hip clicks are benign and not associated with DDH. Unfortunately, the difference between a click and a clunk as noted by the clinically inexperienced may be subjective, and if there is any doubt, such hips should be imaged by ultrasound to exclude significant hip pathology.

Ultrasound screening and DDH

Graf et al. (1999) popularised the use of ultrasound screening in the diagnosis and monitoring of DDH in the 1980s. The advantage of ultrasound is that this should increase the sensitivity of hip joint assessment by reducing the number of false-negative results. This is a dynamic, real-time imaging modality using non-ionising radiation. It is, therefore, safer than conventional X-rays. The disadvantages are that although ultrasound imaging is very sensitive, it may not be specific as there is an increase in the false-positive result rate. It is very operator-dependent with a risk of intra-observer and inter-observer errors (poor Kappa scores). There is a risk of over-treatment secondary to these increased numbers of false-positive cases. Potential false-positive cases include stable minor dysplasia, which in over 90% will spontaneously resolve (Rosendahl et al. 1994, Wood et al. 2000, Sampath et al. 2003), and sonographic hip instability, which may resolve in 70–90% (Gardiner and Dunn 1991, Castelein et al. 1992, Toma et al. 2001). Numerous classification systems are published in the literature (Harcke and Grissom 1986, Zieger et al. 1986, Terjesen et al. 1989, Andersson and Funnemark 1995, Graf et al. 1999). The most commonly used systems are the morphological system of Graf et al. (1999) and the dynamic stress testing system of Harcke and Grissom (1986). In general, both morphological and dynamic assessments are used, specific details of which are not necessary for this chapter on DDH. In general, ultrasound screening is useful in the diagnosis and monitoring of certain physiological and pathological dysplasias, hip instability and irreducibility of the hip joint.

Universal ultrasound screening programmes

These have been advocated mainly in the German-speaking countries of Germany, Austria and Switzerland. The theory is that all cases of dysplasia and instability can be diagnosed early, resulting in identification of all pathological hip abnormalities. These sonographic scans should be done within the first week of life, and 85–98% of the population (Bache et al. 2002, Wirth et al. 2005) can be screened by this method. Advocates highlight the absence of 'late' dislocations and the low open hip joint surgery operative rates (Rosendahl et al. 1994, Graf et al. 1999, Bache et al. 2002). Others have shown that there is not a statistical difference in the open operative reduction of irreducible hip dislocations between clinical screening, selective ultrasound screening and universal screening programmes (Rosendahl et al. 1994, Patel 2001, Shipman et al. 2006). The numbers of false-positive diagnoses may result in over-treatment (Ganger et al. 1991), with up to 9% of the population being treated. Statistically, the low incidence of instability results in huge numbers of normal examinations for every positive instability or irreducible hip discovered. This may not be financially viable, as there will still be cases of irreducibility requiring surgical intervention even after universal ultrasound screening. In a recent universal ultrasound screening study, the operative rate was 0.26 per 1,000 live births (Graf 2007) compared with the 0.5 per 1,000 live births noted in selective ultrasound screening (Paton et al. 1999). However, treatment in the universal ultrasound screening programme included closed reduction methods compared with the selective programme in which the surgery was pure open reduction of irreducible hip joints.

Selective ultrasound screening

The previous British guidelines of 1986 (SMAC 1986) state that 60% of hip dislocations originate from certain risk factors. These risk factors include breech presentation, strong family history (mother and father, first cousins), postural and fixed foot deformities, torticollis of the neck, oligohydramnios, Caesarean section and intrauterine growth retardation. Five- and ten-year reviews (Paton et al. 1999, Paton et al. 2005) confirmed that there were only 30–31% of hip instabilities associated with a true risk factor.

Oligohydramnios, Caesarean section, fixed CTEV and postural TEV have been shown not to be at a significant risk of developing pathological DDH (Paton et al. 1999, Paton and Choudry 2009). In the United Kingdom, 4% of births are by breech presentation (Bache et al. 2002) and in an average district general hospital, this could result in 140–160 breech cases being ultrasounded per year. Selective ultrasound screening may result in 7.4% of the population being screened sonographically (Paton et al. 2005). Family history is often vague and can be difficult to validate as often the mother and father do not know if the problem was a simple click, treated with double nappies or even an open reduction of the hip for irreducibility. This may result in equivocal cases being sent for sonographic screening with little probability of true pathology. There is evidence that congenital talipes calcaneovalgus (CTCV) and metatarsus adductus may have a significant risk of instability (Paton and Choudry 2009). In CTCV, there is a risk of 1:15 and in metatarsus adductus, a risk of 1:25 for irreducible dislocation and instability. The risk for irreducible dislocation and hip instability in breech was 1:70, and in family history, the risk was 1:45 (Paton et al. 2005). If the risk of Graf Type III dysplasia, hip irreducibility and hip instability combined was calculated, in breech, the ratio was 1:27 and in family history, it was 1:15 (Paton et al. 2005). As instability and irreducibility are more common in females, it has been advocated that only females with breech or family history should be screened (Patel 2001).

Ultrasound screening: summary

There is not enough evidence to advocate either a universal or a selective ultrasound screening programme in the United Kingdom. The main problems are that there is a low incidence/prevalence of the condition and the majority of abnormal hips may spontaneously stabilise or resolve without treatment. Treatment may not be effective as there is no evidence-based consensus on when or how the condition should be treated. Treatment has the potential to cause harm, and there is a risk of over-treatment of physiologically abnormal, but not pathological, hip conditions. Statistically, clinical and ultrasound imaging may have a low positive predictive value and pathological DDH appears to be predominantly a disease in women. However, the recent NIPE screening recommendations (see introduction) are a reasonable compromise in this difficult area, where there is an inadequate evidence base.

Ultrasound imaging is useful in monitoring treatment and confirming if clinically abnormal hips are stabilising/resolving or not. Sonography is more useful, accurate and safe than X-rays in the first 3 months of life (McEvoy and Paton 1997).

Treatment of DDH

In neonates, treatment can be subdivided into mobile/dynamic and rigid devices.

Rigid devices

The Von Rosen and Craig splints are the most widely used in the United Kingdom (Jones et al. 2000). These devices hold the hips abducted and flexed in a predetermined position in a 'safe' and stable zone. Wilkinson et al. (2002) showed better results with the Von Rosen splint when compared to the Pavlik splint although this may not be statistically true secondary to confounding factors such as the timing and length of treatment. An alternative is the application of a plaster hip spica, either in a stable position or after a manipulation under anaesthetic and arthrogram under a general anaesthetic (Graf et al. 1999). An arthrogram confirms that congruent reduction of the hip joint is possible without soft tissue interposition. The hip spica is used where there is uncertainty about whether the hip will reduce in other rigid devices, if there is a narrow zone of instability or where it is felt that a dynamic splint is too lax to hold the hip in the reduced position.

Dynamic splintage

The Pavlik harness is the most popular splint in the United States and certain parts of Europe (Figure 6.2). The advantages are that it allows some movement within the hip joints, which may be protective against avascular necrosis. This may be more comfortable than a rigid splint and may have a larger safe zone to protect against avascular necrosis. Avascular necrosis of the head of the hip joint is a risk with any splintage and can occur in up to 16% of cases (Herring 1992,

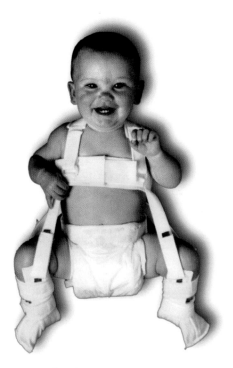

Figure 6.2 Pavlik harness. (Reproduced with kind permission of the Wheaton Brace Company.)

Suzuki et al. 1996). In general, the risk is thought to be 1% (Jones et al. 2000). The long-term effects of avascular necrosis of the hip joint are that this can result in a short femoral neck, hip incongruity and premature osteoarthrosis.

Splintage cannot be used in irreducible hips as the irreducibility is usually secondary to soft tissue interposition. If irreducibility is not identified and splintage is continued, damage to the shape of the femoral head may occur due to indentation of the soft tissues on the soft articular cartilage of the femoral head. In addition, the posterior wall of the acetabulum may be damaged making subsequent open reduction of the hip more difficult (Suzuki 1993). There is a poor evidence base for the use of splintage as no controlled trials have been undertaken, coupled with a high clinical spontaneous resolution rate of instability (Jones et al. 2000, Shipman et al. 2006). There are no robust national recommendations on when a pathological hip dysplasia/dislocation should be splinted and for how long. In several studies, fewer than 10% of unstable hips required splintage and the majority of dysplastic hips resolve (Castelein et al. 1992, Rosendahl et al. 1994, Andersson and Funnemark 1995, Wood et al. 2000).

The optimum time of splintage has not been adequately determined. My personal view would be to splint clinical instability of the hip and Graf Type III dysplasia with a Pavlik harness within 2 weeks postnatally for 6 weeks with an interim ultrasound imaging at 3 weeks to confirm satisfactory progress and to exclude irreducible dislocation. After 6 weeks, the splintage or harnesssplintage the harness is removed and a further ultrasound undertaken 2 weeks later to monitor that the hip joint is reduced and any dysplasia is resolving. Further monitoring by serial ultrasound and later by X-rays is undertaken to confirm resolution of dysplasia or stabilisation of the hip joint. Figure 6.3 shows the UK Screening Committee NIPE process map for Developmental Dysplasia of the Hips.

In the literature, the treatment of instability ranges from splintage immediately (Jones et al. 2000) at 2 weeks (Gardiner and Dunn 1991) to at 6 weeks (Bache et al. 2002). Without a proper controlled trial, it is impossible to judge between these various opinions. However, in the series of Bache, the open reduction rate was extremely low with low splintage rates (0.31%), and this combination of universal sonographic screening and delayed treatment may be a good compromise.

Abnormalities of the foot

The foot is a complex structure designed for propulsion and weight bearing but in the newborn, it has a while to wait before it realises usefulness. Early on, much of the foot is actually cartilage rather than bone, ligaments are supple and this allows any foot deformity to be gently guided into an improved position. As the child grows and later bears weight, the structures respond to the forces put through them, the cartilage is increasingly replaced by bone and the ability

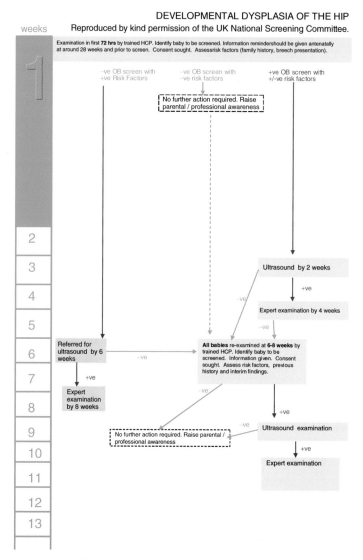

Figure 6.3 Developmental Dysplasia of the hip.

to remodel gradually decreases. Therefore, there is a window of opportunity to correct any major deformity.

The foot, unlike the hand, does not depend on the finesse of individual digit movement for function, but it does require a satisfactory weight-bearing surface and the ability to effectively transfer forces. The feet should also (in our society) be shoe-able. In short, the feet, as a minimum, should allow pain-free walking and running. The bones of the normal foot can be seen in Figure 6.4.

An abnormality in a newborn foot is most likely to be obvious to everyone in the delivery suite. Special tests are rarely required and there should be little delay

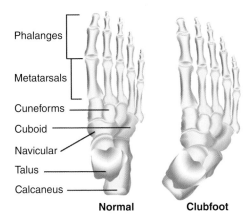

Figure 6.4 The bones of the foot.

in diagnosis and the provision of appropriate information for the most common deformities. The concept of counting the fingers and toes and reporting back to involved family and friends is a traditional one and any divergence from normal can bring devastating and lasting upset. Reliable information given at the time of initial diagnosis is vital.

Clubfoot

This is the most common foot deformity (1:1,000 live births in the United Kingdom) (Wynne Davies 1972) requiring counselling and treatment. It is also known as congenital talipes equinovarus.

- Congenital: From birth
- Talipes: Ankle, foot
- Equinus: Pointing downwards (like a horse's foot)
- Varus: Pointing inwards, towards the midline

It has a higher incidence in boys than in girls, the ratio being 3:1, and around 50% are bilateral. There may be a family history. The incidence of clubfoot is 17 times higher than in the normal population for first-degree relatives and six times higher in second-degree relatives. The risk for a second child in a family where one child is affected but with unaffected mother and father is 1:35 (Wynne Davies 1972, Barker et al. 2003).

The inheritance is polygenic with unknown environmental factors, although maternal smoking, alcohol consumption and intravenous drug abuse have all been mooted (Barker et al. 2003, Dobbs et al. 2006a, 2006b).

Clubfoot can be associated with other conditions including arthrogryposis, spina bifida and Down's syndrome (see also Chapter 7). Other rarer anomalies, some of which may not be fully diagnosed until much later, may be involved or coexist.

Diagnosis

Antenatal diagnosis

Increasingly, clubfoot is diagnosed antenatally. It is not an embryonic malformation and so the earliest it has been seen on ultrasound scan is sixteenth week, although it may not be evident until as late as thirty-second week (Figure 6.5). While antenatal diagnosis can give no indication of the severity of clubfoot including whether it is structural or positional, it does give the mother and father a chance to gain as much information as they would like on the deformity, treatment options and likely outcome. Some centres will have access to prenatal counselling from their local paediatric orthopaedic service. Other agencies and mother and father support groups are accessible through the Internet. A series of surveys (PALS 2003) of mothers and fathers found that their main concern was the lack of information given at diagnosis or that they were given the wrong information about treatment and outcomes for their child. Less commonly, abortion is being suggested or offered after a prenatal diagnosis of clubfoot. This cannot be supported. Accurate information must be given to families at the first diagnosis. Those that are correctly advised and who are able to make a clear treatment plan for their child felt that they could then enjoy the rest of their pregnancy. At delivery, they see all of their new baby rather than just concentrating on their feet and do not have to deal with that particular shock of deformity.

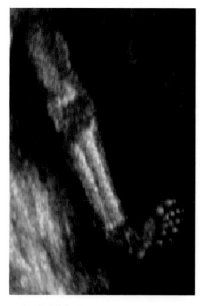

Figure 6.5 Ultrasound diagnosis of clubfoot.

Postnatal diagnosis

A variety of foot deformities are referred to orthopaedic surgeons with the label 'talipes', but some differentiation of the deformity is important in enabling appropriate counselling as soon as possible.

There are three main descriptive areas of the foot: (1) the hindfoot, which consists of the heel (calcaneus/os calcis) and the talus; (2) the midfoot, which is made up of the small tarsal bones, none of which are ossified at birth; and (3) the forefoot, which describes the metatarsals and toes.

Structural clubfoot

Structural clubfoot is a foot positioned pointing downwards and inwards (in a club shape) and is not easily correctible with gentle manipulation. There may be a deep crease above the heel and under the medial arch. The calf will tend to look smaller and thinner than the other side, if the other side is normal (Figure 6.6a).

Anatomically, the hindfoot points inwards and downwards (varus and equinus) (Figure 6.6b) giving the crease above the heel and the forefoot points inwards (metatarsus adductus) giving the crease under the medial arch and a curve to the outer (lateral) edge of the foot (Figure 6.6c).

This foot will require treatment by a specialist unit.

Positional clubfoot

Positional clubfoot has a similar appearance but with less obvious creases and is easily correctible on initial handling. A normal infant's foot can be turned outwards by 50°–70° (Figure 6.7a) and upwards by around 20° (Figure 6.7b). If a foot that looks like a clubfoot will correct this far, then it can be deemed positional and a physiotherapist can advise the mother and father on gentle massage. The foot will quickly improve and there will be no functional deficit.

It is not uncommon for a child to have a structural clubfoot on one side and a positional on the other. It is not clear whether they are degrees of the same entity or not.

In general, massage of the feet prior to an early appointment with a paediatric orthopaedic surgeon will have no ill effects and may well help. Mothers and fathers appreciate the ability to help their child themselves. Some feet will be borderline between positional and structural and will need monitoring.

Treatment

There has been a turnaround in the management of clubfoot in the last decade. Previously, a child with clubfoot would most usually have a period of massage and strapping and then go on to major reconstructive surgery of the foot at around 9 months. This operation was most often a postero–medial release. Now,

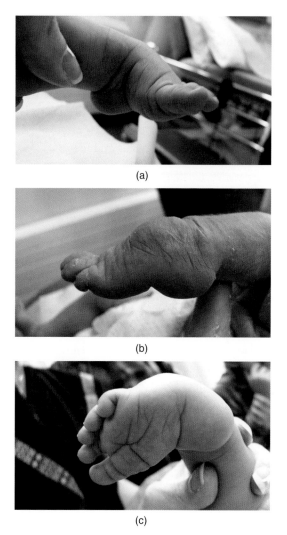

(a)

(b)

(c)

Figure 6.6 Clubfoot.

the mainstay of treatment of clubfoot is the Ponseti method of clubfoot management. The evidence suggests that the Ponseti method gives better functional long-term results than major joint and tendon releasing surgery (Ponseti and Smoley 1963, Cooper and Dietz 1995, Ippolito et al. 2003, Dobbs et al. 2006a, Dietz et al. 2009, Farsetti et al. 2009). The Ponseti method is a technique of gentle manipulation and serial casting at weekly intervals that allows the foot to be gradually corrected over a period of about 6 weeks (Figures 6.8 and 6.9a–c).

Each separate deformity of the foot is corrected in order and the foot position gradually improves. Gentle reshaping of the deformed cartilage in the foot happens during this time and the ligaments are gradually stretched. The foot

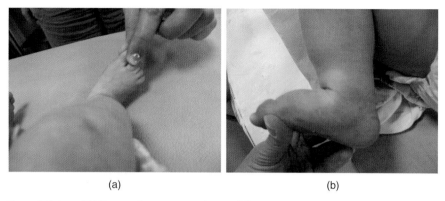

(a)   (b)

Figure 6.7 (a and b) Range of movement of normal foot

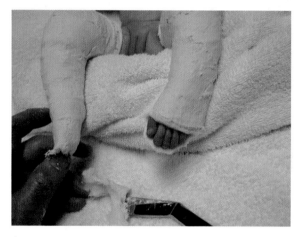

Figure 6.8 Ponseti cast.

moves from its inward facing position to an outwardly turned position, closely resembling the normal foot.

The last thing to achieve is to allow the foot to turn upwards (dorsiflex). The Achilles tendon at the back of the heel tends to prevent this. Therefore, a small procedure under local anaesthetic is needed to cut the Achilles tendon. This heals completely and after 2–3 weeks in a final cast, the foot is fully corrected (Figure 6.10).

Correction is maintained by a period in a foot abduction brace (Figure 6.11a). This is worn full time for 3 months and at night for at least 4 years (Figure 6.11b).

The success rate of the Ponseti method is in excess of 95% and children effectively treated this way learn to walk and run at the same time as any other child and wear normal shoes during the day (Laaveg and Ponseti 1980, Herzenberg et al. 2002, Ponseti et al. 2006, Alves et al. 2009). Long-term studies show no

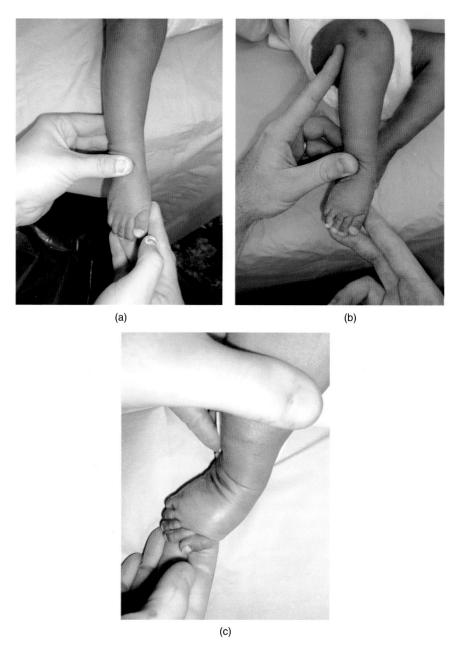

(a)

(b)

(c)

Figure 6.9 (a) Gradual correction – second week. (b) Gradual correction – fourth week. (c) Gradual correction – fifth week.

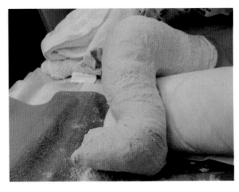

Figure 6.10 Final cast after full correction.

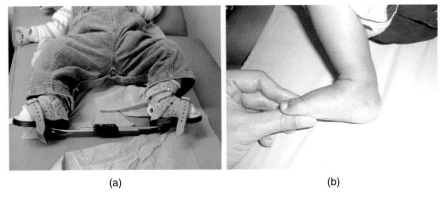

(a)   (b)

Figure 6.11 (a) Foot in abduction brace (one example). (b) Final correction from brace.

discernible difference between people who have had clubfeet treated by the Ponseti method and those who have had normal feet, into middle life.

While the Ponseti method, correctly performed, is an extremely effective way of treating clubfoot, it does involve a partnership between practitioner and mother and father and a considerable commitment from all towards the treatment method. Weekly visits to the hospital for casting, the difficulties of caring for a baby in above-knee casts who cannot be bathed and the parenting skills that in some cases need to be learnt very quickly to enable an infant and family to settle into a routine with the foot abduction brace all put considerable strain on a family. This can be eased with accurate and consistent information across the professionals and support from the treating team and from others, such as situated families.

Children with clubfeet and other complicating conditions may need more intervention and a small number of children will require more extensive surgery (Boehm et al. 2008, Gerlach et al. 2009). However, the Ponseti method should be the first-line treatment for all clubfeet (Figures 6.12 and 6.13).

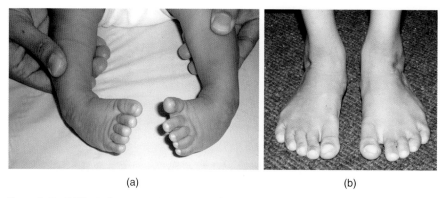

(a)   (b)

Figure 6.12 Child 1 before Ponseti treatment of clubfoot and at 6 years.

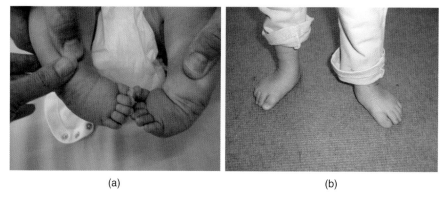

(a)   (b)

Figure 6.13 Child 2 before treatment and at 4 years.

Metatarsus adductus

This is a deformity of the midfoot only; the heel is not affected (Figure 6.14). The front of the foot, the metatarsals, point towards the midline and there is a curve to the lateral border of the foot. This is thought to be purely a 'packaging' problem and can show some variability in presentation. In the vast majority of cases, this is a cosmetic and not a functional deformity. It tends to improve as the child grows and is unlikely to need any treatment other than gentle massage. Occasionally, casting is required in a similar way to the Ponseti method, but as the hindfoot is not involved, no surgery is needed to the Achilles tendon (Ponseti and Becker 1966).

Mothers and fathers should be warned that when their child first starts to walk, the metatarsus adductus may look more obvious. This is related to the increased use of the great toe as a balancing aid while the child first learns to stand up. It settles as walking progresses and muscle control improves. Mothers and fathers will also tend to return for advice after trying to purchase their child's first pair of shoes. A well-meaning shoe store assistant may question any

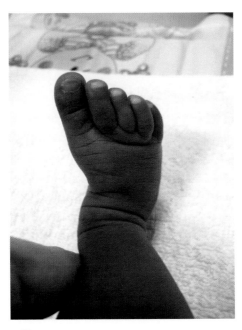

Figure 6.14 Metatarsus adductus.

residual adductus. Reassurance can be given that the foot is entirely correctable and shoe-able without any need for special orthotics.

Calcaneovalgus

This is another deformity supposed to be related only to intrauterine crowding and positioning. In this deformity, the top of the foot lies up against the lower part of the tibia (Figure 6.15). It is more common in babies in the breech position and as such, hip surveillance is also indicated. In most cases, this is a positional deformity and will resolve in the first few months of life. On first examination, the foot should be able to be brought gently into a fully corrected position with neither residual hindfoot nor midfoot deformity. Mothers and fathers can be instructed to perform gentle massage. Occasionally, a plaster cast or two will help correction on its way. This condition should be differentiated from the much more rare and more challenging congenital vertical talus (CVT).

Congenital vertical talus

The incidence of CVT is reported around 1:100,000 but is, in itself, more difficult to diagnose (Figure 6.16). It is sometimes called the 'Persian slipper foot' or 'rocker bottom foot'.

Sixty per cent of these cases will be associated with a neuromuscular abnormality that requires investigation and management. The sex distribution is more

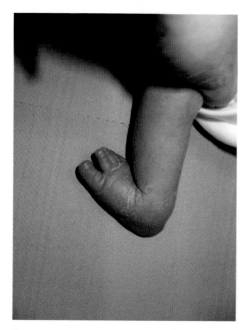

Figure 6.15 Calcaneovalgus.

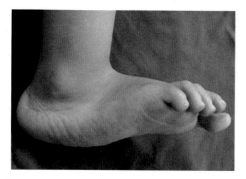

Figure 6.16 CVT in infants. From Ze-Xing Zhu MD, Wei-Lei MD, Yu-Lu Huang MD (2010). The short-term effect of an anchor in treatment of CVT in infants. *Orthopaedic Surgery* **2**(3), 218–222.

equal than in clubfoot. The shape of the foot is caused by tightness of both the hindfoot and midfoot tendons. The Achilles tendon pulls the hindfoot into equinus and the anterior structures, particularly the tibialis anterior tendon, pull the midfoot upwards (Duncan and Fixsen 1999). This gives the classic rocker bottom foot shape. Confirmation of the diagnosis is made by radiology and X-rays of the lateral view of the foot are taken in maximal plantar and dorsiflexion (Figure 6.17).

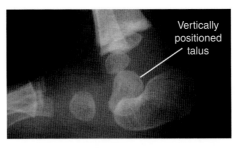

Figure 6.17 X-ray of CVT. From Ze-Xing Zhu MD, Wei-Lei MD, Yu-Lu Huang MD (2010). The short-term effect of an anchor in treatment of CVT in infants. *Orthopaedic Surgery* **2**(3), 218–222.

They show how the midfoot subluxes on the hindfoot. This foot shape is not correctible by manipulation and will require treatment in a specialist unit. The underlying cause is not known but any underlying neuromuscular condition will need to be similarly managed.

The role of manipulation and casting in CVT is less obvious and long-term outcomes as yet unknown (Dobbs et al. 2006b). While it is reasonable to try casting in the first instance, many more patients with CVT will come to more invasive surgery.

Polydactyly

Extra digits vary in anatomy from simple 'nubbins' that can easily be removed with minimal scarring, through partial to full duplications of toes in a variety of locations. Most commonly, they are seen on the lateral border of the foot (post-axial). An example of a 'nubbin' on the newborn hand can be seen in Figure 6.18.

Small accessory digits not involving any osseous component are often treated in the community by tying a length of cotton around the base to occlude the

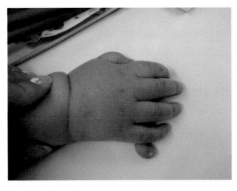

Figure 6.18 Example of nubbin (hand).

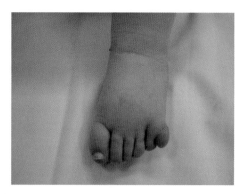

Figure 6.19 Polydactyly.

blood supply, thus allowing the nubbin to infarct and fall off. Some reach surgeons and are removed in theatre with a simple day case procedure.

More complex polysyndactyly involving duplication of bony and soft tissue elements will need greater assessment. The ossification of the bones of the foot is incomplete at birth and so radiological assessment tends to be undertaken nearer the time of planned surgery – usually at around 9–12 months (Figure 6.19).

The surgical goal is to make the foot of a size to fit easily available shoes with comfort and to allow good distribution of forces through the weight-bearing surface. Each case of polydactyly needs to be considered on an individual basis and will require assessment by an appropriate surgeon.

Syndactyly

This is a failure of separation of the toes, which may be full or partial. It is most commonly seen between the second and third toes where it is largely a cosmetic deformity rather than a functional one. The nails may also be fused. Separation is not usually recommended until a child is old enough to be involved in the surgical decision-making. Residual scarring from surgery often makes the decision to leave toe syndactyly alone an easy one (Figure 6.20a and b).

When seen in conjunction with polydactyly, surgical improvement is usually undertaken at around 9–12 months to allow comfortable ambulation and shoe wearing.

Absence or shortening of digits

The absence or shortening of toes presents in a variety of forms. Simple transverse loss at the level of the toe phalanges may be of little or no functional consideration. The effect of the cosmetic deformity on the family and, therefore, the child may be modified by the provision of careful support and advice. The cause tends to remain largely unknown although there may be evidence of amniotic bands. Some amniotic bands need surgical intervention. As the deletion moves

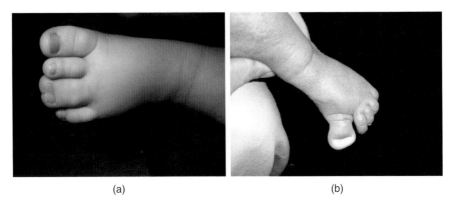

|(a)|(b)|

Figure 6.20 (a) Polysyndactyly of third and fourth toes. (b) Polysyndactyly of the great toe.

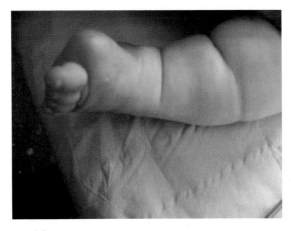

Figure 6.21 Absence of the great toe.

proximally along the foot, the functional capacity is reduced, increasing the need for prosthetics.

The loss of a full toe ray including the metatarsal decreases the functional capacity as the number of lost rays increases.

Both transverse and ray deletions should alert a practitioner to the possibility of other limb deformities that will need careful consideration and may make up part of a syndrome (Figure 6.21).

Conclusion

The diagnosis of DDH is a difficult and controversial subject. Further research is needed in order to establish the natural history of the condition and to assess the effectiveness of the treatments currently advocated. The natural history can only be ascertained by observing the natural history of sonographic abnormalities without splintage. True pathological DDH will then be identified accurately. The effectiveness of splintage as a treatment should be evaluated by a proper multi-centre control trial.

Foot deformities should be easy to diagnose in newborns without resorting to special testing, but may be associated with other abnormalities. Flexibility of the deformity on gentle manipulation will help to determine the type of treatment (if any) that will be required. Clubfoot is the most common foot deformity and is successfully treated by the Ponseti method. Other foot problems may require surgical intervention. Accurate diagnosis and early reliable information are the goals. The main aim of treatment is function and the ability to wear normal shoes.

Hyperextension of the knee – a case study

Maria was a 20-year-old woman (gravida 2 para 1). She had had a previous normal vaginal delivery of a baby girl at term 2 years ago, the baby was fine. Maria had no existing medical conditions and no history of congenital abnormalities on either side of the family.

A review of the antenatal history revealed that Maria had been admitted to hospital at 29, 32, 37+3, 38+2 weeks gestation all due to reduced fetal movements. She had a series of ultrasound scans that all appeared normal. However, due to the reduced fetal movements, she agreed to have an induction of labour at 38+3 weeks, she went on to have an uneventful vaginal delivery. Baby Michael was in good condition at birth (Apgars were 9 at 1 minute, 9 at 5 minutes).

Following delivery, staff became concerned about Michael's legs, as they were both hyperextended at the knee to an angle of around 45°. Michael was seen by the paediatric consultant who initially suspected arthrogryposis; however, after clinical examination, this was ruled out as he could flex the legs back to a neutral position easily. Moreover, there were no other limbs affected as is usually the case in arthrogryposis.

Ehlers–Danlos syndrome was also disregarded as it was thought that this would also affect other joints and the baby's digestive system.

The paediatrician then settled on the diagnosis of Congenital patellar syndrome (absence of knee cap); however, after X-ray and scan, no dislocation or absence of knee cap was seen.

Michael was eventually referred to the local children's hospital and a final diagnosis of uncomplicated hyperextension of the knee was made, which was caused by the position of the baby *in utero*. Michael was treated successfully by having splints fitted to both legs. This was followed by intense physiotherapy.

Think about how you would manage this problem within your Trust.
What information is available for mothers and fathers of these babies?

Look at these resources for more information on congenital knee abnormalities and examination of the hips:

Arthrogryposis http://emedicine.medscape.com/article/941917-overview
Arthrogryposis support group http://www.tagonline.org.uk/
Congenital Ehlers–Danlos syndrome http://emedicine.medscape.com/article/943567-clinical

Ehlers–Danlos support group http://www.ehlers-danlos.org/

Congenital patellar syndrome http://www.rjme.ro/RJME/resources/files/500209291293.pdf

Congenital dislocation of the knee (genu recurvatum) http://www.ncbi.nlm.nih.gov/pmc/articles/PMC3058203/

International Hip Dysplasia Institute http://hipdysplasia.org/for-physicians/pediatricians-and-primary-care-providers/infant-examination/

References

Alves C, Escalda C, Fernandes P, Tavares D, Neves MC (2009) Ponseti method. Does age at the beginning of treatment make a difference? *Clinical Orthopaedic Related Research* **467**, 1271–1277.

Andersson JE, Funnemark P (1995) Neonatal hip instability. Screening with anterior dynamic ultrasound method. *Journal Pediatric Orthopaedics* **15**, 322–324.

Bache CF, Clegg J, Herron M (2002) Risk factors for developmental dysplasia of the hip. Ultrasonographic findings in the neonatal period. *Journal Pediatric Orthopaedics* **11**, 212–218.

Barker S, Chesney D, Mieckybrodzka Z, Mafulli N (2003) Genetics and epidemiology of idiopathic congenital talipes equinovarus. *Journal of Pediatric Orthopedics* **23**, 265–272.

Barlow TG (1962) Early diagnosis and treatment of congenital dislocation of the hip. *Journal of Bone and Joint Surgery* **44-B**, 292–301.

Bialik V, Bialik GM, Blazer S, Sujou P, Wiener F, Berant M (1999) Developmental dysplasia of the hip. A new approach to incidence. *Paediatrics* **103**, 93–99.

Boehm S, Limpaphayom N, Alaee F, Sinclair MF, Dobbs MB (2008) Early results of the Ponseti method for the treatment of clubfoot in distal arthrogryposis. *Journal of Bone and Joint Surgery American Edition* **90**(7), 1501–1507.

Boeree NR, Clarke NMP (1994) Ultrasound imaging and secondary screening for congenital dislocation of the hip. *Journal of Bone and Joint Surgery* **76-B**, 525–533.

Castelein RM, Sauter AJM, De Vlieger M, Van Linge B (1992) Natural history of ultrasound hip abnormalities in clinically normal newborns. *Journal of Pediatric Orthopedics* **12**, 423–427.

Catford JC, Bennett GC, Wilkinson JA (1982) Congenital hip dislocation. An increasing and still uncontrolled disability. *British Medical Journal* **285**, 1527–1530.

Clarke NMP, Harcke HT, McHugh P, Lee MS, Borns PF, MacEwen GD (1985) Real time ultrasound in the diagnosis of congenital dislocation and dysplasia of the hip. *Journal of Bone and Joint Surgery* **67-B**, 406–412.

Clegg J, Bache CE, Raut VV (1999) Financial justification for routine ultrasound screening of the neonatal hip. *Journal of Bone and Joint Surgery* **81-B**, 852–857.

Cooper DM, Dietz FR (1995) Treatment of idiopathic clubfoot: a thirty year follow-up note. *Journal of Bone and Joint Surgery* **77**(10), 1477–1489.

Dietz FR, Tyler MC, Leary KS, Damiano PC (2009) Evaluation of a Disease-specific instrument for Idiopathic Clubfoot Outcome. *Clinical Orthopaedic Related Research* **467**, 1256–1262.

Dobbs MB, Nunley R, Schoenecker P (2006a) Long-term follow-up of patients with clubfeet treated with extensive soft tissue release. *Journal of Bone and Joint Surgery* **88A**(5), 986–996.

Dobbs MB, Purcell DB, Nunley R, Morcuende JA (2006b) Early results of a new method of treatment for idiopathic congenital vertical talus. *Journal of Bone and Joint Surgery* **88A**, 1192–1200.

Duncan RD, Fixsen JA (1999) Congenital convex pes valgus. *Journal of Bone and Joint Surgery British Edition* **81**(2), 250–254.

Engesaeter LB, Furnes O, Havelin LI (2008) Developmental dysplasia of the hip: good results of later total hip arthroplasty. 7,135 primary total hip replacements after developmental dysplasia of the hip compared with 59,774 total hip arthroplasties in idiopathic coxarthrosis followed 0–15 years. *The Norwegian Arthroplasty Register. Journal of Arthroplasty* **23**(2), 235–240.

Farsetti, P, De Maio F, Russolillo L, Ippolito E (2009) Evaluation of a disease -specific instrument for idiopathic clubfoot outcome. *Clinical Orthopoedic Related Research* **467**, 1243–1249.

Ganger G, Grill F, Leodolter S, Vitek M (1991) Ultrasound screening in the neonatal hip; results and experience. *Ultraschall in der Medizin* **12**, 25–30, in German.

Gardiner HM, Dunn PM (1991) Screening for congenital dislocation of the hip. *Lancet* **337**(8749), 1096–1097.

Gerlach DJ, Gurnett CA, Limpaphayom N, Alaee F, Zhang Z, Porter K, Kirchhofer M, Smyth MD, Dobbs MB (2009) Early results of the Ponseti method for the treatment of clubfoot associated with myelomeningocele. *Journal of Bone and Joint Surgery American Edition* **91**(6), 1350–1359.

Graf R (1987) The ultrasound examination of the hip. In: D Tonnis (ed) *Congenital Dysplasia and Dislocation of the Hip in Children and Adults*. Berlin: Springer Verlag, pp. 172–229.

Graf R (2007) Hip sonography: 20 years experience and results. *Hip International* **17**, 8–14.

Graf R, Scott S, Farkas P, Lercher K, Tschauner C, Benaroya A (1999) *Manual for Hip Sonography*. Stolzalpe, Austria: Edition Stolzalpe.

Hadlow V (1988) Neonatal screening for congenital dislocation of the hip. A prospective 21-year survey. *Journal of Bone and Joint Surgery* **70-B**, 740–743.

Harcke HT, Grissom LE (1986) Sonographic evaluation of the infant hip. *Seminars – Ultrasound CT MR* **7**, 3312–3338.

Herring JA (1992) Conservative treatment of congenital dislocation of the hip in the new born and infant. *Clinical Orthopaedics* **281**, 41–47.

Herzenberg JE, Radler C, Bor N (2002) Ponseti versus traditional methods of casting for idiopathic clubfoot. *Journal of Pediatric Orthopedics* **22**, 517–521.

Holen KJ, Tegnander A, Bredland T (2002) Universal or selective screening of neonatal hips using ultrasound? A prospective randomised trial of 15,529 newborn infants. *Journal of Bone and Joint Surgery* **843**, 886–890.

Ippolito E, Farsetti P, Caterini R, Tudisco C (2003) CT study on the effect of different treatment protocols for clubfoot pathology. *Journal of Bone and Joint Surgery American Edition* **85**(7), 1286–1294.

Jari S, Paton RW, Srinivasan MS (2002) Unilateral limitation of abduction to the hip. A valuable clinical sign for DDH? *Journal of Bone and Joint Surgery* **84-B**, 104–107.

Jones D (1998) Neonatal detection of developmental dysplasia of the hip CDH. *Journal of Bone and Joint Surgery* **80-B**, 943–945.

Jones D, Dezateux CA, Danielsson LG, Paton RW, Clegg J (2000) Topic for debate: at the cross-roads – neonatal detection of developmental dysplasia of the hip. *Journal of Bone and Joint Surgery* **82-B**, 160–164.

Klisic PJ (1989) Congenital dislocation of the hip: a misleading term. Brief report. *Journal of Bone and Joint Surgery* **71-B**, 136.

Laaveg SJ, Ponseti IV (1980) Long-term results of treatment of congenital clubfoot. *Journal of Bone and Joint Surgery American Edition* **62**(1), 23–31.

Lehmann HP, Hinton R, Morello P, Santoli J (2000) Developmental dysplasia of the hip. Practice guidelines. Technical report. *Paediatrics* **105**(4), E57.

Lerman JA, Emans JB, Millis MB (2001) Early failure of Pavlik harness treatment for developmental hip dysplasia; Clinical and ultrasound predictors. *Journal of Pediatric Orthopedics* **21**(3), 348–353.

Lloyd-Roberts GC (1955) Osteoarthritis of the hip. A study of the clinical pathology. *Journal of Bone and Joint Surgery* **37B**, 8–47.

Macnicol MF (1990) Results of a 25-year screening programme for neonatal hip instability. *Journal of Bone and Joint Surgery* **72-B**, 1057–1060.

Marks DS, Clegg J, al-Chalabi AN (1994) Routine ultrasound screening for neonatal hip insta-bility. *Journal of Bone and Joint Surgery* **76-B**, 534–538.

McEvoy A, Paton RW (1997) Ultrasound compared with radiographic assessment in develop-mental dysplasia of the hip. *Journal of the Royal College of Surgeons of Edinburgh* **42**(4), 254–255.

Milbrandt TA, Sucato DJ (2004) In: MD Miller (ed) *Review of Orthopaedics*, 4th edn. Philadelphia, PA: Saunders, pp. 182–186.

PALS (2003) PALS Parent Surveys Manchester Ponseti Clinic 2003 & 2009. Available from: http://www.hampshirepartnership.nhs.uk/patients/pals-complaints/nps-2009 (accessed 13 January 2011).

Patel H (2001) Preventative health care 2001 update. Screening and management of devel-opmental dysplasia of the hip in newborns. *Canadian Medical Association Journal* **164**(12), 1667–1677.

Paton RW (2005) Management of neonatal hip instability and dysplasia. *Early Human Develop-ment* **81**, 807–813.

Paton RW, Choudry Q (2009) Neonatal foot deformities and their relationship to developmental dysplasia of the hip: an 11-year prospective, longitudinal observational study. *Journal of Bone and Joint Surgery* **91-B**, 655–658.

Paton RW, Hopgood PJ, Eccles K (2004) Instability of the neonatal hip: the role of early or late splintage. *International Orthopaedics* **28**(5), 270–273.

Paton RW, Hinduja K, Thomas CD (2005) The significance of at risk factors in ultrasound surveil-lance of developmental dysplasia of the hip: a ten-year prospective trial. *Journal of Bone and Joint Surgery* **87-B**, 1264–1266.

Paton RW, Srinivasan MS, Shah B, Hollis S (1999) Ultrasound screening for hips at risk in developmental dysplasia. Is it worth it? *Journal of Bone and Joint Surgery* **81-B**, 255–258.

Ponseti IV, Becker JR (1966) Congenital metatarsus adductus: the results of treatment. *Journal of Bone Joint Surgery American Edition* **43**(4), 702–711.

Ponseti IV, Smoley EN (1963) Congenital clubfoot: the results of treatment. *Journal of Bone and Joint Surgery* **45A**(2), 2261–2270.

Ponseti IV, Zhivkov M, Davis N, Sinclair M, Dobbs MB, Morcuende JA (2006) Treatment of the complex idiopathic clubfoot. *Clinical Orthopedic Related Research* **451**, 171–176.

Robinson R (1998) Effective screening in child health. *British Medical Journal* **316**, 1–2.

Rosendahl K, Markestad T, Lie RT (1994) Ultrasound screening for developmental dysplasia of the hip in the neonate: the effect on treatment rate and prevalence of late cases. *Paediatrics* **94**, 47–52.

Sampath JS, Deakin S, Paton RW (2003) Splintage in developmental dysplasia of the hip: how low can we go? *Journal of Pediatric Orthopaedics* **23**(3), 352–355.

Shipman S, Helfand M, Moyer VA, Yawn BP (2006) Screening for developmental dysplasia of the hip. A systematic literature review for US preventative services taskforce. *Paediatrics* **117**, 557–576.

SMAC (1986) *Screening for the Detection of Congenital Dislocation of the Hip*. London: Department of Health and Social Security.

Suzuki S (1993). Ultrasound and the Pavlik harness in CDH. *Journal of Bone and Joint Surgery* **75-B**, 483–487.

Suzuki S, Kashiwagi N, Kasahara Y, Seto Y, Futami T (1996) Avascular necrosis and the Pavlik harness: the incidence of avascular necrosis in three type of congenital dislocation of the hip as classified by ultrasound. *Journal of Bone and Joint Surgery* **78-B**, 631–635.

Terjesen T, Bredland T, Berg V (1989) Ultrasound for hip assessment in the newborn. *Journal of Bone and Joint Surgery* **71-B**, 767–773.

Toma P, Valle M, Rossi U, Bruneughi GM (2001) Paediatric hip: ultrasound screening for devel-opmental dysplasia of the hip: a review. *European Journal of Ultrasound* **14**, 44–45.

Tönnis D (1987) *Congenital Dysplasia and Dislocation of the Hip in Children and Adults.* Berlin: Springer Verlag, pp. 59–70.

Wilkinson AG, Sherlock DA, Murray GD (2002) The efficacy of the Pavlik harness, the Craig splint and the Von Rosen splint in the management of neonatal dysplasia of the hip. A comparative study. *Journal of Bone and Joint Surgery* **84-B**, 716–719.

Wirth T, Stratman L, Hinrichs F (2005) Evolution of late presenting developmental dysplasia of the hip and associated surgical procedures after 14 years of neonatal ultrasound screening (letter). *Journal of Bone and Joint Surgery* **87-B**, 135–136.

Wood MK, Conboy V, Benson MKD (2000) Does early treatment by abduction splintage improve the development of dysplastic, but stable neonatal hip joints. *Journal of Pediatric Orthopaedics* **20**, 302–305.

Wynne Davies R (1972) Genetic and environmental factors in the aetiology of talipes equino-varus. *Clinical Orthopaedics and Related Research* **84**, 9–13.

Zieger M, Hilpert S, Schulz RD (1986) Ultrasound of the infant hip Part 1, Basic principles. *Paediatric Radiology* **16**, 483–487.

CHAPTER 7

Chromosomal and genetic problems: giving feedback to mothers and fathers

Delyth Webb[1] and Anne Lomax[2]

[1] Warrington Hospital, Warrington, Cheshire, UK
[2] University of Central Lancashire, Preston, UK

KEY POINTS

- Genetic and chromosomal anomalies are individually rare but collectively are commonly encountered at the neonatal examination.

- It is important to have an understanding of the terminology used in genetics in order to interpret both screening results and the level of risk in particular cases.

- An isolated abnormal feature found at the neonatal examination may not be clinically significant but multiple dysmorphic features are highly significant.

- The practitioner should develop an approach to the examination of a newborn in the instance of suspected or definite genetic or chromosomal anomalies.

- History taking prior to conducting the neonatal examination remains implicit to the newborn screening process.

Background

The vast majority of babies examined for their newborn check will be completely healthy. However, on occasion, there may be concerns about a baby from the family history, antenatal screening results or the appearance or behaviour of the baby once born. This chapter aims to help you assess these babies and give initial support and advice to the family. This chapter also discusses some of the basic terminology used in clinical genetics and some of the commoner genetic and chromosomal problems encountered. There are many genetic disorders, and no

---

Examination of the Newborn: An Evidence-Based Guide, Second Edition. Edited by Anne Lomax.
© 2015 John Wiley & Sons, Ltd. Published 2015 by John Wiley & Sons, Ltd.
Companion Website: www.wiley.com/go/lomax/newborn

one performing a newborn check can be expected to know about all of them, but you should develop a strategy for dealing with these situations in an appropriate way.

Useful genetic terminology

Nucleotides: The most basic 'building blocks' of DNA – they are 'read' in groups of three, always in the same direction.

Gene: A row of nucleotides on a chromosome which encodes for a specific piece of RNA – this RNA may be used to produce a protein or to send a message within the cell. Different genes are 'switched' on and off according to their function as the embryo and fetus develops and throughout life.

Chromosome: A collection of DNA – each person should have 22 pairs of autosomes numbered from largest (chromosome 1) to smallest (chromosome 22) and two sex chromosomes (XX or XY). Each chromosome has a short 'p' end and a long 'q' end.

Mutation: A significant change in a gene from the general population. There are several types of mutation – such as a point mutation (a change in one nucleotide, which may be a deletion or substitution) or an inversion or translocation of a larger area of the chromosome. Over recent years, specific genetic mutations have been found for many disorders allowing accurate diagnosis and enabling screening of relatives.

Point mutation: One single nucleotide is changed. This will change the RNA produced and, for example, may change the shape of a protein produced from that RNA so it does not work normally.

Deletion: A part of a chromosome is missing, for example, 5p – causing the loss of a group of genes.

Chromosomal translocation: A chunk of one chromosome is displaced onto another chromosome. This may be 'balanced', that is, does not affect the overall function of any genes or 'unbalanced' in which case some genes are duplicated or missing. Mothers and fathers with balanced translocations are at increased risk of having a child with an unbalanced translocation.

Uniparental disomy: The baby has inherited both sets of one autosome from either mother or father.

Trisomy: The baby has an extra copy of one of the chromosomes. Most trisomies will not develop past the early embryonic stage but some are survivable – the commonest being trisomy 21 (Down's syndrome).

Sex chromosome disorders: The best known of these is Turner syndrome (X0), but extra X or Y chromosomes may occur (XYY, XXX, XXY).

Mosaicism: There is a mixture of more than one cell line. This means that some cells have abnormal chromosomes and others do not. This happens most often in Turner syndrome and can be written as 46XX/45XO.

Modes of inheritance

Autosomal recessive: These disorders only affect the child if they have inherited a mutation in the same gene from both mother and father. Both mother and father will be healthy carriers of the condition. There is 1 in 4 chance for each of their children being affected. Autosomal recessive disorders are common if there are a lot of carriers in the population or if the mother and father are closely related. Most autosomal recessive disorders are severe in that the child would not survive to adulthood without medical support.

Autosomal dominant: In these disorders, a mutation in one autosome causes the condition. These are inherited from an affected mother or father (who has 1 in 2 chance of passing on the condition) or may be a new mutation. These conditions are generally less severe than autosomal recessive disorders.

X linked: These disorders are carried on the X chromosome. Most of these disorders are X-linked recessive, that is, a female baby with the mutation would be a healthy carrier protected by her other normal X chromosome, whereas a male baby with the mutation would be affected, for example, Haemophilia A, Duchenne muscular dystrophy. X-linked dominant conditions also affect female babies – in some of these conditions, male embryos will not survive the early stages of pregnancy.

Fluorescent in situ hybridisation (FISH) test: This is a method of rapid testing for a specific suspected genetic or chromosomal disorder. A gene probe with a fluorescent marker is prepared. This will attach to the area under investigation. Probes for commoner disorders will be available in your local molecular genetics laboratory – rarer disorders will need specialised analysis.

Antenatal screening

Several levels of antenatal screening are now available to expectant mothers and fathers and they should be offered from the first antenatal appointment onwards (see Chapter 1). It is the mother's and father's choice whether or not they take up all or any of the screening offered – they may have personal or religious reasons to reject it. Women who present later in pregnancy may have missed the 'windows' for some screening tests.

Antenatal ultrasound

The 'Booking' scan

The initial ultrasound scan at 11–14 weeks was used until recently mainly to confirm a viable pregnancy and the number of fetuses. Only the most major of structural defects (such as anencephaly) would be visible on the scan. More recently, it has been found that a measurement of nuchal fold thickness (the tissue at the back of the neck) can help identify fetuses with Down's syndrome. This test is not yet universally available and does have limited accuracy.

18–22-week 'anomaly' scan

This scan is designed to pick up structural problems particularly with the heart, brain, bowel and kidneys. Recently, obstetricians have identified 'soft markers' which may be associated with chromosomal disorders, particularly trisomy 21. These include nuchal oedema, multiple choroid plexus cysts, echogenic bowel, ventriculomegaly and renal pelvic dilatation. On finding soft markers, the obstetrician may offer amniocentesis. It must be noted that soft markers are non-specific and are often seen in healthy fetuses. Single choroid plexus cysts are now thought to be a normal variant and may not be reported. The Royal College of Obstetricians and Gynaecologists (RCOG) guidelines quote a Down's syndrome detection rate of 40% for the anomaly scan alone (Royal College Obstetrics and Gynaecologists 2005).

Hormonal screening

This is a test performed on the mother at a known specific gestation assessing hormonal levels in her blood. These may include human chorionic gonadotropin (HCG) and pregnancy-associated plasma protein A in the first trimester, or a combination of alpha-fetoprotein (AFP) and HCG with or without estriol and inhibin A in the second trimester.

Using the hormonal levels, the maternal age, nuchal translucency (if available) and exact gestation, the risk that the fetus has Down's syndrome is calculated. It must be remembered that this test cannot confirm or exclude Down's syndrome – it should be used to guide amniocentesis. This can understandably difficult for a mother to accept if she delivers a baby with Down's syndrome following a reassuring result. In future, there are plans to offer more women nuchal fold testing – combining these tests should improve accuracy but will still not be perfect – the best detection rate will be 70–80% using current techniques.

Antenatal screening for sickle cell and thalassaemia

This screening is now offered in the United Kingdom from the booking appointment. The mother is first tested for carrier status, and if she is positive, the father is screened to see whether he is also a carrier. Carrier status for either of these conditions is usually asymptomatic but may cause mild anaemia. People with sickle cell trait may haemolyse when hypoxic – it is, therefore, important for their anaesthetist to be aware of the condition.

Specific genetic testing: screening of mothers and fathers

Mothers and fathers from families with a high incidence of a particular genetic condition may be offered specific targeted screening for carrier status. This may be offered, for example, if a mother or father's sibling has a recessive condition such as cystic fibrosis. This area is very specialised and a clinical geneticist should be involved at all stages to counsel the mother and father appropriately. If either or neither the mother nor father is a carrier of the condition tested, they can be reassured that the baby is very unlikely to be affected. If both are carriers, early genetic testing of the embryo or fetus can be offered, or in certain cases, *in vitro* fertilization (IVF) with preimplantation diagnosis.

As there are many specific genetic disorders, screening for a specific disorder can only be performed if there is a family history of that disorder, that is, there is no screening test that can exclude all genetic disorders.

Testing of the fetus

There are currently two methods of obtaining fetal DNA – both are invasive.

Chorionic villus sampling

A small sample of placental tissue is obtained by ultrasound guidance either transabdominally or transcervically.

This can be performed from 10 completed weeks of pregnancy for suspected genetic or chromosomal disorders. There is a 3% risk of miscarriage. For example, it may be offered to a mother who has had a previous child with a trisomy or autosomal recessive disorder or if a major anomaly is suspected on the booking scan.

Amniocentesis

A small volume of amniotic fluid is obtained under ultrasound guidance. Fetal cells are extracted and analysed. This test is safer for the fetus than chorionic villus sampling with a 0.5–1% miscarriage risk. It may be offered from 14 weeks' gestation in high-risk women.

Postnatal screening via the newborn blood spot test

Neonatal blood spot screening is carried out at around a week of age. Obviously, this is later than the newborn check, but it is useful to be aware of the conditions tested for in your area of the country. The decision to implement screening is based on early detection of conditions which benefit from treatment prior to the onset of symptoms and are common enough for screening to be economically viable.

The current national screening programme includes testing for hypothyroidism, phenylketonuria, cystic fibrosis, medium-chain acyl-CoA dehydrogenase deficiency (MCADD) and sickle cell anaemia. In some areas, screening for Duchenne muscular dystrophy also occurs (UK NSC 2008).

Congenital hypothyroidism: This is not strictly a genetic disorder, although there may be increased risk with a family history. There is an incidence of about 1 in 4000. Newborns with hypothyroidism may be asymptomatic, although sometimes they present with hypoglycaemia or prolonged jaundice. Untreated hypothyroidism leads to developmental delay and short stature. Treated individuals usually grow and develop within the normal range. Screen-positive individuals are referred to a paediatric consultant.

Phenylketonuria: This is an autosomal recessive disorder with an incidence of 1 in 10–15,000. There is a deficiency of the enzyme phenylalanine hydroxylase, which breaks down the amino acid phenylalanine found in various foods including formula and breast milk. There are no symptoms in the newborn. Untreated individuals suffer from mental retardation, and children of mothers with phenylketonuria, which is poorly controlled in pregnancy, will have poor *in utero* brain development. The treatment is a lifelong specialised diet. Positive screening tests will be passed straight on to a paediatric metabolic consultant.

Cystic fibrosis: This is also an autosomal recessive disorder with an incidence of about 1 in 2000. It causes malabsorption of fats (leading to diarrhoea and failure to thrive) and progressive lung disease. Screening for cystic fibrosis has been implemented recently, using a pancreatic enzyme immunoreactive trypsinogen (IRT). If levels are elevated, the blood spot is screened for the common gene mutations. Suspected cases are notified to the local paediatrician, who will see the mother and father and arrange a confirmatory sweat test at 4 weeks of age. Although cystic fibrosis is not curable, there is a significant benefit in life expectancy if treatment with antibiotics and pancreatic enzymes is started before the onset of symptoms. Mothers and fathers should be aware that some screening results may come back initially positive when their child does not have the condition (Simms et al. 2005).

Sickle cell disease: This is caused by mutations in the genes producing haemoglobin. These mutations are relatively common in people of African or Indian ancestry as carriers are relatively protected from malaria. People with sickle cell disease develop anaemia due to rapid red cell breakdown and blockage of small blood vessels particularly within the spleen. This leads to increased risk of bacterial infections. If sickle cell disease is detected in the newborn, the baby will be referred to a haematologist who will monitor anaemia and treat with regular antibiotics. Population screening for sickle cell disease by blood spot analysis has recently been introduced in parts of the United Kingdom (UK NSC 2008).

MCADD: This is an autosomal recessive metabolic disorder that causes difficulty in processing stored fats into energy. The incidence is about 1 in 12,000. It presents with life-threatening hypoglycaemia after prolonged fast or illness. If diagnosed, it can be managed by giving regular feeds and monitoring blood sugars. The NHS has introduced blood spot screening for acylcarnitine, which will pick up MCADD and several other rarer metabolic disorders. Abnormal screening results are reported to a metabolic consultant, who will arrange further investigation (UK NSC 2008).

Duchenne muscular dystrophy: This is an X-linked recessive disorder leading to progressive muscular weakness. Affected boys may present with delay in walking. Diagnosis may not occur until the child is 2 or 3 years old. There is no treatment that significantly prolongs life. Postnatal blood spot screening measuring levels of creatinine kinase is possible. This has been available in Wales and other selected areas of the world (Parsons et al. 2003) but is not currently recommended by the UK National Screening Committee. The rationale for early detection would be to inform future pregnancies rather than to treat the affected child and is ethically controversial (Kemper et al. 2005).

The rationale for early detection would be to inform future pregnancies rather than to treat the affected child and is ethically controversial (Kemper et al. 2005).

Ways in which actual or suspected genetic or chromosomal anomalies may present on the newborn check

Several different circumstances may lead the examiner to suspect a genetic or chromosomal disorder:
- Concerns from antenatal screening tests
- Family history
- Appearance of the baby – 'dysmorphic features'
- Poor feeding and/or low tone on examination
- Small for dates/small head circumference

Problems detected on antenatal screening

A definite or possible chromosomal or genetic disorder may be identified from the triple test or from the anomaly ultrasound scan performed around 20 weeks' gestation. This may lead to significant anxiety on the part of the mother and father around the newborn examination. It is important to find out the results of the triple test and antenatal ultrasound scan from the maternal notes prior to examining the baby and to determine whether chorionic villus sampling or an amniocentesis has been performed. Ask the mother and father if there is anything they are still worried about from the screening tests. For example, they may have been told about 'soft markers' on the antenatal ultrasound or given a borderline high triple test result leading to concerns about Down's syndrome.

In many cases, reassurance can be given, once the examination has been completed. If, unsure, ask an experienced paediatrician to see the baby prior to discharge home.

Family history of genetic disorders

Some families will have a history of a common or rare genetic disorder. They may ask about this on the newborn check for the first time. In many cases, the risk of their baby being affected is low, even if they have had a previous child with a chromosomal disorder.

Many disorders are not detectable on the newborn examination – if you are asked about a disorder that you are not familiar with, ask for advice. Look up the condition on the 'Contact a Family' website (for useful websites, see Appendix 1), which will not only give you more information about the condition's genetics and clinical features but will also lead you to an appropriate support group.

It is useful to obtain a basic family tree initially as this will help determine whether the baby is at risk. Mothers and fathers who have previously had an affected child with an inherited disorder are at much higher risk than those whose sibling or cousin has had an affected child, unless the family is interrelated. In most conditions, screening of an apparently well child should only be carried out by a clinical geneticist following counselling of the family; this issue would need to be discussed with the paediatrician responsible for the baby. The exceptions would be those conditions now covered in the routine screening tests as mentioned previously.

Problems visible at birth or on first-day check: dealing with dysmorphic baby

At times, you may be asked to examine a baby about whose appearance the midwife or mother and father have concerns. Alternatively, unusual facial features or other minor anomalies may be noted during a routine newborn check.

As with all babies seen on the first-day check, assess the baby's level of activity and muscle tone (newborn behavioural aspects are also discussed in Chapter 8). Ask or observe how the baby is feeding and whether the baby is vomiting. Also ask mother if she had any specific concerns about the baby during pregnancy or since birth.

Measure the baby's head circumference and plot it on a growth chart. Symmetrical growth retardation is associated with chromosomal disorders (although most small babies are healthy) (see also Chapter 3).

If you see one unusual feature on examination, for example, a single palmar crease (Figure 7.1), is this isolated or are there other unusual findings? Many healthy babies will have an isolated abnormality; the more there are, the more likely there is an underlying condition.

If there are concerns about the baby's facial features, look at the rest of the baby. Is anything else unusual? Does the baby look like his mother or father?

If in doubt, ask an experienced person to assess the baby as well (without forgetting to obtain consent from the mother and father first). You will develop your own communication style over time – it is important to try and tailor this

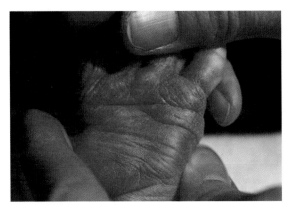

Figure 7.1 Simian crease. (Reproduced with kind permission of Dr David Clark.)

to the mother and father's needs, trying to avoid unnecessary anxiety but not falsely reassuring them.

Studies of mothers and fathers of children with Down's syndrome show that they prefer to hear the news together without other relatives in the room, from a person who will be caring for their child in the future and who has a positive attitude towards the condition. However, they do not appreciate being 'kept in the dark' (Skotko 2005). It is likely that the same circumstances would apply whatever the disorder. Communicating with the mother and father in cases of congenital abnormalities is discussed more fully later on in this chapter.

It is reasonable for you when examining a baby who you suspect of having any genetic disorder, to explain that you would like a more senior member of staff to check over the baby without being more specific. Try to make sure the second check is done in a timely manner and that ideally the second person is senior enough to discuss the condition further with the mother and father. With a confirmed diagnosis, mothers and fathers appreciate written information about the condition and contact details for other mothers and fathers of children with the condition. Support groups are available now even for very rare conditions – you may find these via the 'Contact a Family' database (details can be found in Appendix 1). Many of these support groups also provide information for professionals caring for affected children.

Commoner specific genetic and chromosomal disorders

Trisomy 21 (Down's syndrome)

Trisomy 21 is the most common chromosomal disorder occurring in about 1 in 800–1000 births. Attitudes towards the care of babies and children with trisomy 21 have changed hugely in the last few decades; the emphasis is now on early detection and treatment of any associated medical disorders in order to optimise the child's potential and quality of life.

In view of this change in attitudes, an increasing number of women are opting out of antenatal screening or choosing to continue with their pregnancy with a suspected or confirmed diagnosis of Down's syndrome.

In most cases, babies with suspected or confirmed Down's syndrome can stay on the ward with their mother. There is no contraindication to breastfeeding, although extra support may be needed, and associated medical conditions should be anticipated.

A suspected or confirmed diagnosis of Down's syndrome is still very distressing for most families and each family will have different attitudes and emotional responses to the diagnosis. Early involvement of the paediatric consultant who will provide ongoing support to the child and family is ideal.

Causes of Down's syndrome

The most common cause of Down's syndrome is non-disjunction – that is, an extra copy of chromosome 21 is present in the ovum (or sperm) at the time of fertilisation. The risk of this happening increases with maternal age although most babies with Down's syndrome are born to young women. A small proportion of Down's syndrome is due to translocation – this is usually inherited with one parent having a balanced translocation so there is a much greater risk of recurrence with future pregnancies or within the family.

Clinical features

Many of the clinical features seen in Down's syndrome can be found in healthy babies. However, the greater the number of these features seen, the more likely that the baby has Down's syndrome. In the United Kingdom, about two-thirds of babies who reach the threshold for blood testing for Down's syndrome actually have the condition (Hindley and Medakkar 2002).

Muscle tone: Almost all babies with Down's syndrome have low muscle tone on examination. This is rarely severe enough to affect feeding significantly, so if the baby is not feeding well, suspect other associated problems.

Skin: The skin often feels soft and doughy with a mottled appearance known as cutis marmorata, which means marbled skin (see also Chapter 3).

Facial features: The bridge of the nose is usually flat, with skin folds at the inner corner of the eyes (epicanthic folds). The irises may have pale flecks within them known as Brushfield spots. The baby's mouth is relatively small compared to the tongue, causing the tongue to protrude (Figure 7.2). When the baby grimaces or cries, vertical creases may be seen in the mouth and eyes (these are relatively specific to Down's syndrome).

Head shape: The head circumference is often on a lower centile than the weight. The occiput may be flat and continuous with the neck (brachycephaly). There is often excess skin at the back of the neck.

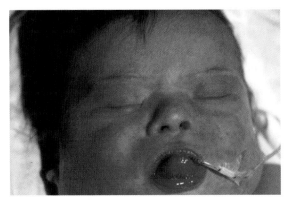

Figure 7.2 Down's syndrome. (Reproduced with kind permission of Dr David Clark.)

Hands and feet: One of the best-known features of Down's syndrome is the single palmar crease (Simian crease) (Figure 7.1). This is present in 5% of the normal population so is not discriminatory unless seen with other features. The hand is often broad and short, and there may be incurving of the little finger (clinodactyly). The feet may also have a single plantar crease and a large gap between the first and second toes (sandal gap).

Medical problems seen in Down's syndrome

Babies with Down's syndrome may have a combination of medical problems or none at all. This is not predictable by the appearance of the baby – so a high index of suspicion is needed until each problem can be ruled out.

Cardiac

The most common cardiac defects in Down's syndrome are septal defects – atrial, ventricular or atrioventricular. These rarely cause any problems in the first few weeks of life, but are more likely to require surgery in the first year of life than in children without Down's syndrome due to the risk of high pulmonary arterial blood pressure.

Other problems such as Fallot's syndrome, pulmonary atresia can occur – these cause cyanotic heart disease presenting with severe cyanosis when the duct closes – pulse oximetry and ideally an echocardiogram should be performed prior to discharge if Down's syndrome is strongly suspected. Assessment of the cardiovascular system and common cardiac abnormalities are discussed more fully in Chapter 2.

Gastrointestinal

The common structural gastrointestinal abnormalities are duodenal atresia and Hirschsprung's disease. About 1 in 10 babies with Down's syndrome will have one of these problems.

Duodenal atresia is a blockage of the second part of the duodenum. Babies with this problem will be poor feeders and will develop vomiting (which may be bile stained) in the first 48 hours of life. As the blockage is high in the gut, the baby may pass meconium normally.

Hirschsprung's disease is a lack of sympathetic nerve cells at the distal end of the bowel, making it unable to relax normally. Babies with Hirschsprung's disease usually have delay in passing meconium but may initially feed normally.

Therefore, when looking after a newborn with trisomy 21, it is essential to ensure that they are feeding normally without vomiting and have passed meconium. If this is not the case, a plain x-ray will exclude duodenal atresia and may show dilated bowel loops in Hirschsprung's disease.

Hearing

Children with Down's syndrome are at increased risk of both sensorineural and conductive hearing loss. Sensorineural hearing loss can be identified on the initial hearing screen, but conductive hearing loss develops over time due to 'glue ear'. Newborns with Down's syndrome should be referred to the audiologist for ongoing screening.

Development

Almost all babies with Down's syndrome will have low muscle tone. Therefore, there is usually a delay in reaching motor milestones (sitting, walking) but they will be achieved in time. Physiotherapy assessment may be helpful for some babies.

Speech delay is often an issue – this is often more of a delay in expressive speech than understanding. Early speech therapy support and teaching of simple sign language such as Makaton can help support development of a preschool child with Down's syndrome, whether or not there are any hearing problems.

Children with Down's syndrome usually fall in the category of mild-to-moderate learning difficulty. A proportion of children with Down's syndrome now attend mainstream school.

Other medical issues

There is an increased risk of congenital cataract in Down's syndrome – if any concerns about the red reflex, ask for ophthalmological review (see also Chapter 4).

There is also an increased risk of congenital hypothyroidism, but this will be detected by the routine blood spot screening at 6 days.

Confirming trisomy 21

Trisomy 21 can be confirmed by genetic analysis of blood. Many genetic laboratories offer rapid analysis via a FISH test (which has a probe for chromosome

21 and has been mentioned earlier in this chapter) within 72 hours. This allows mother and father the option of staying in hospital if they wish to, until the diagnosis is confirmed or excluded.

Checking the baby with antenatally diagnosed Down's syndrome

Ideally, a baby with known Down's syndrome should be checked by a consultant paediatrician as the mother and father will often have many questions and ongoing follow-up will be planned. When performing the initial check, be aware of the potential cardiac and gastrointestinal problems.

Actions prior to discharge home in suspected or known Down's syndrome

It is important to ensure that the baby is well prior to discharge home – a baby who is feeding well and passing meconium is unlikely to have duodenal atresia or Hirschsprung's disease.

The peripheral oxygen saturation should be checked even if it is not routine in your hospital. Ideally, an echocardiogram should be performed prior to discharge; if this is not possible, it should be arranged as an urgent outpatient investigation. The baby's mother and father should be informed of who to contact in an emergency if the baby becomes unwell in the first few weeks of life. There is a large UK support group, the Down's Syndrome Association, who produce excellent information for mothers and fathers and can offer other mother and fathers as a source of support (see Appendix 1).

Trisomy 13, 18

Trisomy 13, Patau syndrome, and Trisomy 18, Edward's syndrome, are rarer and more severe than Down's syndrome. Many of the babies die within the first week of life. In both conditions, there is severe microcephaly and abnormal hand and foot shape. Cardiac and gastrointestinal malformations are common. Severe hypotonia will be evident at delivery, and these babies will be admitted to the neonatal unit immediately after birth as they will appear unwell. Therefore, if antenatal scans, particularly of 'soft markers', have raised the possibility of either of these syndromes and the baby appears healthy and is feeding well, it does not have either of these syndromes.

Turner syndrome (XO)

Turner syndrome is the complete or partial absence of the second sex chromosome. It occurs in 1:2000 live female births, but causes up to 10% of miscarriage as 99% of Turner's pregnancies will spontaneously miscarry. Turner syndrome is sporadic – there is no increased risk in older women or with family history.

The main issues with Turner syndrome are later endocrine problems – short stature and ovarian failure – but structural cardiac and renal defects also occur. Most girls with Turner syndrome lead a full and productive life.

Antenatal diagnosis

Turner syndrome is associated with abnormal triple test results and is often picked up coincidentally on chorionic villus sampling (CVS) or amniocentesis. There is sometimes increased nuchal fold translucency or cystic hygroma picked up on early scans. There may be polyhydramnios, hydrops and/or renal anomalies visible on the anomaly scan.

Features visible on the newborn examination

Many girls with Turner syndrome appear healthy at birth. In some babies, there will be some typical clinical features – these are a short webbed neck with a low hairline, low set ears, lymphoedema of hands and feet and widely spaced nipples (Figures 7.3–7.5).

Postnatal management

Even in babies who have been diagnosed by amniocentesis or CVS, postnatal chromosomal analysis should be done as mosaicism is common. As with Down's syndrome, an initial FISH test can be done followed by more detailed analysis.

Screening for associated problems

Congenital heart disease occurs in about 30% of girls with Turner syndrome, most commonly coarctation of the aorta or bicuspid aortic valve, so an echocardiogram should be performed in the first week of life.

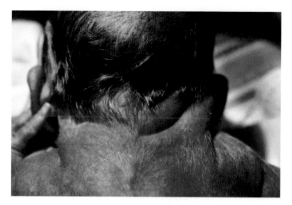

Figure 7.3 Webbing of the neck in Turner syndrome. (Reproduced with kind permission of Dr David Clark.)

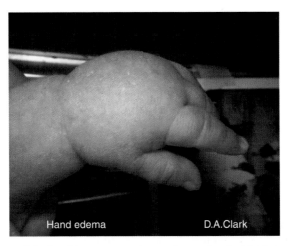

Figure 7.4 Oedema of the hand in Turner syndrome. (Reproduced with kind permission of Dr David Clark.)

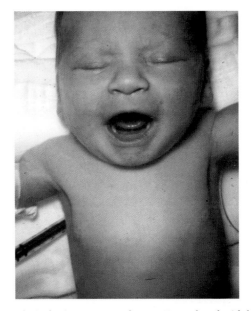

Figure 7.5 Widely spaced nipples in Turner syndrome. (Reproduced with kind permission of Dr David Clark.)

Hearing problems are common, both sensorineural and conductive, so a hearing screen should be performed.

Renal malformations such as horseshoe kidney are also common; these can be detected by postnatal ultrasound.

There is an increased risk of congenital dysplasia of the hip – the hip examination should be performed and the baby placed on the high-risk pathway.

Ongoing follow-up of hearing and growth throughout childhood should be arranged with the paediatrician (Saenger et al. 2001). Recommendations for follow-up are available from the Turner syndrome society website (see Appendix 1).

DiGeorge syndrome/velocardiofacial syndrome

Velocardiofacial syndrome is a group of disorders due to a deletion in the short arm of chromosome 22 (22q11.2). Some people with this chromosomal problem will be generally healthy, but have typical facial features that become more obvious in adulthood – a long face with a high broad nose and small chin. Some individuals will have Pierre Robin syndrome (posterior cleft palate and small chin). Others have DiGeorge syndrome, which is characterised by cardiac problems (most commonly aortic arch abnormalities and Tetralogy of Fallot), thymic deficiency and hypocalcaemia. This is the second common cause of congenital heart disease with an incidence of 1 in 1,800. Ninety per cent of DiGeorge is due to a new mutation, but the babies may have a mother or father with velocardiofacial syndrome. If there is a family history of velocardiofacial syndrome, there should be a low threshold for echocardiogram.

Prader–Willi syndrome

Prader–Willi syndrome is a condition in which there is a lack of the paternal copy of part of chromosome 15. This may be due to a deletion of this part of the chromosome or inheritance of only the maternal copies of chromosome 15. Babies with Prader–Willi syndrome exhibit low birth weight with hypotonia and a poor suck, usually needing tube feeding. Children with Prader–Willi usually have learning difficulties and develop obesity during childhood due to hypothalamic malfunction.

Gene disorders

Osteogenesis imperfecta

This term covers a group of inherited conditions of varying severity, the milder of which are autosomal dominant and the more severe being autosomal recessive. This condition is not usually detectable at birth but may be suspected from a family history or the detection of bowing of long bones on antenatal scan. If suspected, these babies need careful handling for clothing and nappy changes (avoid lifting by the chest or limbs) and should not have their hips examined on their newborn check. They require early support from a specialist physiotherapist and paediatric orthopaedic surgeon. Specific advice on initial care of these babies is available from the Brittle Bone Society (see Appendix 1).

Achondroplasia

Achondroplasia is the most common cause of short-limbed dwarfism. It is autosomal dominant, occurring in about 1 in 15,000 to 1 in 40,000 births. The affected gene has been identified on chromosome 4 and codes for fibroblast growth factor 3, which controls cartilage growth. Seventy-five per cent of children with achondroplasia are born with a new mutation, almost always the same point mutation. Mothers and fathers with achondroplasia have a 50% chance of having a child with achondroplasia if either mother or father is affected. If both mother and father are affected, they have a 25% chance of their child inheriting both genes, which causes a lethal form known as thanatophoric dysplasia.

The diagnosis may be suspected antenatally due to short limbs seen on ultrasound – this picks up one-third of cases but is non-specific for achondroplasia. Amniocentesis will confirm the diagnosis and may be used to exclude thanatophoric dysplasia (Trotter et al. 2005).

Features at birth

A newborn with achondroplasia will have a head circumference on a significantly higher centile than its weight. The newborn's forehead may be prominent. The proximal limbs will be short compared to the trunk and the digits short and wide.

Medical issues

People with achondroplasia have a normal intelligence and life expectancy. A proportion of infants and children with achondroplasia will develop hydrocephalus or spinal cord compression. An initial cranial ultrasound will exclude this at birth. The head growth should be monitored in childhood on the achondroplasia centile chart. There is also a risk of spinal cord compression. Motor milestones are delayed and physiotherapy support is useful to guide positioning in infancy to avoid problems with spinal development. Due to small airways, there is a higher risk of glue ear and asthma. It is likely that the main concern for a new mother or father will be their child's long-term growth and height. Average adult height is about 4 ft. Leg lengthening is available in adolescence but this decision should be agreed with the child. Support from other people with achondroplasia and their families is invaluable.

Epidermolysis bullosa

Epidermolysis bullosa (EB) is a group of genetic disorders affecting the structure of the skin. The commonest is epidermolysis bullosa simplex (EBS), which is usually autosomal dominant, with an incidence of about 50 per million. There are more severe forms of EBs and also junctional and dystrophic EBs, which are autosomal recessive. They all present with blistering on minimal trauma, which may be visible from birth. If suspected, dermatology assessment and referral to the national EB support nurses based at Great Ormond Street in London should be arranged. Trauma to the skin should be avoided and dry dressings may be helpful. Blisters should be popped with a sterile needle to halt progression. Further information is available from DebRA (see Appendix 1).

Inborn errors of metabolism (IEM)

These are a group of disorders in which the newborn is unable to convert food (milk) into usable energy. There is a mutation in one of the genes coding for a specific enzyme in a metabolic pathway. These disorders are usually autosomal recessive so are common in interrelated populations. Most infants with IEM will appear well at birth, with normal birth weight. Once feeding is introduced, they develop hypoglycaemia and acidosis due to toxic by-products of the blocked pathway. They may have signs similar to sepsis – sleepiness or irritability, vomiting and increased respiratory rate. A low blood sugar and metabolic acidosis on blood gas will lead the examiner to suspect the diagnosis. Initial treatment is with intravenous glucose and discontinuation of feeds. Advice from a paediatric metabolic consultant should be sought.

Feedback to the mother and father in cases of congenital abnormality

Screening of the newborn can potentially improve the quality of a baby's life through early diagnosis of serious conditions, and in some cases, the screening process can be life saving. However, there are an irreducible number of false positives (babies diagnosed as having the condition when they do not) and false negatives (babies diagnosed as not having the condition when they do) (UK National Screening Committee 2008).

Clearly, a false-positive result can cause unnecessary stress. Conversely, a false-negative result can destroy the mother and father's expectation of having the perfect child, particularly if the pregnancy has progressed uneventfully to term. Medical screening has led to fewer babies now being born with major congenital abnormalities. Many mothers and fathers will simply not have considered the fact that their baby may be malformed. It is, therefore, imperative that mothers and fathers hold realistic expectations of the outcome of screening in the newborn and be given information about the limitations of this process in the antenatal period (DH 2009).

Screening focuses on reducing risk; it does not provide a foolproof guarantee of diagnosis (NHS National Down's Screening Programme for England). The responsibility for educating mothers and fathers about newborn screening will be placed with the health-care professionals they come into contact with around the time of birth. It is questionable how much of this information they are able to understand or even remember. Each Trust will give out its own version of written material to support the screening process (Kemper et al. 2005); however, the UK National Screening Committee have produced a leaflet for mothers and fathers which supports the newborn screening event. It is intended to be used to maintain consistency of information nationwide. (A copy of this leaflet can be found in Appendix 2.)

The practitioner must be suitably equipped to inform the mother and father in an effective and knowledgeable way that their baby has a congenital abnormality. Information given to the mother and father should include clear explanations of the malformation, delivered in a way in which they can understand. It is important that the professional is able to understand and respond appropriately to the range of behaviours demonstrated by the mother and father who are receiving bad news.

The role of the father in this situation can also get easily overlooked. All too often during this type of encounter, the needs of the father may be relegated whilst the practitioner, unintentionally in most cases, focuses on the needs of the mother. It is important to try to establish how the father perceives his role in the care of the infant. Does he feel marginalised by the whole experience? How far does he feel he is able and willing to share parental responsibility in caring safely and effectively for the baby? Health-care professionals can play an important part in helping fathers expand their parenting role by establishing a relationship that is based on trust and respect. They need to be aware of the impact that the baby will have on family dynamics and the factors that can affect parenting capacity within the wider context (DH 2009). A leaflet to help guide professionals on including fathers in care has been written by Fisher (2007) and can be found at the Fatherhood Institute's website: www.fatherhoodinstitute.org.

The website contains a wealth of information on approaches to supporting the role of the father in the transition to parenthood, as well as legislative and policy frameworks that are currently in place to ensure health and other professionals engage with fathers.

For further information regarding breaking unexpected news, see the webpage that accompanies this book.

Conclusion

Only a few of the many genetic disorders have been addressed within this chapter. There are various ways in which these conditions can impact on the newborn examination. Many conditions will not be identifiable immediately and need specialist assessment and support. However, as one of the first people examining the baby, your role in the newborn check is essential in both identifying whether there appears to be a problem present and ensuring that the mother and father receive appropriate information, support and advice.

Case study: Mowat–Wilson syndrome

Trudi was a gravida 4 para 3 and was known to have learning difficulties. She was found to be a gestational diabetic and at 38 weeks gestation had an induction of labour. She was admitted to the delivery suite in established labour accompanied by her partner and very quickly progressed to full dilatation.

The head delivered quickly but then progress was delayed for quite some time and shoulder dystocia was suspected. As the baby's head slowly emerged, the midwife noticed a 'pointy' chin. The baby girl was delivered normally. Baby Karen was in good condition at birth and cried immediately, Apgars 9 at 1 minute and 10 at 5 minutes. However, Trudi immediately pushed Karen away when skin-to-skin contact was offered. At 20 minutes old, the midwife noticed that Karen had developed deep sternal recession. She was transferred to the resuscitaire where general observations and pulse oximetry were carried out.

Heart rate: 120 beats per minute

Respiration rate: 45 breaths per minute

Temperature: 36.6 °C

Colour: centrally pink.

Pre- and post-ductal oxygen saturations: 98% and 99%, respectively.

The general morphology of the infant made the midwife suspicious, but at this stage she said nothing. Dad remarked that the baby looked just like their middle daughter. At this point, Trudi turned her back and appeared not to want to make eye contact with Karen, she also refused to breastfeed. The midwife and attendants sensed that the mother knew something was 'not right'.

The midwife performed an initial examination of the baby. She found that Karen's eyes were wide set and the bridge of her nose thick set and bulbous. The sternal recession persisted. The midwife looked back in the maternal notes but could not find any significant information.

The paediatrician was called and he performed a full examination of the baby. Oxygen saturations continued to fall within normal limits. The paediatrician agreed that the baby should be monitored, and Karen was transferred to the Special Care Baby Unit. Over the next few hours, the abdomen became more swollen. By midday the following day, the abdominal girth had grown by 5 cm and Karen was transferred as an emergency case to the local children's hospital for surgery to the colon. After weeks of screening and investigations, it was discovered the baby had Mowat–Wilson syndrome complicated with Hirschsprung's disease.

Afterwards, the midwife commented that this was a notable example of how the mother appeared to intuitively know something was wrong, despite suffering from learning difficulties.

How would you deal with this situation within your Trust?

How would you support the parents?

Look here for more information on Mowat–Wilson syndrome:

http://ghr.nlm.nih.gov/condition/mowat-wilson-syndrome

http://www.mowatwilson.org/

Read these articles:

http://www.ojrd.com/content/pdf/1750-1172-2-42.pdf

http://jmg.bmj.com/content/40/5/305.full

Look here at the parent support group for Mowat–Wilson syndrome:

http://www.mowatwilsonsyndrome.org.uk/

Mowat–Wilson Syndrome Foundation
http://www.mowat-wilson.org/
Family support
Read Julie Campbell's story about her son with Mowat–Wilson syndrome.
http://www.mowatwilsonsyndrome.org.uk/julias-story.htm
See Appendix 1 for more information on chromosomal abnormalities.
Also visit the companion website to find more information on safeguarding issues.

References

DH (2009) *The Healthy Child Programme. Pregnancy and the First Five Years of Life*. London: Department for Children, Schools and Families.

Fisher D (2007) Including new fathers: a guide for maternity professionals. Available from: www.fatherhoodinstitute.com (accessed June 2010).

Hindley D, Medakkar S (2002) Diagnosis of Down's syndrome in neonates. *Archives Disease in Childhood. Fetal and Neonatal Edition* **87**, F220–F221.

Kemper AR, Fant KE, Clark SJ (2005) Informing parents about newborn screening. *Public Health Nursing* **22** (4), 332–338.

UK Screening Committee (2011). Recommendation on Down's Syndrome Screening in Pregnancy. Available at: http://www.screening.nhs.uk/downs. Last accessed February 2015

Parsons EP, Bradley DM, Clarke AJ (2003) Screening for Duchenne muscular dystrophy. *Archives of Disease in Childhood*. **88**: p273.

Royal College Obstetrics and Gynaecologists (2005) Statement on antenatal screening for Down's Syndrome. Available at: http://www.rcog.org.uk/what-we-do/campaigning-and-opinions/statement/rcog-statement-antenatal-screening-down%E2%80%99s-syndrome (accessed August 2014).

Saenger P, Albertsson Wikland K, Conway GS, Davenport M, Gravholt CH, Hintz R, Hovatta O, Hultcrantz M, Landin-Wilhelmsen K, Lin A, Lippe B, Pasquino AM, Ranke MB, Rosenfeld R, Silberbach M (2001) Recommendations for the diagnosis and management of turner syndrome. *Journal of Clinical Endocrinology and Metabolism* **86**, 3061–3069.

Simms EJ, McCormick J, Mehta G (2005) Newborn screening for cystic fibrosis is associated with reduced treatment intensity. *Journal of Pediatrics* **147**(3), 42–46.

Skotko B (2005) Mothers of children with down syndrome reflect on their postnatal support. *Pediatrics* **115**, 64–77.

Trotter TL, Hall JG; and the Committee on Genetics for the American Academy of Pediatrics (2005) Health supervision for children with achondroplasia. *Pediatrics* **116**, 771–783.

UK NSC (2008) *Newborn and Infant Physical Examination: Standards and Competencies*. London: NHS.

CHAPTER 8

Newborn behavioural aspects

Jeanette Appleton

Trainer, Brazelton Centre in Great Britain, Cambridge, UK

KEY POINTS

- The addition of a behavioural approach to the newborn examination is recognised as being of significant benefit to the infant, mother, father and professionals.

- By highlighting behavioural cues, the health-care professional can show mother and father that their infant is someone who can communicate their needs and preferences.

- The more the mother and father see and learn about their infant, the more realistic and appropriate they will be in their care giving, interactions and expectations.

Introduction

Newborn behavioural status and its significance in the newborn examination are discussed in this chapter in the context of the trainee practitioner or health-care professional working with the newborn infant. The reader is encouraged to make use of the references at the end of the chapter to further develop their knowledge and to spend time observing baby behaviour to develop their skills in behavioural observation.

The examination of the newborn infant used to be a system of procedures undertaken by the doctor within 72 hours of birth to ensure that the infant is healthy and also to screen for certain conditions. It is now recognised that this time provides an early and important opportunity to introduce mothers and fathers to their baby at a time when they are open to forming new attachments, not only with their child, but also with health-care professionals (Sparrow, 2010). Guidelines published by National Institute for Health and Clinical Excellence (NICE) lay out a framework whereby the health-care professional can collaborate with the mothers and fathers with the aim to promote the child's development and well-being (NICE, 2014; DH, 2007). Organisations including 'Parenting UK' have produced National Occupational Standards for working with mothers which provide a model for service providers and individuals whose role involves working with mothers and fathers. These resources provide the practitioner with

---

Examination of the Newborn: An Evidence-Based Guide, Second Edition. Edited by Anne Lomax.
© 2015 John Wiley & Sons, Ltd. Published 2015 by John Wiley & Sons, Ltd.
Companion Website: www.wiley.com/go/lomax/newborn

a model to develop skills in collaborative working (Parentline Plus, 2006; UK National Screening Committee, 2008).

This chapter outlines and describes the range of behaviours and the developmental abilities of the newborn infant and shows how a sensitive health-care professional can combine the newborn examination with the opportunity to show mothers and fathers that, contrary to centuries of opinion, the newborn infant is not a *'blooming, buzzing, confusion'* (James, 1890). Conversely, mothers and fathers can be shown that, according to the paediatrician and psychoanalyst Donald Winnicott, 'In each baby there is a vital spark and this urge towards life, growth and development is a part of the baby, something the child is born with' (Winnicott in Davis and Wallbridge, 1980). Donald Winnicott also commented 'that there is no such thing as a baby', meaning that a baby cannot exist outside a relationship with a carer, usually the mother. A brief overview of the process through which women and men become mothers and fathers is also included in this chapter, to inform practice in communication and promote collaborative working. Mothers and fathers can be empowered in their care-giving skills when a sensitive professional shows them the range of newborn behaviours and explains how they can support their infant's development (Klaus et al., 1995; Wolke et al., 2002).

Before continuing to read this chapter, it may well be useful, if not necessary, for you to put on a different set of 'glasses', so that you can *see* the newborn baby as an individual who has a unique range of behavioural cues, which have been developing throughout pregnancy.

Fetal development

Infant development does not start at birth but is an ongoing process from conception, and this process evolves from the simple to the complex. This is seen in the autonomic system where the organs develop from basic structures to the more specialised, rather than forming in 'miniature' and growing. From as early as 8 weeks, jerky motor movements of the limbs can be seen, and by 20 weeks, all the motor movements of the fetus are observed and practised. This period of practice appears to promote joint and motor development as well as to develop co-ordination (e.g. the infant is able to bring their hand to their mouth). Recent research provides new evidence that this exploratory movement may also be important as part of preparation for self-other awareness (Piontelli, 2010). Studies of twins *in utero* show a sensitivity of one twin to the other in the manner in which they touch, demonstrating a sense of 'social awareness' (Delafield-Butt and Trevarthen, 2012).

The mother will report periods of infant activity (awake) and inactivity (sleep) from about 20 weeks, and by 36 weeks, these periods of awake and sleep are more focused. The five senses develop *in utero* and these senses appear to be important to the establishment of breastfeeding, the recognition of the mother and social community. This can be seen in the development of the olfactory system where from as early as the twelfth week of gestation, the fetus has an experience of the taste of amniotic fluid, which is similar to colostrum, breast milk and breast skin. This link would indicate a developmental process for promoting the establishment of breastfeeding, essential to the survival of the infant in times and situations where bottle-feeding is not an alternative. Babies are able to recognise their mother's voice from 20 weeks and are able to recognise the language their mother speaks from other language (Hepper, 2005; Delafield-Butt and Trevarthen, 2012). These skills promote mother–baby attachment and support the theory of the baby being a social baby.

The challenge at birth is for the baby to integrate all these skills that are essential to their development. Brazelton describes this as being the 'newborn developmental agenda' and highlights four developmental tasks: autonomic, motor, state and social interaction (Brazelton and Nugent, 2011).

Babies are ready to engage and interact with the world as soon as they are born. The key factor is for the baby to be able to integrate these developmental tasks as they adapt to the extra-uterine environment and continue their developmental progress after birth (Nagy, 2011).

The mother and father

The fifth aim of the NICE guidelines is to 'consider good practice in communication between health-care providers and women' (NICE, 2006 p. 13). In order to achieve this objective, it is helpful to understand the process by which women and men adapt to their new role of a mother or father.

With the birth of the baby, the practitioner is able to register the exact time at which the baby was born. However, the process is not so simple for the mother. The process through which women become mothers is explored in the book, *The birth of the mother*, Stern *et al.* (1998). This starts as early as the third year, when it is generally accepted that girls develop an awareness of their gender identity and that they have a potential future role as a mother. The girl is often given her first doll at this age and will model parenting behaviour. It is through these behaviours the girl develops notions and ideas of what it means to be a mother. By the beginning of puberty, girls start to consider the reality of motherhood seen in behaviours, such as choosing names for future babies or by deciding on a career instead of motherhood. When the female becomes pregnant, the mother-to-be considers what they will be like as a mother and also what the child will be like. However, there are several scenarios being considered at the same time. In a way there are three pregnancies taking place; to some degree, there are two fantasy babies that emerge from the moment they are aware of the pregnancy. The first will be the longed-for baby who will have positive characteristics of beauty, talent, intellect or sporting ability and the second will be the feared-for baby who could be ugly, unlovable, disabled or difficult. As the pregnancy reaches the sixth to seventh month, these two fantasy babies will be at their most intense. It is appropriate to pause for a moment and consider those women who have a premature baby, particularly at the period of around 26–30 weeks gestation. They give birth to what most mothers would describe as the feared-for baby. Health-care professionals who care for these mothers will want to consider the implications of this situation within the context of bonding and attachment and support the new mother appropriately. Over the remaining 2 to 3 months of the full term pregnancy, these fantasy babies will diminish and the mother is ready for the real baby that is born at 40 weeks.

At birth, the mothers and fathers are ready to reshape their image of the infant based on the child that they have, rather than the hopes and fears felt during pregnancy. The newborn examination is an opportunity for the practitioner to emphasise the individual characteristic of the newborn infant and highlight these behaviours to the mothers and fathers.

The mother–fetus relationship has been studied for more than 25 years and a number of scales developed to measure the mother's relationship with the unborn child, which is a key developmental task in the successful psychological adjustment for all pregnant women (Van den Burgh, 2009). The framework of a prenatal relationship may assist in understanding why some pregnant women change their behaviour to improve their health while others are reluctant to persist in practices including alcohol and drug use. Included in the NICE guidelines are standards of care for screening those women who have a combination of recognised risk factors such as unplanned pregnancy, illicit drug use, adolescence, advanced maternal age or maternal depression (NICE, 2014).

The father has never been the focus of the same level of research and insight, and as recently as three decades ago, the father's role would be best described as traditional. This role was mainly that of provider and disciplinarian and there was not the intimate emotional relationship with his child or children, and he was not involved in direct childcare other than entertaining the children.

Currently, the mother and father appear to have a more egalitarian approach to parenthood and the father is expected to take on more duties at a practical level as well as be more emotionally involved. In addition, discipline is a more shared responsibility with the mother. This increased level of involvement extends to the preparation for the birth of the baby. The Fatherhood Institute's The Dad Deficit

(2008): 'The missing piece of the maternity jigsaw' report provides an insight into current attitudes of fathers. The survey shows that an increasing number of fathers regularly attend antenatal classes and antenatal scans. Seventy per cent of fathers aged 18–34 attended 'most' or 'all' of the antenatal scans, compared to 45% of fathers older than 55 years of age. A third of younger fathers had stayed overnight in the maternity ward when their child was born, compared with 21% of fathers in the overall survey. The Fatherhood Institute also provides guidelines for maternity professional to enable units to better meet the needs of fathers (The Fatherhood Institute, 2007, see also Chapter 7).

While these findings might indicate that the younger fathers are more involved with services, the findings also indicate that younger fathers want to play a greater role in the birth of their baby and are less satisfied when this goal is not realised. Interestingly, the 2008 survey revealed that three-quarters of those polled felt that information provided by services was directed more towards mothers than fathers. Children's centres have proactively taken measures to ensure that services are responsive to supporting fathers in their role as a parent and in their relationship with their partner or ex-partner and more generally to promote the role of fathering (Department for Children, Schools and Families, 2007). The practitioner is in a position to encourage this greater involvement by ensuring that the father is included throughout the pregnancy and is notified of the timing of the newborn examination. This can also be facilitated by simple practical measures (e.g. ensuring adequate seating for all mothers and fathers) and a more personal approach, including addressing the father by name, engaging him directly in conversation and through regular eye contact. These steps may seem both obvious and trivial but, on a busy shift, it is these aspects that are frequently omitted or forgotten and yet they can have a real impact on the father as he adjusts to his new role (Murray-Smith, 2013).

The practitioner will also appreciate the needs of the single mother who may be bringing up the baby on her own. Stern and Bruschweiller-Stern (1998) showed that a new mother will receive and need the affirmation of up to 10 other mothers to support her in her new role as a mother. These supporters will include a close female friend who has had a baby, her mother and other female relatives who are experienced mothers. Considering this information, the practitioner may consider it appropriate to invite the new single mother to have a supporter with her during the newborn examination, and this could be her close female friend or her mother.

It is important to remember that while the newborn examination is a routine procedure to the practitioner, for the mothers and fathers, this is part of the wonderful event, that is, the birth of a new baby. Although this will not be found on an official list of things to do, it is important to congratulate the mothers and fathers and remember this throughout the examination; in so doing, you will convey to the mothers and fathers your understanding and appreciation that this is an important occasion.

Feedback to mothers and fathers

Anticipatory guidance provides a framework for providing feedback, supporting the new mother and father and promoting the objective of collaborative working between the health-care professional and the mothers and fathers. The more the mothers and fathers see and learn about their infant through observing their baby's behaviour, the more realistic and appropriate they will be in their care giving, interactions and expectations. The practitioner first needs to listen to the mothers and fathers and assess their level of understanding of the baby and his needs and their role as the baby's main caregiver (see also Chapter 7). At this level, active listening is a skill that all health-care professionals should aim to acquire and develop; there is an opportunity in the interview prior to the newborn examination to move away from a 'check box' or 'tick list' approach, by asking open-ended questions that allow the parent to voice their expectations, fears and anxieties as new mothers and fathers. The practitioner can invite the mothers and fathers to comment about the baby's ability to sleep, feed, as well as what they have observed of the baby's physical appearance. These questions could include the following:

- 'What have you learnt about your baby when you have been watching him?'
- 'How does your baby like being cuddled … on your shoulder or in your arms?'
- 'What does your baby do to show you he needs a feed?'
- 'How does your baby sleep … what position does he like?'
- 'What does he do as he wakes up?'
- 'How does your baby like to be held when he is upset?'
- 'What does your baby like you to do most of all?'

By providing the mothers and fathers with good, non-verbal feedback through eye contact, appropriate body language and by summarizing their comments, the practitioner can enable the mothers and fathers to learn about themselves and their relationship with their baby (Sparrow, 2010).

These questions, regarding the observations of mothers and fathers, are non-threatening and allow the practitioner to assess the mother's and father's and baby's relationship and areas of strength and sensitivity. Practitioners are advised to use descriptive phrases when talking to the mothers and fathers about their baby and to avoid labels such as 'good', and 'naughty', when discussing baby behaviour. Babies are not able to express these traits of good or bad behaviour, and these labels are not helpful in terms of discussing the baby's behaviour and the development sequelae. It may be that babies who sleep for prolonged periods are often described as 'good babies' and while the sleepy baby may be less challenging to a parent, the sleepiness may in fact indicate difficulty in achieving an alert state due to a self-regulatory dysfunction.

Using anticipatory guidance, the health-care professional is encouraged to describe the infant's behaviour and its meaning in constructive terms with the aim to support the baby's development. A baby who is able to sleep, make a smooth transition to a bright alert state and is able to focus and follow a face and voice is an organised baby who really enjoys watching and listening. A baby who wakes easily due to a sound in the room, who fusses, has no energy to feed and cannot achieve a restful sleep needs help and support to organise his world.

If, during this time of listening to the mothers and fathers, information is disclosed, which indicates a specific problem (e.g. feeding), a follow-up session should be arranged for further discussion. It is important that on topics such as feeding, consistent advice is given by all the staff. A concerned mother or father often asks the same question of several professionals and conflicting advice, or advice based on personal experience, could only confuse the mother or father and may also undermine the credibility of the health-care staff. When discussing any aspect of the baby's care such as breastfeeding, crying or sleeping, it is important to consider how vulnerable the mother may be feeling; a light remark or joke, in an attempt to diffuse a tense situation, is not appropriate. The practitioner also needs to consider cultural issues and avoid statements of judgement as to which behaviours are positive and preferred.

Mothers and fathers should always be encouraged to be present during the newborn examination. The practitioner also needs to consider the situation where mothers and fathers may be reluctant to engage with the health professional due to a previous negative experience which has resulted in a lack of trust.

The concept of behavioural states

In order to understand and observe newborn behaviour, it is important to appreciate the six levels of sleep and alert behaviour. The concept of states of alertness may be new to the practitioner, and therefore requires explanation, as it is the key to observing the infant's behaviour. In the Newborn Behavioural Assessment Scale (Brazelton and Nugent, 2011) and also in the Newborn Behavioural Observations (Nugent et al., 2007) are descriptions of six stages of behavioural states of alertness as observed in the newborn infant. These states are a continuation of the states of alert and sleep behaviour mentioned earlier in fetal development. It is important that health-care professionals examining the newborn infant are familiar with these states and are able to use this information to help mothers and fathers care for their baby, for instance, highlighting how to support the infant to achieve an alert state for feeding (see Table 8.1). Studies have indicated that where the fetus has been exposed to alcohol, tobacco, cocaine and marijuana, infants were observed to have poorer state regulation, attention and responsiveness. There may also be cumulative social and emotional developmental effects (Tronick, 2005; Shankaran, 2007).

In the first few days of life, the baby may be unable to organise a smooth transition from one state to the next; some babies may remain in a light sleep

Table 8.1   States of sleep and alertness.

State 1: Deep sleep	Regular breathing, eyes closed and no eye movements, no spontaneous movements except startles
State 2: Light sleep	Eyes closed, rapid eye movement often observed under closed lids, low activity level, sucking movements can occur and breathing may be irregular
State 3: Drowsy	Eyes may open but dull and heavy lidded, dazed look, closed or fluttering eyelids, variable activity level, the infant's responses often delayed and motor activity at a minimum
State 4: Alert	Bright-eyed look, infant seems focused on visual or auditory stimuli, activity is at a minimum
State 5: Fussing	Eyes open, considerable motor activity, brief fussy cries
State 6: Crying	Intense crying which is difficult to break through with stimulation, motor activity high

Adapted from Brazelton and Nugent (2011) and Nugent et al. (2007).

or drowsy state as the extra-uterine environment is over-stimulating and they respond by shutting out and conserving their energy through a low-level alert state. These babies can often be slow to feed and have difficulty latching on to the breast. Other babies appear over-alert and cannot achieve a restful sleep, fussing and crying for several hours. Both these behaviours require support to assist the baby to self-regulate its state. One technique that can be employed, to provide this support, is to swaddle the baby in a light sheet and, if required, administer gentle vertical rocking. This strategy of swaddling can help to calm the fussing or crying baby and enable the baby to achieve a restful sleep; the same swaddling and rocking technique can also enable the sleepy baby to come to an alert state and, if required, take a feed (Figures 8.1 and 8.2).

During the newborn examination, it is likely that the infant will cry. It is useful to note at what stage this occurs, whether early on in the examination, or after a challenging manoeuvre such as the examination of the hips. Mothers and fathers are often concerned when the baby cries, especially in the first few

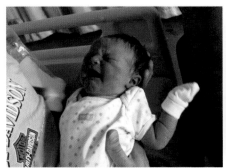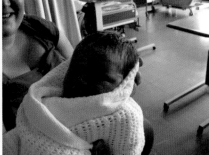

Figure 8.1 The crying infant consoled when swaddled.

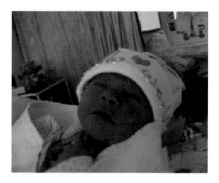

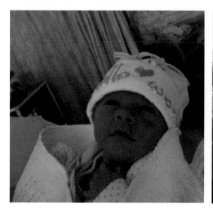
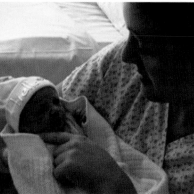

Figure 8.2 Swaddling supports the baby to enable it to come to an alert state and interact with the parent.

days before they have learnt the meaning of each cry, i.e. the hungry cry, the tired cry, the dirty nappy cry and the bored cry. An infant who is irritable and prone to excessive crying is the most common reason for seeking medical advice in the first few months of life (Oberklaid, 2000). Not only does this behaviour cause distress to the mothers and fathers, it also decreases the parent's confidence in their parenting skills. Most mothers and fathers of the newborn infant will use picking-up and rocking as a consoling technique for irritable or crying behaviour. However, some infants are able to console themselves if given sufficient time and others can often be consoled without the necessity of being picked up. The practitioner who is able to demonstrate an effective set of strategies to console a crying infant is able to resource the new mothers and fathers and give them confidence and is a powerful tool to support their baby (Bruning and McMahon, 2009). Improved relationships between mothers and fathers and the infant are also known to have a positive impact on subsequent infant development (Balbernie, 2001). Local NHS initiatives include the distribution of a leaflet and DVD at the booking-in appointment, which includes information to promote improved parent–infant relationships, including soothing strategies and time-out signals (Pennine Care NHS Foundation Trust, 2013).

Consoling strategies

If the baby starts to cry during the newborn examination, the infant should be given the opportunity to self-console; allow the baby to have up to 15 seconds in which to stop crying. During this time, there is an opportunity to listen to the cry and comment to the mothers and fathers appropriately, once again by using descriptive terms such as whether the cry is strong, rhythmic, sustained or intermittent. The baby should be observed to see if he tries to bring his hands to the mouth or focus on an object in the room in an attempt to self-soothe. These attempts to self-soothe should be highlighted to the mother and father. Hands-to-mouth movements are frequently jerky and uncoordinated in the first days of life. Mothers and fathers may try to cover the baby's hands with mittens, as they see the baby's actions as negative and liable to cause scratch marks on the infant's face. By explaining the function of bringing the hand to the mouth and sucking as self-regulatory behaviour, which assists the baby to self-soothe, the practitioner can help mothers and fathers to make informed decisions about the use of mittens.

If the baby continues to cry, then the following approach is recommended:

- Place your face in front of the baby's and engage their gaze. Mothers and fathers are amazed when a simple action such as this calms their baby.
- If the baby continues to cry, then start talking to them in a voice that the baby can hear over their own cries.
- If they are still crying, then place your hand on their abdomen while continuing to talk and look at them.
- Give each stage time to work (approximately 10 seconds) before moving onto placing your hands over their arms and legs to calm the motor activity.
- It is only at this stage that you pick up the baby, if it is still crying, and hold it in your still arms. Some babies prefer to be held on the shoulder and others horizontally, so confirm this with their mothers and fathers.
- Rocking the baby vertically, in a manner that is more than gentle but not too vigorous, is often the 'on–off switch' of a crying baby.
- However, there are some babies who require more support such as swaddling or the use of a pacifier, or both. Mothers who are breastfeeding may not want to use a pacifier, in which case you can facilitate the baby to suck on his fist by gently placing your finger in his fist, so that the grasp reflex is initiated, then guide their hand to their mouth. Swaddle the baby in a light sheet and ensure that the mothers and fathers realise that the baby should not be allowed to sleep swaddled as this may result in the baby becoming too hot.

Some practitioners, when confronted by a baby who is crying inconsolably, might consider continuing the examination as quickly as possible so that it can be completed. This is not appropriate, as the inconsolable infant is expressing a degree of stress or sensitivity and requires support; continuing with the examination without first consoling the baby would be not in the infant's best interest. Infants whose mothers misuse substances, such as alcohol and barbiturates, during pregnancy exhibit excessive or shrill crying that is difficult to console. For these infants, swaddling and then slowly and rhythmically moving the baby up and down is a more effective and successful consoling strategy. This head-to-toe movement is soothing to the baby's neurological system, as is keeping the baby away from the examiner's body (Hudak and Tan, 2012).

The newborn infant's smile

It has been generally considered that the baby's first smile is observed at around 6 weeks of age. However, smiles have been observed in the uterus. Most early smiles have been dismissed as wind, but if the corners of the baby's mouth are turned up, associated with a bright-eyed look and occur in conjunction with the sound of a familiar voice, or looking at a familiar face, is it not more likely that this is a social smile? How the mother responds to her baby, when smiling or crying, is important in understanding the mother–baby attachment process (Nagy and Molnar, 2004). Mothers report how their baby's smile makes all the work of being a mother worthwhile (Strathearn et al., 2008).

Behaviours indicating sensitivity and stress

Each baby will have a threshold, in terms of how they respond to stimulation, both from the environment and activity and how they organise and self-regulate during situations such as the newborn examination. Once that threshold has been exceeded, the baby may exhibit behaviours during the newborn examination that indicate signs of sensitivity, which can precede more overt stress behaviours such as crying. These signs of sensitivity can be observed in the autonomic, motor, state or social interaction systems. If observed and acknowledged by the examiner, these opportunities can be used to highlight the infant's needs and demonstrate the appropriate supporting strategies to the mothers and fathers. A parent who is able to observe their infant's increasing sensitivity, whether during a feed, as the infant wakes, during a nappy change or bath, is more able to provide support to the infant's attempts to organise and self-regulate. The practitioner will want to include comments regarding the infant's efforts to self-soothe and self-regulate so that the mothers and fathers

Table 8.2   Range of behaviours as observed in the autonomic system.

Stable behaviour	Signs of sensitivity	Signs of stress
Even pink skin colour	Subtle colour changes such as	Noticeable colour changes
Smooth pattern of breathing	paling, webbing, acrocyanosis	such as reddening
(between 40 and 60 breaths	around the mouth, eyes	Breathing shallow, with
per minute (bpm))	or nose	pauses
Absence of tremors, startles,	Rapid breathing above 60 bpm	Vigorous hiccoughs
twitches	Occasional startles, tremors or	Spit up
	twitches	Significant number of startles
	Bowel movements	or tremors
	Yawns, series of sneezes	

Adapted from Brazelton and Nugent (2011).

can understand the active role that a newborn infant plays in organising their world. These self-soothing behaviours include:

- Bringing hands to the face
- Bringing hands to the mouth
- Inserting hands into the mouth
- Sucking on fingers or fist
- Grasping a blanket or finger of a career.

The autonomic signs of sensitivity (see Table 8.2) include changes in the colour of the skin; these may be subtle such as a webbing or marbling of the skin, pale skin colour and the more dramatic signs of stress such as reddening of the whole body, which takes some time to resolve. The infant may be observed to increase or decrease their rate of respiration when sensitive and when stressed their breathing may become shallow with pauses. Occasional twitches, sneezes or hiccoughs are early indications of sensitive behaviour, and when the infant is stressed, these become significant. One sneeze alone is not a sign of sensitivity, it is when a meaningful cluster of signs has been observed that the practitioner employs strategies to support the infant. Mothers and fathers generally misunderstand the significance of sneezing and hiccoughing as a sign of sensitivity; the response to an infant sneezing is likely to result in the adult responding with 'Bless you' and cooing noises, and to a bout of hiccoughs by picking up and rubbing its back. A more appropriate response to both behaviours would be to consider placing a still hand on the baby's head or chest; this still touch provides positive support to the infant and assists in the process of self-regulation (Brazelton and Nugent, 2011).

Each infant has its unique individual repertoire of behaviours and by observing the infant's early signs of sensitivity, the practitioner can highlight to the mothers and fathers the trigger for the behaviour, whether it was undressing the baby, placing the baby in a prone position or examining the hips. The practitioner can then model the supporting strategy, such as giving a rest period, vertical

Table 8.3 Range of behaviours as observed in the motor system.

Stable behaviour	Signs of sensitivity	Signs of stress
Relaxed tone	Jerky movement of limbs	Arching movements of trunk
Ability to bring hand to mouth	Flaccid or hypertonic tone	Stretching movements of arms
Sucking	Uneven tone	Leg bracing
Smooth movements of legs and arms		Disorganised activity
		Baby feels limp

rocking or swaddling. This anticipatory guidance should continue throughout the examination with the aim of enabling the mothers and fathers to see these behaviours, not as random events, but as their infant's efforts to self-regulate and organise their interaction with the extra-uterine world and their key carers.

The range of stable, sensitive and stress behaviours that can be observed in the motor system are shown in Table 8.3. Once again, the practitioner can comment during the examination on the positive aspects of stable behaviour such as infant's relaxed muscle tone, the quality of movements and if sensitive signs are observed, such as jerky movements or altered muscle tone and this can be highlighted to the mothers and fathers. Signs of stress, including arching, stretching of the arms or leg bracing may be misunderstood by mothers and fathers and if not supported can result in a crying infant, or one who becomes limp and unresponsive. Early maternal infant interactions are known to frame future relationships, so the practitioner is in a position to support families through sharing knowledge of the range of infant behaviours. Sharing rather than teaching is the key to empowering mothers and fathers; this can be achieved by including the parent in the observation, reflecting back their own observations and encouraging the mothers and fathers to contribute their thoughts and feelings (Brazelton and Nugent, 2011).

As mentioned earlier, the concept of the states system is that of a hierarchy with state and social interaction systems supported by the autonomic and motor states. The newborn examination is increasingly undertaken in the first 24 hours of life, due to the reduced length of hospital admission on postnatal wards. The optimum time for observing newborn behaviour is after 72 hours, when the infant is more able to organise smooth transition from one state to the next. During the examination, the baby may close their eyes in an attempt to self-regulate by reducing the level of stimulation; mothers and fathers often misinterpret this as the baby going to sleep. Shading the baby's eyes with a hand, talking quietly or remaining silent often results in the baby being able to open their eyes and regain an alert state. Some babies become locked into eye-to-eye contact and their expression becomes one of wide-eyed or panicked alertness; it is important that the practitioner withdraws their gaze to release the infant from this overwhelming interaction. The practitioner can highlight all the behavioural

Table 8.4 Range of behaviours as observed in the state and social interaction systems.

Stable behaviour	Signs of sensitivity	Signs of stress
Able to maintain a robust sleep state	Shutting out by closing eyes, baby is not asleep	Inconsolable crying
Able to move from sleep to awake with a smooth transition	Averting eye gaze	Cannot be aroused
	Fussing/irritable	Very irritable
Bright-eyed and alert	Difficult to console	Constant averting of eyes
Focused gaze	Wide-eyed hyper alert look	Panicked alertness
Able to self-quiet when alert		Twitching eye movements
		Setting sun eyes

signs of sensitivity and stress within the social interaction system, as the mother and father may misinterpret these behaviours as a rejection of themselves by their infant (see Table 8.4).

Where the baby shows stable behaviour, the examination can continue uninterrupted. However, if the baby shows any of the signs of sensitivity, then the examiner will want to respond, whether by altering the pace of the examination, the volume of their voice or by giving a short rest period. If the baby shows only an isolated sign such as one sneeze, then this can be ignored, as one type of behaviour in isolation does not constitute sensitivity. Should the baby display any of the stress behaviours, then this would indicate the need for a break while the baby recovers their stability. This use of short breaks can assist mothers and fathers in their care giving, such as when dressing the infant or giving a bath. If the care-giving activity is paced according to the infant's ability to self-regulate, then the mother and father and infant are more likely to have positive and enjoyable experiences.

Learning how to identify the range of infant behaviours requires time, and the practitioner should allocate time for watching the babies during normal care-giving activity to help develop skills in behavioural observation. It is important to become totally familiar with these behaviours and their meanings. It is also important to consider the impact of any activity or event that occurred just before the signs of sensitivity or stress are observed. In this way, the trainee can identify the potential relationship between the activity or impact of the environment and the behavioural response of the baby.

Preparations before the newborn examination

In order to elicit the best behaviour of the infant, it is important to consider the timing of the newborn examination. Where possible, the baby should not be examined soon after a feed, as the baby is often sleepy and also is more liable to spit up (posset). For obvious reasons, the period just before a feed should also be avoided, as the baby is likely to cry. Half-way between feeds is the ideal time, when the baby has the opportunity to show his full range of behaviours from sleep to awake. Newborn babies are still adjusting to the extra-uterine environment, so the room should be prepared by closing any blinds to reduce the light level; bright lights should be avoided. It is the usual convention for any examination for the room to be brightly lit, often with overhead fluorescent lights. If the use of a bright light is required for a specific manoeuvre, then it is possible to use a spotlight that is directed away from the baby's face, or the baby's eyes should be shaded, using a hand or asking the mothers and fathers to use their hands. The temperature of the room should be at around 22–27 °C as the baby will still be organising self-regulation of their body temperature; when the baby is undressed for examination of the hips, a cold room may be stressful.

Describing newborn behaviour during the examination

Before the examination of the newborn infant begins, it is important to take a few moments to observe the state of alertness of the infant. The practitioner then has an opportunity to discuss these states and their significance to care giving, including feeding, consoling or helping the baby to go to sleep. Mothers and fathers will have observed their baby as it sleeps and wakes and guidance can be given regarding the quality of the sleep and the significance of deep sleep in relation to the baby's growth. The practitioner can also ask the mothers and fathers if they have noticed whether a noise or change in light levels has disturbed the baby's sleep and the baby's ability to shut out noise and light in order to protect their sleep at this stage.

This skill of shutting-out is called habituation (Brazelton and Nugent, 2011). It enables the baby to focus on the main task in hand, such as sleeping or feeding. By being able to select what stimulation to respond to and what to ignore, the baby is developing a key tool for future learning.

If the baby is asleep, observe whether the baby reacts to the touch of the stethoscope and how they show any disturbed behaviour. Is it a significant startle or just a small movement of the legs? The level of reaction can be explained to the mothers and fathers in the context of the baby's ability to maintain their sleep state.

The sleeping baby will usually wake when they are undressed, often with stretching movements of the arms and legs and the baby may fuss or cry. Encourage the mothers and fathers to place a finger in their baby's hand or place a still hand on the baby's head; these techniques show the mothers and fathers how a simple step can help them to calm their baby and support the baby's transition from a sleep to an alert state.

During the examination of the infant's hips, there is an opportunity to show the mothers and fathers the powerful soothing effect of sucking behaviour. The manoeuvre required to assess the development of the hip joint is quite challenging for the baby, and by bringing the baby's fist to their mouth or by using a pacifier, the baby can be supported; and the jittery or tense movements of the baby, often observed at this stage of the examination, can be avoided. This is also an opportunity to comment to the mothers and fathers on the quality of the muscle tone and to demonstrate the baby's ability to stand and also his walking reflex. Mothers and fathers see these reflexes as skills and will often beam with pride as the practitioner elicits this reflex.

When examining the eyes, the practitioner can engage with the infant's gaze and demonstrate how newborn can track a face both horizontally and also vertically. Not all newborn babies are able to track a moving face with smooth and co-ordinated eyes movements. If the baby loses track of the moving face, he may need to be given time to re-focus. If you want to be sure that you are showing the mothers and fathers the baby's capability to focus and follow visually, make sure that you do not talk or make any sounds at the same time. As many mothers and fathers think a newborn baby is blind at birth, this can be a moment of significant recognition for the parent that their baby is able to see. One mother commented following a behavioural observation that they had a new respect for their baby as a result of learning how the baby could track a face (Johnson and Johnson, 2004).

Babies are able to recognise their mother's voice from the third trimester (Hepper, 2005) and, through preverbal memory, is able to recognise the language their mother speaks from other languages (Moon et al., 1993). The examiner could demonstrate this during the assessment by asking the mother to talk to her baby, while out of the line of the baby's vision. Most babies will turn their heads towards the mother in response to hearing her voice. This is an opportunity to reinforce to the mother that her baby knows who she is (DeCasper and Fifer, 1980). By 7–10 days of age, babies who have been cared for consistently by their mother will also recognise her face (Bushall, 2003).

Babies will also use their gaze to engage with mothers and fathers. However, for some babies this may be an overwhelming experience and they may consequently avert their gaze. The mother may misinterpret this as the baby's rejection of her and this behaviour needs to be explained within the context of the sensitive baby who requires support for social interaction. Supporting the baby's alert behaviour can be achieved by:

• Reducing the level of stimulation by just talking or just looking
• Reducing the light or noise levels in the room

- Looking just over the baby's head
- Using still hands to contain the baby's arms and legs
- Providing a rest period
- Swaddling him with a light sheet.

Once the examination is over, it is usual for the mothers and fathers to want to hold their baby. This provides an opportunity to review the behaviours observed. In the very busy schedule of the current-day postnatal ward, this golden moment can so often be easily missed.

Documentation

After completion of the newborn examination, the practitioner will document the findings in the neonatal records. The behavioural component should be included in this report because it will help to inform future episodes of care.

The practitioner can include comments regarding the strengths and sensitivities of the infant using the framework of the autonomic, motor, state and social interaction systems. Although it is not usual nursing practice to include comments made by the mothers and fathers, in behavioural observations, it is everyday practice to add parent's observation of their baby and what they view as their baby's strengths and sensitivities.

Postgraduate training

There are formal postgraduate training opportunities for health-care professionals who wish to develop their skills in newborn behavioural observation. The Brazelton Centre (UK) currently has two programmes of training in behavioural observation. The Newborn Behavioural Assessment Scale (NBAS) developed by Dr Brazelton in the early 1970s has been used extensively in clinical and research practice and the Newborn Behaviour Observation (NBO) was introduced in 2008. The training includes formal workshops followed by self-directed learning, leading to certification. Health-care professionals completing the training are able to use their skills in behavioural observation, not only for the purpose of assessment, but also to provide sensitive everyday care giving to empower mothers and fathers and promote collaborative working.

The organisation 'One Plus One' runs course for health-care professionals to develop their listening and communication skills. These are available as workshop study days or as a training pack for use within the workplace. The courses are accredited by the Royal College of Nursing (RCN). The 'One plus One' website has a range of current research articles and policy news which will be of interest to health-care professionals working with new families (http://www.oneplusone.org.uk/).

Conclusion

In an age where smaller families are the norm, many new mothers and fathers may have little or no experience of caring for a baby, and new mothers and fathers are less likely to have local support from their extended family. These factors and the shorter hospital admissions post-delivery place greater emphasis on practitioners to ensure that the new mothers and fathers are as fully prepared as possible to care for their infant. The addition of a behavioural component to the newborn examination is gaining in recognition as being of significant benefit to the mothers and fathers. These behavioural observations provide a key opportunity to introduce the mothers and fathers to their baby as an individual who is an active participant in the parent–infant relationship and who can communicate with them his needs and preferences; however, this can only be effectively realised if his carers understand this language of infant behaviour.

Neonatal behavioural aspects

Case study one

Baby Stephen is having a full examination by the midwife; the mother and father are present during the examination. The mother comments that Stephen baby cries frequently and is rarely awake long enough for a full feed. The examiner observes the baby before beginning the examination, noting the baby's pale colour and heavy-lidded eyes and then Stephen sneezes a few times and sighs. This meaningful cluster of signs of sensitivity guides the examiner to use a quiet voice and smooth, gentle handling during the examination. Modelling this way of handling the baby provides insights for the mother and father to better support their baby and promote alert behaviour.

During the hip examination, Stephen starts to fuss then cry; the examiner uses this opportunity to show the mother and her partner strategies to console their baby. The examiner places a still hand on Stephen's tummy and though the crying continues, the intensity lessens. The examiner suggests to the mother to give the baby her finger to suck on or to place the baby's hand near their mouth to encourage sucking. This soothes Stephen and the crying stops. The mother observes that her baby does not need to be picked up each time he cries.

Case study two

Molly has Down's syndrome, diagnosed soon after delivery, and the mother and father have had a consultation with a paediatrician to discuss the implications of the diagnosis. During the newborn examination and by observing her behaviours, the mother and father can be shown Molly is an individual. This allows them to explore the baby's strengths and sensitivities and helps them support her development.

During the examination of head, neck and eyes, the examiner engages Molly by looking at her. Once the baby focuses on his face, the examiner moves his head to one side and then the other. Molly initially follows but then turns away; he gives the baby time to recover and waits for the baby to look back. The examiner explains to the mother and father that Molly needed a short break as it had been hard work to focus and follow a face. This break allows her time to self-regulate. Consequently, Molly can re-engage and start looking at and following the examiner's face. At this point, the mother speaks and Molly turns to look at her. The examiner highlights this response and comments that the baby really knows her mother's voice and prefers to look at her.

Small insights such as described above can have a profound effect on the mother and father as they realise that their baby has 'skills' and behaviours that can guide them as they work out their baby's needs, whether it is around feeding, playing, sleeping or needing to be consoled.

Look here for more resources on understanding neonatal behaviour

Here, you can look though a learning module on 'Understanding behavior in term infants'.
http://www.marchofdimes.com/nursing/modnemedia/othermedia/states.pdf
Infant reflex and cues
http://www.marchofdimes.com/nursing/modnemedia/othermedia/infantBehavior.pdf
Look here for more information on the Brazelton Assessment Score.
http://www.brazelton-institute.com/intro.html
http://www.brazelton.co.uk/scale.html
http://www.waimh.org/Files/Signal/Signal_2004_12_3-4.pdf
Watch the video
http://www.youtube.com/watch?v=tqc8gKuXs3s
Information for mothers and fathers on newborn development.
http://www.pamf.org/children/newborns/development/
Test your knowledge on behavioural characteristics of the newborn.
http://quizlet.com/10094435/behavioral-characteristics-of-newborn-flash-cards/

References

Balbernie R (2001) Circuits and circumstances: the neurobiological consequences of early relationship experiences and how they shape later behaviour, *Journal of Child Psychotherapy* **27**, 237–255.

Brazelton, TB. and Nugent JK (2011) *Neonatal Behavioural Assessment Scale* 4th edn. Clinics in Developmental Medicine No 190 London: MacKeith Press.

Bruning S McMahon C (2009) The impact of infant crying on young women: a randomised controlled study. *Journal of Reproductive and Infant Psychology,* **27**, 206–220

Bushall IWR (2003) *Newborn Face Recognition. The Development of Face Processing in Infancy and Early Childhood.* O Pascalis. A Slater 41.54. New York: Nova Science Publishers Inc.

Davis M, Wallbridge D (1980) *A Boundary and Space: Introduction to the Work of D.W. Winnicott,* London: Karnac

DeCasper AJ and Fifer WP (1980) Of human bonding: newborns prefer their mothers' voices, *Science,* **208**, 1174–1176

Delafield-Butt JT, Trevarthen, C (2012) Ontogenesis of human communication: biological foundations of language. In P Cobley, PJ Schultz (eds) (2014) *Handbook of Communication Science.* Gruyter.

Department for Children, Schools and Families (2007) *Every Parent Matters.* London: Department for Children Schools and Families.

Department of Health Publications (2007) *Birth to Five,* London: TSO Publications Centre.

Hepper P (2005) Unravelling our beginnings. *The Psychologist,* **18**, 474–477

Hudak ML, Tan RC (2012) Neonatal drug withdrawal, *Pediatrics* **129**(2) e540–e560.

James W (1890) *The Principles of Psychology,* p462. New York: Holt.

Johnson and Johnson Pediatric Institute and the Brazelton Centre in Great Britain (2004) *More than Words Can Say: Understanding a baby's language through the Neonatal Behavioural Assessment Scale. DVD.* Cambridge: Brazelton Centre.

Klaus MH, Kennell JH, Klaus PH (1995) Bonding, building the foundations of secure attachment and independence. Reading, MA: Addison-Wesley.

Moon, C., Cooper, R.P. and Fifer, W.P. (1993). Two-day-olds prefer their native language. *Infant Behaviour and Development* **16**, 495–500.

Murray-Smith J (2013) Epilogue: the spare room: a father confronts his fatherhood, *The Baby as Subject: Clinical Studies in Infant-Parent Therapy* P Campbell, F Thomson-Salo (ed), London: Karnac.

Nagy E (2011) The newborn infant: a missing stage in developmental psychology. *Infant and Child Development,* **20**(1), 3–19.

Nagy E., Molnar P (2004) Homo imitans or homo provocans? Human imprinting model of neonatal imitation. *Infant Behavior and Development* **27**, 54–63.

NICE (2006) *Postnatal Care Guidelines Routine Postnatal Care of Women and Their Babies.* London: NICE, p14.

NICE (2014) Post Natal Care guideline CG37. Available at: https://www.nice.org.uk/guidance/cg37 (accessed February 2015).

Nugent JK, Keefer CH, Minear S, Johnson LC, Blanchard Y (2007) *Understanding Newborn Behaviour & Early Relationships.* Baltimore: Brookes Publishing.

Oberklaid F (2000) Editorial comment. 'Persistent crying in infancy: a persistent clinical conundrum', *Journal of Paediatrics and Child Health* **36**, 297–298.

Parentline Plus, The Centre for Parent and Child Support, 'One Plus One' (2006) *How helping works: Towards a Shared Model of Process.* London: One Plus One.

Pennine NHS Foundation Trust (2013) *Getting it Right from the Start: Understanding Your Baby* 3rd edn. Hyde: Stockport NHS Foundation Trust.

Piontelli A (2010) *Development of Normal Fetal Movements: The First 25 Weeks of Gestation,* Italia: Springer-Verlag.

Shankaran et al. (2007) Taeusch W, Ballard R, Gleason C. *Avery's Diseases of the Newborn,* 9th edn. Philadelphia: Elsevier Saunders.

Sparrow, JD (2010) *Nurturing Children and Families: Building on the Legacy of T. Berry Brazelton: Chapter 2. Aligning Systems of Care with the Relational Imperative of Development.* Oxford: Wiley-Blackwell.

Stern D, Bruschweiller-Stern N, Freeland A (1998) *The Birth of a Mother.* London: Bloomsbury.

Strathearn L, Li J, Fonagy P, Montague PR (2008) What's in a smile? Maternal brain responses to infant facial cues, *Pediatrics* **122**, 40–51.

The Fatherhood Institute (2007) Including New Fathers: A Guide for Maternity Professionals, (Online), Available: http://www.fatherhoodinstitute.org.

The Fatherhood Institute (2008) *The Dad Deficit: The Missing Piece of the Maternity Jigsaw,* Abergavenny: DHA Communications.

Tronnick (2005) cited in La Sala G.B, Fagandini. P,Lori.V,Monti. F, Blickstein. I.(Eds) *Coming Into The World: A Dialogue Between Medical and Human Sciences.* De Gruyter.

UK National Screening Committee (2008) Newborn and Infant Physical Examination: Standards and Competencies, (Online), Available: http://newbornphysical.screening.nhs.uk/competencies.htm (March 2008).

Van Den Burgh BR (2009) A review of scales to measure the mother-foetus relationship. *Journal of Reproductive and Infant Psychology* **27**(2), 114–126.

Wolke D. Dave S, Hayes J, Townsend J, Tomlin M (2002) Routine examination of the newborn and maternal satisfaction: a randomised controlled trial. *Archives of Disease in Childhood. Fetal and Neonatal Edition* **86**(3), F155–F160.

CHAPTER 9

Examination of the newborn: professional issues in practice

Norma Fryer[1] and Claire Evans[2]

[1] Retired Senior Lecturer

[2] Warrington and Halton Hospitals NHS Foundation Trust Warrington, Cheshire, UK, Seconded post as Implementation Lead with the UK NSC NIPE Programme Centre, Public Health England, London, UK

KEY POINTS

- The enhancement of midwives' role to carry out the initial assessment of newborns has embraced the use of previously untapped midwifery skills and greater multi-professional collaboration through compliance of agreed national standards.

- The professional demands of role enhancement involve appropriate preparation and scrutiny of practice. The Nursing and Midwifery Council (NMC), as the regulator for practice, defines the benchmarks for conduct performance and ethics through its new Code, which became effective 31 March 2015. A fair and proportionate system of revalidation for all nurses and midwives will be complete by the end of 2015.

- Service providers have a responsibility to promote multidisciplinary collaboration in the approach to newborn service provision and a need to provide safe and effective outcomes for mothers and babies. This will in turn reduce those cases that may require recourse from the courts or professional regulator.

Introduction

Previously, the expansion of roles for midwives to carry out the initial assessment of newborns was one of a number of initiatives to expand the midwife's role (Michaelides 1998, Hayes et al. 2003). Others included ventouse extractions (Lewis 1998) and ultrasound scanning (Morrell 2002, Gargan 2010). This saw the beginning of a move to utilise previously untapped midwifery skills.

Initial reactions to role changes raised some concern that the move was more of a reaction to demands on the service, rather than a proactive measure to enhance the professional profile of nurses and midwives (NHS Executive North West Regional Professional Forum Group 1996). In reality, the enhanced role for midwives improves the continuity and consistency of care for women and

---

Examination of the Newborn: An Evidence-Based Guide, Second Edition. Edited by Anne Lomax.
© 2015 John Wiley & Sons, Ltd. Published 2015 by John Wiley & Sons, Ltd.
Companion Website: www.wiley.com/go/lomax/newborn

their babies in the immediate post-partum period (NHS Quality Improvement Scotland 2008, Lomax and Evans 2005, Dermott et al. 2006, Baker 2010).

Many government initiatives have raised the importance of 'high-quality education' and systems, to ensure that individuals have the requisite skill to identify concerns and respond appropriately (DH 2007a). The *NHS Knowledge and Skills Framework* (DH 2004a), *Agenda for Change* (DH 2004b), *Maternity Matters: Choice, Access and Continuity of Care in a Safe Service* (DH 2007b) and the Skills for Health Framework (DH 2006) set the scene for a more structured model to ensure quality and safety. The greater utilisation of experience and skills of all health-care workers led to the introduction of a decisive set of competencies relating to a range of clinical health-care activities, which have influenced the generation of new national policies, standards and educational programmes.

The adaptation of such competencies for use by midwives seeking to enhance their own role in the care of the newborns is now evident in the *Skills for Health Maternity and Care of the Newborn* (DH 2009a) competency framework. In addition, as part of The Healthy Child Programme (DH 2009b), the work of the National Screening Committee (NSC) (UK NSC 2008a) forms part of the wider agenda to improve quality and safety. The introduction of national guidance and standards on the antenatal and newborn screening programmes is also framed through a specific set of competencies relating to the newborn examination (UK NSC 2008a). When these competencies are mapped against the NMC's professional framework, it is clear that they bear a strong resemblance to, and reflect the essence of the principles set out in the NMC's Code (NMC 2010a), which defines the professional benchmarks for conduct, performance and ethics required from all nurses and midwives. The NMC (2015) have recently published a revised Code of practice which came into effect 31 March 2015 and can be found at http://www.nmc-uk.org/The-revised-Code/.

In April 2013, the UK National Screening Programmes became part of Public Health England. Public Health England is the expert national public health agency working on behalf of the Secretary of State to protect health and health inequalities and promote the health and well-being of the nation. More information on Public Health England can be found here: https://www.gov.uk/government/organisations/public-health-england and also on the website that accompanies this book.

The standards set out within the UKNSC's document *Newborn and Infant Physical Examination* (NIPE) (UK NSC 2008b) are currently being reviewed and remain, for now, in the developmental phase. They will be available to view at http://newbornphysical.screening.nhs.uk/ as soon as they are re-launched. They will also appear on the website that accompanies this book.

This review is part of the UKNSC's response to the National Service Specification 21 NIPE Screening Programme (DH 2013a). The service specification will ensure consistency in approach to the newborn examination and will be used to control the monitoring and provision of services across England. It represents the service that should be provided when the NIPE Programme Team have completed the current review. The NIPE Programme Team are also influenced by the Section 7a Agreement (NHS 2013) which allows responsibility for commissioning some of the public health budget to be passed to NHS England. It also ensures that decisions are made by those with subject expertise, that a collaborative and strategic leadership approach is adopted and that programme boards are in place.

Other influences affecting professional competency and conduct have come into focus with the Francis Inquiry (DH 2013b). Between 2005 and 2008, patients at Mid Staffordshire NHS Foundation Trust experienced appalling suffering due to substandard care. The interests of patients were not put first and their concerns were not listened to. Alongside this, Jane Cummings Chief Nursing Officer for England introduced a new vision for the nursing profession in the form of the '6 C's in nursing': Care/Compassion/Competence/Communication/Courage and Commitment. She believes that a nursing profession built on these concepts will be one that focusses on quality, safe and effective care and good patient experience (DH 2013c).

Following on from this in July 2013, the NMC published a formal response to the report on the Francis Inquiry. The response emphasised the need to embed care and compassion as well as competence in clinical skills into standards for nurse and midwifery education. They emphasised the importance of registrants maintaining safe and effective practice throughout their career. They pledged to develop effective ways to deal fairly and promptly with registrants who fail to demonstrate the values of care and commitment within the profession (NMC 2013). To that end, the NMC is currently in the process of revising the revalidation of registrants to assess their continued fitness to practice. The NMC has embarked on a public consultation on how revalidation can be applied in practice and is planning to develop a fair and proportionate system of revalidation by the end of 2015 (NMC 2013). See also 'How the Code will work with the new revalidation model' at http://www.nmc-uk.org/Nurses-and-midwives/Revalidation/Revalidation-professionalism-and-the-Code/

Moreover, the publication in April 2014 of the draft law commission bill: Regulation of Health and Social Care Professionals (Law Commission 2014) set out a new clear and consistent legal framework to enable regulators to uphold their duty to protect the public. The NMC have welcomed the draft Bill and believe that if it were implemented, they would be able to make fundamental changes to the way in which they regulate the profession and protect the public (NMC 2014).

The neonatal examination: competence for practice

The daily assessment of newborns is not, in itself, a new activity for midwives, in the same way that reporting deviations from the norm is integral to the mid-wives' role and is at the heart of multi-professional collaboration. However, new knowledge and skill are required to assess additional clinical indices on low-risk women and their babies (DH 2010) with a prerequisite for more advanced clinical judgement, without endorsement from the paediatrician.

The assessment and examination of the newborn are the first of many formal and informal 'screening' activities the baby is likely to encounter. Whilst the informal observations will become an integrated feature of parenthood, the contribution from health-care practitioners has wider professional short- and long-term implications. What has become clear from the national agenda for health over the last 20 years is the growing emphasis on providing national standards and recognised competencies that seek to enhance quality and reduce risk.

In brief, they relate to the assessment of the health and well-being of babies and agreed courses of action. Significance is placed on the involvement of mothers and fathers in discussion both during and after the assessment. Particular emphasis is given to the legislation and professional directives relating to confidentiality, information sharing, the rights of mothers, fathers and babies, anti-discriminatory practice, valid consent and appreciation of child protection legislation. Weight is given to the 'ethics' concerning 'consent and confidentiality' and that of respect for the rights and responsibilities of women to make informed choices.

The relationship and communication with mothers and fathers and any sub-sequent liaison with other health professionals highlight placing the individual needs of the woman and baby at the centre. Special attention is given to the need for effective record keeping again with an understanding of any legal and professional considerations and national and local policies and standards.

See the website that accompanies this book for more information on safe-guarding and the neonatal examination.

The Code and the newborn examination process

Examination of *The Code* (NMC 2015) and how it may be used to articulate the key professional considerations relating to the examination of the newborn may best be done through the NSC *Newborn and Infant Physical Examination Standards and Competencies* (UK NSC 2008b). In broad terms, there are six competencies mapped against the *Skills for Health* (DH 2006) and Knowledge and Skills Frame-work (DH 2004b) with benchmarks and guidance from which programmes should be delivered and practitioners appraised. These are summarized below:

UK NSC newborn and infant physical examination standards and competencies 1–6

- Impact of antenatal and intrapartum events on newborn health status
- Environmental safety
- Informed decision making
- Holistic and systematic examination
- Records and effective communication and referral processes
- Maintenance and development of professional competence

Source: Adapted from UK NSC (2008b).

It is easy to see the underlying moral values and shared philosophy that *The Code* brings to these competencies. Its tenet is to define what the public can expect in order to be able to trust practitioners with their care and well-being and directs practitioners towards the application of some key principles relating to conduct and performance and more importantly, a sound moral context from which all care should be provided. The overall premise contained within the NSC standards is one that aims to raise the quality of examinations and commands significant attention to the 'competence' of the practitioner.

> *All health-care practitioners working within the NHS should be working to the level of competency as defined by their professional qualification and should ensure that if they do not have the appropriate competency for a particular aspect of care, that they make an appropriate referral.*
>
> UK NSC (2008b), p. 5

Whilst overall responsibility and accountability for the quality of newborn screening is directed firmly at the hands of Directors of Public Health (UK NSC section 7.3), it also acknowledges the need for effective multidisciplinary collaboration emphasising the importance of appropriate training and education (section 7.6). The link with the NMC Code is an explicit requirement in that it suggests providers of the service should ensure that 'the scope of practice and competencies are commensurate with professional legal and ethical codes/guidance for practice' (Section 7.2).

Consent in practice

The ethico–legal consideration awarded to the matter of consent in health care has taken on much greater emphasis in recent times. Governments (DH 2001, 2009c), regulators (NMC 2008a, 2010a), professional organisations and lay groups alike have all been subjected to its importance.

The revised guidance from the Department of Health on Consent for Treatment (DH 2009c) presents a useful overview of the legal consequences and potential action that could be taken against an individual or employing body who fails to adhere to the position relating to informed consent. It states that:

> *While there is no English statute setting out the general principles of consent, case law ('common law') has established that touching a patient without valid consent may constitute the civil or criminal offence of battery.*
>
> *DH (2009c)*

Midwives must be aware that the examination of babies at any time demands that clear information be given to the mother and father to obtain 'proxy' consent, being mindful of how to respond should a mother or father raise any objections. The babies' interests will always be at the forefront of any disputes between mothers and fathers and professionals, and it is important for midwives to be mindful of potential challenges. The role of advocate for the baby is a central precept for the midwife (NMC 2008b, 2012) and may apply equally to the mother who may face complex social and/or personal difficulties disclosed during the examination.

Again, guidance from the Department of Health urges as good practice, involvement from appropriate health-care personnel within the multidisciplinary team and the patient's family where possible, as imperative in the decisions made.

Griffiths (2008b) states that if a midwife thinks the best interest is not being recognised, she has a professional and legal duty to challenge the proxy decision-maker. Although it may be unusual for this to occur before or during the newborn examination, it is nonetheless something that should be considered especially in those circumstances where the capacity of the mother or father is in doubt. The ultimate decision to overrule a mother or father may ultimately need to be settled through the courts, or may be resolved with the assistance of the Independent Mental Capacity Advocate whose role would be to ensure that the rights of mothers and fathers, families and the child are given appropriate consideration (DH 2009c).

Confidentiality in practice

The NSC Competencies 2 and 3 (see current UKNSC document at http:// newbornphysical.screening.nhs.uk/standards) identify benchmarks relating to the emotional status of mother and father and the need for effective communication of sensitive and confidential information between parent and examiner; this supplements those relating to safety, comfort and timing of the examination. The sometimes complex issues surrounding confidentiality require midwives to understand when and to whom information may need to be disclosed, both in relation to the assessment itself and what may be revealed by the mother or father during the process.

The legal position relating to confidentiality is complex and despite the fundamental ethico–legal principle supported by the regulator and the employer, it requires sound understanding, sensitive judgement and personal integrity in order for it to be appropriately honoured in practice. Griffiths (2008c) summarises the key points relating to the duty of confidentiality stating that it is subject to the protection of third parties, where children are uniquely placed. Griffiths (2008d) reminds us that the public interest to protect vulnerable adults and children outweighs the duty to maintain confidentiality and that disclosure of information may be necessary in the interest of justice and safety.

In practice, if a mother or father during the process of examination of the baby imparts information that may raise concerns about the potential safety of the baby or other children within the family, protection of that child and/or other children has priority. A midwife would, therefore, be legally and professionally obliged to disclose this information. The right to confidentiality does, however, take precedence in all other circumstances and any breaches that do not relate to the protection of a third party may lead to legal proceedings and or action by the employer or NMC (Griffiths 2008c; NMC 2008c, 2010a).

The NSC framework champions multidisciplinary working with a requirement to exercise professional autonomy in deciding whether or not to undertake the examination or to refer to a more appropriately qualified member of staff (NSC Competencies 1, 3, and 6). Pointers to ensure a safe environment to minimise risk (NSC Competency 2) and the need for robust referral systems provide the indices of good professional practice as does effective feedback to mothers and fathers, reflected in the first section of *The Code* (NMC 2015) Sections 1–5.

The mandate here to provide high standards of care using the best available evidence is a familiar call to all health-care practitioners. The importance of keeping clear and accurate records has gained a specific place in the current Code (NMC 2015, Section 10) and midwives must be mindful of the supplementary directives within the *Midwives Rules and Standards* (NMC 2012) and NMC Guidance on Record Keeping (NMC 2010b). In summary, the NMC states that:

> *You have a duty to keep up to date with and adhere to relevant legislation case law and national and local policies relating to information and record keeping.*
>
> *NMC (2010b), p. 9*

and that:

> *... [o]ther people will rely on your records at key communication points, especially during handover, referral and in shared care.*
>
> *NMC (2010b), p. 9*

It is obvious that the principles contained within *The Code* are implicit in all six NSC competencies. This includes explicit reference to the provision of high standards (NSC Competencies 4, 5 and 6), knowledge of and familiarisation with equipment (NSC 1.4), the safety of the environment (NSC 2.4, 2.5) and a directive to apply 'current evidence based practice as integral to effective decision making' (NSC 3.2, 3.6). The need for effective and sensitively written records is again a major feature of good practice (NSC 5) whilst the instruction to maintain competence places personal accountability with each practitioner to do so (NSC 6.1)

Both the legal and the professional mandates relating to the maintenance of high standards emphasise the commitment to accept personal responsibility for maintaining skills and competence at all times. In addition, the NMC reminds midwives that both the PREP requirements (NMC 2011) and the annual monitoring of midwifery practice by Supervisors of Midwives (NMC 2012) Rule 12: para 2b) are endorsed with legal authority.

The link here with the NSC Competency Framework is perhaps self-evident in that such ideals are, or should be, integral to the relationship with mothers' families and babies. However, the skills required in decision making (NSC 1.3, 3.7), competence and working within boundaries (NSC 1.3, 4.15, 6), aspects relating to confidentiality and sensitivity (NSC 2.3), consent (3.6), records (NSC 5) and all elements relating to the relationship with mothers and fathers (NSC 3; 4.1) serve only to reinforce how the client/practitioner relationship must be fortified by trust.

Role of the employer

In order to capture the employer's position and responsibility in supporting a midwife who has embarked on any role enhancement, consideration should be given to the prevailing climate that surrounds the NHS agenda.

The national NIPE (UK NSC 2008b) document has provided a formalised governance pathway through proposed quality assurance measures. With the appointment of a lead clinician for the examination of the newborn in each Trust, the responsibility for evaluating and monitoring the service provided and the assurance that health-care professionals undertaking the examination are appropriately trained and competent rests in part with this person. This does not, however, detract in any way from the personal accountability that lies with the individual and/or those responsible for managing midwifery services. What is important is the additional audit activity required and the need for improved communication between commissioners and service providers.

Local policies to direct practice

Local policies and guidelines supporting practice must incorporate the national standards that demonstrate clear referral pathways. Other directives such as

'Public health functions to be exercised by NHS England, Service Specification 21, NHS Newborn and Infant Physical Examination Screening Programme' (DH 2013a) need to be taken into consideration in order to adequately govern and monitor the provision of this service nationally.

The adoption of such standards across the country will promote a much more consistent approach on how the examination is conducted and equity in the level of referral services available to the neonate. Prompt referral for the neonate is implicit in the diagnostic process and a robust evidence base must underpin all local guidelines. This includes national policy and guidance, particularly those from the NSC and the National Institute for Health and Care Excellence (NICE).

As discussed in Chapter 1, the history-taking perspective and the newborn examination have embraced a new and much more extensive health-care agenda. This has implications for the remit of the practitioner where further direction is needed and to some degree delineation of professional roles. It must be clear within local documentation when it is necessary for a senior paediatrician to conduct the newborn examination or review the baby. The referral process must be comprehensible to ensure that appropriate and timely referrals are made to the correct department or individual for expert opinion.

Midwives and neonatal nurses must be aware of the examinations that they cannot perform. This will vary between maternity units based upon local agreement with paediatric medical collaboration. For more examples of individual Trust's exclusion criteria, see the website that accompanies this book.

Risk management

Examination of the newborn in the past featured within the post-natal and newborn care standard of the National Health Service Litigation Authority (NHSLA 2012) Clinical Negligence Scheme for Trusts (CNST) Maternity Standards. This reflects the level of risk that the examination poses within maternity services. Unfortunately, a minority of babies are still discharged home with an anomaly not detected at the time of the routine examination, for example, a cleft palate. In a large retrospective audit review, approximately 28% of clefts are missed on the first-day examination (Bannister 2008).

Suboptimal practice is inversely related to competence and calls into question ongoing education and updating for all health-care professionals. This lies at the centre of maintaining fitness to practice and self-audit. Any level of risk must be identified and incident reporting mechanisms in place to escalate any incident where lessons can be learned in line with local Risk Management Policy.

Clinical audit must, therefore, feature as a key performance indicator for quality measurement. It is useful for all practitioners to be familiar with the audit process and contribute to local audit activity. Following the introduction of the national NIPE standards, the NIPE SMART (Screening Monitoring and Reporting Tool) IT system has been developed to record and monitor the coverage of the newborn examination at both local and national levels. The system also houses the functionality to monitor referral outcomes mapped to the four screening elements of the NIPE Standards. In addition, the system provides data through predefined or specified search fields that support varied levels of newborn examination local audit activity.

The use of the NIPE SMART system is recommended in the DH Public health functions to be exercised by NHS England, Service Specification 21, NHS Newborn and Infant Physical Examination Screening Programme' (DH 2013a). Most importantly, the NIPE SMART provides a 'failsafe' to ensure that the newborn population within maternity services receives a newborn screen examination in line with the national NIPE Standards. It is implicit within the 'failsafe' process that any newborn that is 'missed' whereby the newborn examination is not performed, then such an incident is reportable and should be investigated. The NIPE SMART is also compliant with the national quality assurance framework through the provision of KPI data attached to the national NIPE Standards. The KPI data is now reportable to the national Screening Quality Assurance Teams and of interest to local Commissioning Groups.

The NIPE Screening Programme is currently rolling out across England. The Programme aims at improving service performance, promote timely referral pathways and programme delivery of the newborn examination with a robust 'failsafe 'process firmly embedded within maternity services provision.

The newborn examination practitioner: education and competence

Underperformance with the newborn examination is directly related to the level of experience and competence of the examiner. As with any skill acquisition, exposure to the skill and continued practice are necessary to gain experience, confidence and competence. From a localized qualitative study, Steele (2007) reported a decline in the number of midwives undertaking the newborn examination upon completion of the former English National Board (ENB) N96 programme. Undefined roles, workloads and lack of support from management were cited as the root causes. Similarly, McDonald (2008) conducted a local audit of midwives, neonatal nurses and health visitors who conducted the discharge examination of babies. Contributory factors cited were excessive workload pressures, lack of time as well as litigation fears. More local and national audit activity is needed to qualify these findings and establish trends. Simms and Mitchell (2012) also support this assertion.

The newborn examination demands a practitioner who has not only excellent clinical skills but also sound decision-making abilities. The NIPE

Programme provides an educational e-Learning resource for all health professionals who perform the newborn examination at http://newbornphysical.screening.nhs.uk/elearning

The module is accessible by password only but provides an excellent visual and interactive overview of the newborn examination particularly of the four screening elements of the newborn examination. Completion of the module is a useful learning resource particularly for doctors in training that can complement the Induction Programme content for the newborn examination.

Recommendations for practice

There are viable options to be considered to assist practitioners with the maintenance of their skills in conducting the newborn examination. Firstly, the facilitation of the examinations in a clinic setting would engage all health-care disciplines in the examination on a rota basis. A daily clinic would have an allocated health-care professional to take a lead role and in that way, all disciplines could experience equity in exposure to the examinations on a fairly regular basis. The workload of the newborn examinations would be fairly distributed overall, negating the need for junior doctors to feel overloaded. Ultimately, not only the quality of the examination would improve but also morale and motivation amongst all practitioners would be more likely to increase. Alternatively, midwives and/or neonatal nurses could be allocated 1 day on a rota basis to undertake the newborn examinations alongside the doctors in training. Overall, these initiatives strengthen collaborative working relationships. However, such approaches do require a structured workforce and resource planning to be successful. The roll out of the NIPE Programme will be an important focus for some maternity units with a restructuring of newborn examination service.

There is increasing educational activity provided across the country to support and update the newborn examination practitioners. This could be viewed as a healthy indication that there is demand for updates in relation to growing performance. Updating activity should be a prerequisite of the maternity unit Training Needs Analysis and a register maintained of all practitioners within the maternity unit, who are competent to conduct the newborn examination. Annual assessment of newborn examination practitioners should be considered as a performance measure. Evidence of the assessment can be used by midwives at the annual supervisory interview and for neonatal nurses, through the personal development review (PDR). The number of examinations conducted to maintain and demonstrate competence should be agreed on an individual basis and local need. A similar assessment document could be used to assess junior doctors. Such a mechanism may highlight the failings in the systems, which limit skill exposure for practitioners that may have consequences for the newborn.

Clinical effectiveness

The concept of Practice Development Groups is not new to health-care disciplines, but it is a very inclusive way of disseminating information and monitoring clinical effectiveness in a non-threatening environment. The remit of the examination of the newborn practice development group would embrace all aspects of the clinical service, would be multidisciplinary and provide the all-important peer support. The aims of the group could include the following:

• Audit activity
• Standardisation of best practice approaches
• Mentorship responsibilities
• Peer assessment
• Dissemination and discussion from current evidence reviews to support practice
• Feedback from educational updates
• Identification of local training needs
• Clinical debate and case reviews.

This list is not exhaustive and may be tailored to the local needs of each Trust. However, its benefits are far reaching in terms of clinical effectiveness and monitoring how well the service is performing as well as identifying its limitations. What is important is that it would promote collaboration in the approaches to newborn service provision that could balance the need to provide safe and effective outcomes for mothers and babies and minimise or avoid those that may require recourse from the courts or professional regulator. For further guidance on the wider issues relating to structures and processes for effective implementation of screening programmes within Trusts, see *Part 7: Roles and Responsibilities for Service Commissioning and Provision, Newborn and Infant Physical Examination Standards and Competencies* document (UK NSC 2008b) together with External Quality Assurance Process for Antenatal and Newborn Screening Programmes – Guidance for Providers and Commissioners (UK NSC 2014).

Conclusion

The introduction of the newborn examination as a part of the midwives' role has become part of a move towards greater multidisciplinary working and collaboration with other health-care practitioners. As a means to provide midwives with an opportunity to enhance their own role and position, the focus is to improve care programmes and outcomes for mothers and babies with potential benefits for health service provision overall.

Historically, the role of the midwife has been the subject of much discourse with the introduction of 'new' roles often widely debated and challenged from within the profession itself. What is clear is that in seeking such opportunities, midwives must have a clear understanding of their professional mission to ensure the safety and well-being of mothers and babies. Whilst the legal framework for care is often less clear and often misunderstood, at its heart it has the same fundamental aim to protect mothers and babies from harm and provides its own guidance on how this may be fulfilled.

The NMC as the regulator for midwives and nurses has its own statutory functions with methods in place to guide, monitor and scrutinise practice, which includes structures and processes that drive its own fitness to practise framework. Likewise, the legal system holds a unique position in using its statutory authority to remind health-care professionals to practice lawfully. Finally, the employer has commitment to ensure that robust systems are in place to facilitate effective processes and outcomes for care and that the fitness for purpose of its employers is appropriately monitored and managed.

At the time of some uncertainty, midwives should see the enhancement of their role as an opportunity to develop skills that will encourage positive relationships with other health-care groups that will forge the shared values and commitment of health-care programmes rather than separate out the roles of each group. Furthermore, maybe the time has come for understanding the important role of regulation in both legal and professional terms and the governance framework of the NHS and will be something that is welcomed rather than feared in the future.

Examination of the newborn: professional issues – a case study.

Julie was a 25-year-old woman (gravida 3 para 2). She had an uneventful antenatal history, and her pregnancy had been free of complications. There was no family history of congenital heart disease.

Julie had a spontaneous vaginal delivery of a male infant she named Callum. Callum weighed 3.5 kg (Apgars were 8 at 1 min and 9 at 5 min). Shortly after birth, Julie gave Callum his first feed and he took a small amount by bottle.

As she had requested a 6-hour discharge, the midwife undertook the full newborn examination when Callum was approximately 6 hours old. When the midwife auscultated the heart, a soft murmur could be heard. Callum had no other symptoms and pulse oximetry revealed pre- and post-ductal saturation readings of 98%. All other aspects of the examination were within normal limits, and the midwife had checked that no risk factors for infection were present. The midwife referred Callum to the duty paediatrician but she was unable to come straight away due to an emergency situation on the neonatal unit. The midwife explained her findings to the mum and the requirement for Callum to be seen by the paediatrician.

At 6 hours old, his mum was ready to leave the ward. Her partner had arrived and they seemed in a rush. The midwife called the paediatrician again but none were available at that time due to other priorities.

Julie and her partner refused to wait and began to pack her things. The midwife explained the risks to Callum if they left without him being re-examined but the mother and father were determined to go.

Here's what the midwife did next:
- She made sure the mother and father understood the risks involved in leaving the hospital with Callum.
- She explained the signs to look for should Callum's condition deteriorate and made sure the mother had emergency contact numbers.
- She arranged for the mother and father to be seen at the paediatric outpatient's clinic as soon as possible.
- She informed the paediatric staff.
- She informed her manager and supervisor of midwives.
- She completed all the relevant documentation including a Trust incident form.

  Think about how you would deal with a situation like this in your Trust. What does your Trust policy say about this?

Look here for some resources on dealing with professional issues surrounding the newborn examination.

Nursing and Midwifery Council (NMC): http://www.nmc-uk.org/

Look here to see the latest hearings and outcomes for professional misconduct from the NMC: http://www.nmc-uk.org/hearings/

Tengnah GR, Patel C (2010) *Law and Professional Issues in Midwifery.* Exeter: Learning Matters.

Hutchinson A (2010) Critical reflection on a midwife's development and practice in relation to examination of the newborn. *Midwives Magazine:* December 2009/January 2010.

Lumsden H (2008) Health visitor's role of the physical examination of the 6-8week event. *Journal of Health and Social Care improvement* June 1–6. Available from: http://www.wlv.ac.uk/pdf/jun2008_HLumsden.pdf (accessed February 2015).

Mitchell M (2003) Midwives conducting the neonatal examination: part 1. *British Journal of Midwifery* **11**, 1, 16–21.

Mitchell M (2003) Midwives conducting the neonatal examination: part 2. *British Journal of Midwifery* **11**, 1, 80–84.

Steele D (2007) Examining the newborn: why don't midwives use their skills? *British Journal of Midwifery* **15**, 12, 784–752.

See this link for a power point presentation on Professional Roles and Responsibilities and the Neonatal Examination. http://www.anglia.ac.uk/ruskin/en/home/microsites/postgraduate_medical_institute/news/raising_the_profile.Maincontent.0017.file.tmp/The%20Midwives%20Statutory%20Role%20-%20Bev%20Lynn.pdf

References

Baker K (2010) Midwives should perform the routine examination of the newborn. *British Journal of Midwifery* **18**(7), 416–421.

Bannister P (2008) Management of infants born with a cleft lip and palate. Part1. *Infant* **4**(1), 57–60.

Dermott K, Bick D, Norman R (2006) *Clinical Guidance and Evidence for Post Natal Care of Recently Delivered Women and Their Babies.* London: National Collaborating Centre for Primary Care and Royal College of General Practitioners.

DH (2001) *Reference Guide to the Consent for Examination and Treatment*. London: DH.

DH (2004a) *NHS Knowledge and Skills Framework*. London: DH.

DH (2004b) *Agenda for Change*. London: DH.

DH (2006) *Skills for Health: Learning for Change in Healthcare First Report to the Department of Health and the NHS*. London: DH. Available from: http://www.skillsforhealth. org.uk/~/media/Resource-Library/PDF/glossary09.ashx (accessed July 2010).

DH (2007a) *Trust, Assurance and Safety: The Regulation of Health Professionals in the 21st Century*. London: The Stationery Office.

DH (2007b) *Maternity Matters: Choice, Access and Continuity of Care in a Safe Service*. London: DH.

DH (2009a) *Skills For Health Maternity*. London: Department of Health. Available from: http://www.skillsforhealth.org.uk/ (accessed August 2014).

DH (2009b) *The Healthy Child Programme: Pregnancy and the First 5 Years of Life*. London: Department of Health. Available from: https://www.gov.uk/government/publications/healthy-child-programme-pregnancy-and-the-first-5-years-of-life (accessed August 2014).

DH (2009c) *Reference Guide to Consent for Examination or Treatment*. London: Department of Health on Consent for Treatment.

DH (2010) *Midwifery 2020. Delivering Expectations*. London: Department of Health. Available from: https://www.gov.uk/government/uploads/system/uploads/attachment_data/file/216029/dh_119470.pdf (accessed August 2014).

DH (2013a) *Public Health Functions to be Exercised by NHS England, Service Specification 21. Newborn and Infant Physical Examination Screening Programme*. London: Department of Health. https://www.gov.uk/government/uploads/system/uploads/attachment_data/file/256488/21_nhs_newborn_and_infant_physical_examination.pdf (accessed April 2014).

DH (2013b) The Francis report. http://www.midstaffspublicinquiry.com/report (accessed April 2014).

DH (2013c) The 6 C's of nursing. Department of Health. http://www.google.co.uk/url?sa=t&rct= j&q=&esrc=s&source=web&cd=1&cad=rja&ved=0CC8QFjAA&url=http%3A%2F% 2Fwww.changemodel.nhs.uk%2Fdl%2Fcv_content%2F30520&ei= wCqGUvzzDeaU0AXplYDAAw&usg=AFQjCNGA6uRFX1weZRdNEAqA1pinerY71A&bvm= bv.56643336,d.d2k

Gargan P (2010) Implications of ultra sound scanning for midwives. *British Journal of Midwifery* **18**(7), 429–435.

Griffiths R (2008a) Guide to the Mental Capacity Act (2005): determining best interests. *British Journal of Midwifery* **16**(5), 327–328.

Griffiths R (2008b) Guide to the Mental Capacity Act (2005): decision making capacity. *British Journal of Midwifery* **16**(4), 262–263.

Griffiths R (2008c) Midwives and confidentiality. *British Journal of Midwifery* **16**(1), 51–53.

Griffiths R (2008d) Disclosing patient information. *British Journal of Midwifery* **16**(2), 126–127.

Hayes J, Dave S, Rogers C, Quist-Therson E, Townsend J (2003) A national survey of the routine examination of the newborn. *Midwifery* **19**(4), 277–284.

Law Commission (2014) Regulation of Health Care Professionals. Available from: http:// lawcommission.justice.gov.uk/docs/lc345_regulation_of_healthcare_professionals.pdf (accessed August 2014).

Lewis P (1998) Boundaries to practice: when is a midwife not a midwife? *RCM Midwives Journal* **2**(2), 60–61.

Lomax A, Evans C (2005) Examination of the newborn: the franchise experience integrating theory and practice. *Infant* **1**(2), 58–61.

McDonald S (2008) Examining a newborn baby: are midwives using their skills. *British Journal of Midwifery* **16**(11), 722–724.

Michaelides S (1998) Examination of the newborn. *MIDIRS Midwifery Digest* **8**: 93–96.

Morrell M (2002) Should midwives carry out ultra sound scans? *British Journal of Midwifery* **2**(5), 202–208.

NHS Executive North West Regional Professional Forum Group (1996). *Professional Boundaries between Medical and Nursing Staff and the Future Strategy for Nursing.* London: NHS Exec.

NHS Quality Improvement Scotland (2008) Best Practice Statement. NHS Quality Improvement Scotland.

NHS (2013) NHS Public health functions agreement 2014-15. Public health functions to be exercised by NHS England. NHS England 2013. Available from: https://www.gov.uk/government/uploads/system/uploads/attachment_data/file/256502/nhs_public_health_functions_agreement_2014-15.pdf (accessed August 2014).

NHSLA (2012) Clinical negligence scheme for trusts. *Maternity Clinical Risk Management Standards 2010/11.* London: NHS Litigation Authority. Available from: http://www.nhsla.com/NR/rdonlyres/786ACCA2-5145-4461-8B47-5A13117DEF3C/0/CNSTMaternityStandards201011.doc.

NMC (2008a) *Consent: Advice Document.* London: NMC.

NMC (2008b) *Advocacy and Autonomy: Advice Document.* London: NMC.

NMC (2008c) *Confidentiality: Advice Document.* London: NMC.

NMC (2010a) *The Code: Standards for Conduct Performance and Ethics.* London: NMC. Available from: http://www.nmc-uk.org/Documents/Standards/The-code-A4-20100406.pdf (accessed August 2014).

NMC (2010b) *Record Keeping: Guidance for Nurses and Midwives.* London: NMC.

NMC (2011) *The PREP Handbook.* London: NMC.

NMC (2012) *Midwives Rules and Standards.* London: NMC.

NMC (2013) Our response to the Francis report. Available from: http://www.nmc-uk.org/About-us/Our-response-to-the-Francis-Inquiry-Report/ (accessed August 2014).

NMC (2014) *NMC Welcomes Publication of a Bill that Could "Revolutionise Healthcare Regulation.* NMC: London.

NMC (2015) *The Code: Standards for Conduct Performance and Ethics.* NMC: London. Available from: http://www.nmc-uk.org/The-revised-Code/ (accessed February 2015).

Steele D (2007) Examining the newborn: why don't midwives use their skills? *British Journal of Midwifery* **15**(12), 748–752.

Simms, M., Mitchell, S. (2012) Seamless service? Midwives report job satisfaction from carrying out the examination of the newborn. Yet the numbers actually doing so are low. *Midwives* **3**, 48–49.

UK NSC (2008a) *Ante Natal and Newborn Screening Programmes: Newborn and Infant Physical Examination Standards and Competencies.* London: NSC. Available from: www.screening.nhs.uk/home.htm (accessed July 2010).

UK NSC (2008b) *Newborn and Infant Physical Examination: Standards and Competencies. Part 7: Roles and Responsibilities for Service Commissioning and Provision.* London: NHS, pp. 36–41. Available from: http://newbornphysical.screening.nhs.uk (accessed July 2010).

UK NSC (2014) External quality assurance process for antenatal and newborn screening programmes - guidance for providers and commissioners. Available from http://newbornphysical.screening.nhs.uk/ (accessed August 2014).

Useful website addresses

Chromosomal and genetic problems

Achondroplasia
The Achondroplasia Society – www.achondroplasia.co.uk
Little People of America – www.lpaonline.org – useful support for achondroplasia and other short stature

Cystic fibrosis
Cystic Fibrosis Trust – www.cftrust.org.uk

DiGeorge syndrome
Max Appeal – www.maxappeal.org.uk – support for DiGeorge and velocardiofacial syndromes

Down's syndrome
Down's Syndrome Association – www.downs-syndrome.org.uk; information, booklets, helpline and contacts for local support group

Duchenne muscular dystrophy
Duchenne Family Support Group – www.dfsg.org.uk

Edwards' and Patau's syndrome
S.O.F.T. UK – www.soft.org.uk – information and support for families affected by Edwards' and Patau's syndromes

Epidermolysis bullosa
DebRA – www.debra.org.uk; includes contact details for the EB nursing team

Examination of the Newborn: An Evidence-Based Guide, Second Edition. Edited by Anne Lomax.
© 2015 John Wiley & Sons, Ltd. Published 2015 by John Wiley & Sons, Ltd.
Companion Website: www.wiley.com/go/lomax/newborn

Inborn errors of metabolism and MCADD

CLIMB – www.climb.org.uk for family support

Mowat-Wilson Syndrome Support Group

http://www.mowatwilsonsyndrome.org.uk/

Osteogenesis imperfecta

Brittle Bone Society – www.brittlebone.org – UK support

Osteogenesis Imperfecta Foundation – www.oif.org – advice leaflets on handling affected infants

Prader–Willi syndrome

The Prader–Willi Syndrome Association UK – www.pwsa.co.uk – parent and professional support

Sickle cell disease

Sickle Cell Society – www.sicklecellsociety.org – advice about sickle cell disease including for carriers

Thalassaemia

UK Thalassaemia Society – www.ukts.org – patient and professional advice

Turner syndrome

Turner Syndrome Support Society – www.tss.org.uk – parent support and information for professionals including health checklist

Savage M – Diagnosing Turner Syndrome – downloadable booklet available from Turner Syndrome Support Society website

General websites

Contact A Family – www.cafamily.org.uk – for links to UK-based support groups for genetic and other disorders in childhood

NHS Newborn and physical Examination Programme: http://newbornphysical.screening.nhs.uk/

Royal College of Obstetricians and Gynaecologists Green Top Guideline No. 8 2005. Amniocentesis and Chorionic Villus Sampling. Available from: www.rcog.org.uk

Ultrasound Screening (supplement to ultrasound screening for Fetal Abnormalities) RCOG Working Party 1998 explains antenatal ultrasound and includes an information leaflet for mothers and fathers. Available from: www.rcog.org.uk

Learning resources

Fetal Anomaly Screening Scan – Online resource: http://www.fetalanomaly .screening.nhs.uk/fetalanomalyresource/

If you are a member of the Royal College of Midwives (RCM), you can access the learning module on Genes and Chromosomes called 'Its in the Genes' (access via i learn link on RCM webpage): https://www.rcm.org.uk/

For more information on this resource, look here: https://www.rcm.org.uk/ content/it%E2%80%99s-in-the-genes

Also visit the NHS National Genetics and Genomics Education Centre to access modules on genetics and inheritance http://www.geneticseducation.nhs.uk/ mededu.

NIPE Information leaflet for mothers and fathers

An introduction to physical examinations of newborn babies and those aged six to eight weeks

What is the physical examination?

When your baby is born, the midwife will carry out some checks. You will then be offered a more detailed physical examination of your baby **within 72 hours of birth and again at six to eight weeks old.** These examinations include a screening examination to find those babies who may have a problem with their eyes, heart, hips and, in boys, testicles. Your baby will experience a lot of physical changes in the first two months of life and this is why the examination is repeated at six to eight weeks.

This section gives you information about:

• why the physical examinations are carried out;
• who will carry them out;
• where the examinations will be carried out;
• how the examinations are carried out;
• how to prepare for the examinations;
• what the results may mean for parents and babies;
• what happens after the examinations;
• where the results will be recorded; and
• where you can go for more information and advice.

Why should I have my baby examined?

The purpose of the examination is to identify babies more likely to have conditions that need to be investigated. However, screening will not always pick

Examination of the Newborn: An Evidence-Based Guide, Second Edition. Edited by Anne Lomax.
© 2015 John Wiley & Sons, Ltd. Published 2015 by John Wiley & Sons, Ltd.
Companion Website: www.wiley.com/go/lomax/newborn

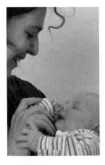

up every problem. Some conditions may only become apparent after several weeks or months and a few may still not be found at the six to eight week check.

The physical examinations can help identify health concerns at an early stage. Most babies who have the physical examinations will be healthy and will not have any health problems. In some cases the findings may suggest a problem, but further investigations often show there is nothing to be concerned about. Most of the problems babies have are minor and do not need treatment.

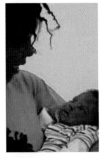

Health professionals such as GPs, midwives or health visitors are happy to see parents who may have worries about the health and development of their babies.

For the small number of babies who do have serious problems, there are a lot of benefits of having these identified as soon as possible. Early treatment can improve the health of the baby and prevent disability. If further investigations or treatments are needed, an appointment with a specialist will be arranged.

It is recommended that you have your baby examined, but if you are not sure, discuss it with your midwife or other health professional. Also if you think your baby might not have been examined, speak to your midwife, health visitor or GP.

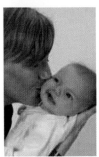

Who will do the examinations?

A doctor, midwife, health visitor or nurse will carry out the examinations. All health professionals carrying out the examination have been specially trained.

Where will the examinations be carried out?

Depending on the health professional doing the examination, and the age of the baby, the examinations may take place in a hospital, GP's surgery, clinic, children's centre or at home.

How are the examinations carried out?

The health professional will introduce themselves and explain the examination. They will ask you about your pregnancy, and the birth, and will check your family history. They will also ask you about your own health and how you are feeling. This is an opportunity for you to talk about the general care of your baby and aspects such as feeding, crying or sleeping and to discuss anything that might be worrying you.

The examinations are normally done when your baby is calm and comfortable. The health professional will carry out an overall physical examination which includes a head-to-toe examination of your baby, looking at their development, feeding, weight, alertness and general wellbeing.

The health professional will look at your baby's eyes, heart, hips and, in boys, his testicles. They will listen to your baby's heart with a stethoscope and will look at your baby's eyes using an instrument called an ophthalmoscope.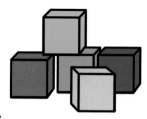

Other parts of the examination involve gently handling your baby and moving their legs to check the hips. This should not hurt, although testing your baby's hips can sometimes be a little uncomfortable. If necessary, you can comfort your baby during and after the examination.

How can I prepare for the examinations?

You will be with your baby during the examination but you do not need to prepare anything special. Your baby will need to be undressed for part of the examination, but will be kept warm.

For the six to eight week examination it will be useful for you to think about the growth and development checklist in your baby's child-health record (sometimes known as the 'red book') before talking with your health visitor or doctor.

The checklist asks you to think about a number of questions and discuss them at the 6-8 week examination.

The checklist asks you to think about the following.

• Whether you feel well yourself

• Any worries you have about feeding your baby

• Any concerns you have about your baby's weight gain

• Whether your baby watches your face and follows it with his/her eyes

• Whether your baby turns towards the light

• Whether your baby smiles at you

• Whether you think your baby can hear you

• Whether your baby is startled by loud noises

• Any problems you have looking after your baby

• Whether you have any worries about your baby

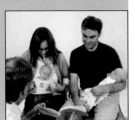

What the results may mean for parents and babies

This section contains general information about conditions that may be found by the physical examination. It is not possible to go into detail here about further referrals or treatments in this booklet. If there is a problem, what happens next will depend on what has been found during the examination. The health professional will be able to discuss this with the parent. Most babies will benefit from the treatments available.

As well as an overall physical examination, the following four
screening examinations will be carried out.

Eyes:

The health professional will examine the baby's eyes, focusing on how
they look and move. If the eye looks cloudy, this may mean the baby
has a cataract and this may affect how well
the baby can see. Babies who may have
problems will be referred to an eye specialist
(an ophthalmologist). About two or three in
10,000 babies have eye problems that need
treatment.

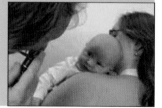

Heart:

A general examination of the baby's heart is done by listening with a
stethoscope. Sometimes murmurs are picked up. This can be worrying for
the parent. A murmur is an extra noise made by blood as it passes through
the heart. Murmurs are common in babies and do not necessarily mean that
there is a heart problem. In nearly all cases
the heart is actually normal. If the health
professional finds something that suggests
there may be a heart problem, another
examination and further tests will be
arranged. Around one in 200 babies have a
heart problem that needs treatment.

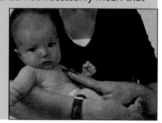

Hips:

Babies can be born with hip joints that are not formed properly. If
untreated this can lead to a limp and joint problems. Babies who could
benefit from further investigation may
have an ultrasound scan of the hips
followed by an appointment with a
specialist to check the hips again. About
one or two in 1,000 babies have hip
problems that need treatment.

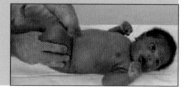

Testicles:

Baby boys will be checked to make sure their testicles are in the right place. It can take several months for them to drop down into the scrotum. If this does not happen, a specialist may advise a small operation when the boy is one or two years old. About one in 100 baby boys have problems that need treatment.

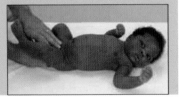

What happens after the examinations?

The health professional who does the examination will discuss the results with you immediately. If the examination shows that everything seems to be all right with your baby, there will be no need for any further action.

The examination may highlight concerns with your baby. If this is the case, the health professional will either ask to see you and your baby again, or will offer you an appointment with a specialist. The specialist will give you a detailed explanation about the concerns identified, any further investigations and possible treatment.

Waiting to see the specialist can be an anxious time. Don't hesitate to talk to your midwife, GP or health visitor about your concerns.

Where will the results be recorded?

The outcome of the examination carried out within the first 72 hours of birth will be recorded in both your maternity notes and in your baby's child-health record.

The outcome of the six to eight week examination will be recorded in your baby's child-health record. You need to keep this record safe and take it with you whenever you and your baby see a health professional.

Additional information leaflets for parents can be found on the NIPE website at: http://newbornphysical.screening.nhs.uk/leaflets

Glossary of terms

Developmental dysplasia of the hip: a spectrum of hip disease ranging from dysplasia of the hip to irreducible hip dislocation.

Dislocation of the hip joint: a separation of the hip joint surface which can be (i) irreducible – a fixed separation, or (ii) reducible (dislocatable) – a dynamic process of dislocation. Stress on the hip joint that can result in reduction of the joint clinically.

Dysplasia of the hip joint: an abnormality of the development of the morphological (shape) of the acetabulum without subluxation or dislocation of the hip joint.

Hip spica: a rigid plaster cast including both hip joints, legs and around the lower abdomen and spine. Used as a splintage. Method after open or closed reduction of the hip joint.

Incidence: the number of new cases recorded over a specific time period (i.e. 1 year).

Instability of the hip joint: a clinical diagnosis of a reducible or subluxable joint. Tested by Ortolani or Barlow manoeuvres.

Negative predictive value: True negative ÷ (True negative + False negative); a measure of when the test is negative if the disease is not present.

Ortolani test: a clinical test of hip joint reducibility.

Pavlik harness: a dynamic device used to hold the hips in flexion and abduction in a safe and stable position encouraging stabilisation of a reducible hip joint.

Positive predictive value: True positive ÷ (True positive + False positive); a measure of when the test is positive if the disease is present.

Prevalence: the number of cases recorded in the community at a specific moment in time.

Sensitivity: True positive ÷ (True positive + False negative); an assessment of the false-negative rate.

Specificity: True negative ÷ (True negative + False positive); an assessment of the false-positive rate.

Subluxation of the hip joint: a 'partial' dislocation with some contact between the hip joint surfaces, usually with poor congruity; (i) irreducible – a fixed separation; (ii) reducible – can be reduced.

Examination of the Newborn: An Evidence-Based Guide, Second Edition. Edited by Anne Lomax.
© 2015 John Wiley & Sons, Ltd. Published 2015 by John Wiley & Sons, Ltd.
Companion Website: www.wiley.com/go/lomax/newborn

Ultrasound imaging: a diagnostic method that uses high-frequency sound transmitted and received to image the structures of the hip joint.

Von Rosen splint: a rigid device used to hold the hips in flexion and abduction encouraging stabilisation of a reducible hip joint.

Index

Note: Page numbers in **bold** represent figures.

A

abdominal examination
  abnormalities, 125
  approach to, 124–25
  bowel obstruction, 126–27
  necrotising enterocolitis, 127–28
achondroplasia, 187
acne (neonatal), 78–79, **79**
acrocyanosis, 74–75
adrenal hyperplasia, congenital, **137**, 137–38
alcohol, 12, 13, **21**
alertness, states of, 198–201, **199–200**
amniocentesis, 175
Andersson, O., 40
androgen insensitivity syndrome, **137**, 138–39
ankyloglossia (tongue-tie), 109, 120–121
anomaly scan, 18–22 week, 174
antibiotics, NICE guidance, 10
antidepressant medications, 18–19
aortic stenosis, **45**, 48, **51**, **58**
Association of Tongue Tie Practitioners (ATP), 109
asthma screening, 17
atopy screening, 17
atrial septal defect, **45**, **51**
atrioventricular septal defect, **45**, **51**, **58**
attachment behaviours, 19
autosomal dominant inheritance, 173
autosomal recessive inheritance, 173

B

Babinski reflex, 95, **96**
Barlow, T. G., 145
Barlow test, 146
BCG vaccination resources, 26
Beckwith–Wiedemann syndrome, **51**, 108
Bedford, C., xiii–xiv
behavioural status
  alertness, states of, 198–201, **199–200**
  case studies, 209–10
  consoling strategies, 201–2
  documentation, 208
  examination, describing behaviours during, 206–8
  examination preparations, 205–6
  facial recognition, 207

  fetal development, 193–94
  mother and father, 194–97
  mother and father, feedback to, 197–98
  overview, 192–93, 209
  postgraduate training, 208
  resources, 210
  self-soothing, 203
  sensitivity, stress, 202–5, **203–5**
  smiles, 202
  sucking, 95–96, 207
  swaddling, 199, **199–200**, 201
benzodiazepines, 19
Bialik, V., 142
bicuspid aortic valve, **45**
bifid uvula, 108
Billings, J. A., 3
Blake, D., 20, 21
blood circulation
  fetal, 36–38, **37**
  postnatal, 38–39
blood gases measurement, 64
blood glucose monitoring, 10
blood pressure measurement, 55–56
body mass index (BMI), raised, 8
Booking scan, 173–74
Bornstein, M. H., 8
bowel obstruction, 126–27
Brazelton, T. B., 194
breastfeeding, 109, 121, 180, 194, 201
breathing movements, 34, 40–41, 52
breech presentation, 8
bruising (ecchymosis), 77
Bruschweiller-Stern, N., 194, 196

C

café-au-lait spots, 82
calcaneovalgus, 161, **162**
Candida infection, 82
capillary haemangioma (strawberry naevus), 84, **84**, 119, **119**
caput succedaneum, **105**
carbamazepine, 18
cardiac screening
  abnormalities, origins, 36

cardiac screening (*continued*)
   abnormality detection, 55–61, **58–59**
   blood pressure measurement, 55–56
   cord clamping, delayed, 39–40
   echocardiography, 57, **59**, 60, 61
   electrocardiography, 57
   examination generally, 44
   examination process, 49–55, **51**, **54–55**
   extrauterine life transition, 36
   fetal circulation, 36–38, **37**
   follow-up, 57
   heart auscultatory areas, **48**, 66
   heart development, 34–36, **35**
   heart murmurs, **47**, 47–48, 52–53, 66
   heart sounds, 46–47
   history taking, 8, 15–17, **16**, 25, 49–50
   hypoglycaemia/hypoxia/hypothermia impacts,
      42–44, **43**
   NIPE process map, 53, **54**
   overview, 32
   postnatal circulation, 38–39
   pulse oximetry, 53, 56, 59–61
   resources, 65–66
   tools, 48–49, **49**
   ultrasonography, 57–59, **58**
   see also congenital heart defects (CHD)
cardiomyopathy, dilated, **58**
cardiomyopathy, hypertrophic, **58**
cataracts, congenital, **115**, 115–16, 182
cavernous haemangioma, 84
cephalhaematoma, **105**
chest wall transillumination, 64
Chlamydia, 117
chorionic villus sampling, 175
chromosomal translocation, 172
chromosome, 172
circulation
   fetal, 36–38, **37**
   postnatal, 38–39
cleft lip, palate, xiv, 19, 107–8
clubfoot
   bone anatomy, **153**
   diagnosis, **154**, 154–55, 166
   foot abduction brace, 159, **159**
   overview, 153
   Ponseti cast, 156–59, **157–60**, 166
   positional, 155, **156**
   range of motion, normal foot, **157**
   structural, 155, **156**
   treatment, 155–60, **156–60**, 166
coarctation of the aorta (CoA), **45**, **51**, 53, 56, **58**,
      184
The Code, 216–20
competency framework initiatives, 213–15
confidentiality, 218–20
congenital adrenal hyperplasia, **137**, 137–38
congenital cataracts, **115**, 115–16, 182
congenital glaucoma buphthalmos ('ox eye'), 118,
      119
congenital heart defects
   abnormality detection, 55–61, **58–59**
   case study, 65

incidence, 45–46, **45–46**
   origins, 34
   presentation, 45–46, **46**, **51**
   resources, 65–66
   screening, 8, 15–17, **16**, 25, 44
   see also cardiac screening
congenital hypothyroidism, 176
congenital talipes calcaneovalgus, 149
congenital vertical talus, 161–63, **162–63**
consent, 217–18
consoling strategies, 201–2
cord clamping, delayed, 39–40
cord intact resuscitation, 40
cradle cap (seborrhoeic dermatitis), 79, **79**
craniosynostosis, **105**
craniotabes, **105**
Cri du chat syndrome, **51**
Cross, K. W., 62
Crossland, D. S., 56
cryptorchidism (testes, undescended), **130**,
      130–134, **133**, 139–40
Cummings, J., 215
cutis aplasia, 105, **106**
cutis marmorata, 75, **75**
cyanosis, **45**, 50, 181
cystic fibrosis, 127, 176
cystic hygroma, 110, **110**
cytomegalovirus (CMV), 117

D
deletion, 172
depression, material, 18–19
developmental dysplasia of the hip.
      see hip dysplasia
DH National Service Specification 21 Newborn and
      Infant Physical Examination Screening
      Programme, xiii
DiGeorge syndrome, **51**, 186
digits, absence/shortening of, 164–65, **165**
disclosure, 218–20
domestic abuse, **21**
double inlet left ventricle, **58**
double outlet right ventricle (DORV), **45**, **58**
Down's syndrome (trisomy 21), **51**, 108, **115**,
      179–83, **181**
drug abuse, 13–14, **21**, 26
Duchenne muscular dystrophy, 177
ductus arteriosus, 37, **37**, 39, 53
ductus venosus, 36, **37**
Dunn, P. M., 145
duodenal atresia, 126, 181, 182
dynamic splintage, **150**, 150–151, **152**

E
early-onset sepsis, 9–10
ear position, **106**, 106–7
Ebstein's anomaly, 15, 18, **45**, **58**
echocardiography, 57, **59**, 60, 61
Edward's syndrome (trisomy 18), **51**, 183
electrocardiography, 57
epidermolysis bullosa, 187–88

epispadias, **130**, 137
erythema toxicum neonatorum, 77, **78**
Evans, C., xiii
exchange transfusion, 91
eye examination
   anatomy, **111**
   behavioural status, 207
   capillary haemangioma (strawberry naevus), 84,
      84, 119, **119**
   congenital cataracts, **115**, 115–16, 182
   congenital glaucoma buphthalmos ('ox eye'),
      118, **119**
   embryology, 111
   history taking, **16**, 25–26, 112
   injury, non-accidental, 118
   leukocoria, 114, **114**, 117, 118
   nasolacrimal duct obstruction, 120
   NIPE process map, 112, **113**
   ophthalmoscopy, 114
   overview, 110–111
   persistent hyperplastic primary vitreous
      (PHPV), 117
   physiology, 111–12
   ptosis, 119–20
   retinoblastoma, 116
   retinopathy of prematurity, 110, 118
   strabismus, 120
   TORCH infections, 116–17

F
fetal anomaly screening, **6**, 11–14
fetal circulation, 36–38, **37**
fetal DNA, obtaining, 175
Finigan, V., 109
fluorescent in situ hybridisation (FISH), 173
fluoxetine, 18
foot abduction brace, 159, **159**
foot abnormalities
   bone anatomy, **153**
   calcaneovalgus, 161, **162**
   clubfoot, **153–54**, 153–60, **156–60**, 166
   congenital vertical talus, 161–63, **162–63**
   digits, absence/shortening of, 164–65, **165**
   metatarsus adductus, 160–161, **161**
   overview, 151–53, 165–66
   polydactyly, 163–64, **163–64**
   polysyndactyly, 164, **165**
   range of motion, normal, **157**
   syndactyly, 164, **165**
foramen ovale, 37, **37**
Francis Inquiry, 215

G
Gardiner, H. M., 145
gastrointestinal obstruction, 126–27
gene, 172
genetic, chromosomal problems
   achondroplasia, 187
   anomaly scan, 18–22 week,174
   antenatal screening, 173–74, 177
   background, 171–72
   Booking scan, 173–74

DiGeorge syndrome/velocardiofacial syndrome,
   186
Down's syndrome (trisomy 21), **51**, 108, **115**,
   179–83, **181**
dysmorphic baby examination, 178–79, **179**
Edward's syndrome (trisomy 18), **51**, 183
epidermolysis bullosa, 187–88
family history/tree, 178
feedback to family, 188–89
fetal DNA, obtaining, 175
hormonal screening, 174
inborn errors of metabolism (IEM), 188
inheritance modes, 173
mothers/fathers screening, 174–75
Mowat–Wilson syndrome, 190–191
osteogenesis imperfecta, 186
Patau syndrome (trisomy 13), **51**, 183
postnatal screening, 175–77
Prader–Willi syndrome, 186
sickle cell, thalassaemia screening, **5**, 174
terminology, 172
Turner's syndrome, **51**, 183–86, **184–85**
ultrasonography, 173–74
genital examination
   androgen insensitivity syndrome, **137**, 138–39
   approach to, females, 132–33
   approach to, males, 129–32, **130–131**
   congenital adrenal hyperplasia, **137**, 137–38
   development, sex determinants, 128–29, **129**
   deviations, male, **130**
   epispadias, **130**, 137
   history taking, **16**, 26
   hydrocele, **130**, 131–32, 136
   hypospadias, **130**, 132, **136**, 136–37, 139–40
   inguinal hernia, **130**, 130–132, **135**, 135–36
   overview, 128
   resources, 140
   testes, undescended (cryptorchidism), **130**,
      130–134, **133**, 139–40
   testicular torsion, 134, **135**
genitalia, ambiguous, **130**, 137
gestational age assessment, 91–94, **93–94**
glaucoma, congenital, 118, **119**
glucose levels, 42–44, **43**
Gnanalingham, M. G., 60
Gonorrhoea, 117
Graf, R., 142, 147
grasp reflex, 95, **95**
Griffiths, R., 218
Grissom, L. E., 147
group B haemolytic streptococcus, 9–10
growth charts, 97–99, **98**
growth restriction, 11

H
habituation, 206
Harcke, H. T., 147
Harlequin sign, 75
head and neck examination
   cleft lip, palate, xiv, 19, 107–8
   ear position, **106**, 106–7
   facial features, 105–6

head and neck examination (*continued*)
   fontanelles, sutures, 105
   hearing tests, 107
   malformations, **105**
   mouth, 107
   neck, 109–10
   nose, 107
   process, 104–5
   scalp, 105
   tongue-tie (ankyloglossia), 109, 120–121
hearing tests, 107
heart assessment. *see* cardiac screening
heart auscultatory areas, **48**, 66
heart development, 34–36, **35**
heart murmurs, **47**, 47–48, 52–53, 66
heart sounds, 46–47
hepatitis B screening, **5**, 11
heroin withdrawal, 14, 26
herpes (neonatal), 81–82
hip dysplasia
   Barlow test, 146
   classification, 142–43, **143**
   clinical hip joint instability, 145
   clinical screening, 145–47
   consequences, 143–44
   definition, 142
   dislocation, 143, **143**
   dynamic splintage, **150**, 150–151, **152**
   incidence, 144
   knee hyperextension, 166–67
   Ortolani test, 146
   resources, 166–67
   risk factors, 8
   screening, **16**, 25
   subluxation, **143**
   treatment, 149–51
   treatment algorithm, **152**
   ultrasonography, 147–49
Hirschsprung's disease, 127, 181, 182
history taking
   alert indicators, **9**
   cardiac screening (*see* cardiac screening)
   delivery mode alerts, 8–9
   depression, material, 18–19
   documentation, 23–24
   eye examination (*see* eye examination)
   genital examination (*see* genital examination)
   information interpretation, 22–23
   intrapartum history, 8
   limitations, **24**, 24–25
   location importance, 23–24
   maternal medical records evaluation, 4–10, **9**
   metabolic disease screening, 11, 26
   NIPE screening elements, **16**
   NIPE SMART, xiii, 17, 221–22
   NSC Antenatal Screening Programme, **5–7**,
      10–14, **18**, 26
   objectives, characteristics, 2–3
   overview, 1–2, 25
   parental dialogue, involvement, 20–22, **22**
   process generally, 4
   psychosocial, safeguarding agenda, 17–20, **18**, **21**

resources, 25–26
risk factors generally, 14–15, **16**, **18**
screening tools, 4, **5–7**
serology investigations, **5–6**, 10–11
ultrasonography, **6–7**, 11
HIV screening, **5**, 11
Holt–Oram syndrome, **51**
Howard, F. M., 2
hydrocele, **130**, 131–32, 136
hypoglycaemia/hypoxia/hypothermia impacts,
   42–44, **43**
hypoplastic left heart, **45**, **51**, **58**
hypoplastic right heart, **45**, **58**
hypospadias, **130**, 132, **136**, 136–37, 139–40
hypothyroidism, 108

I
impetigo, 80, **81**
inborn errors of metabolism, 188
infection
   Candida, 82
   screening, 9–10
   TORCH, 116–17
informed consent, 217–18
inguinal hernia, **130**, 130–132, **135**, 135–36
intestinal malrotation, 126
iron deficiency anaemia, 40

J
jaundice
   assessment, 11, 26, 88–89
   case study, 99–100
   categorisation of, 87–88
   causes, 75
   dangers of, 87
   early, 89
   haemolytic, 89–91
   management of, 90–91
   overview, 85
   physiological, 77, 90, 99–100
   physiology of, 85–87, **86**
   prolonged/late onset, 90
   resources, 100
   see also skin
Jones, D., 146

K
Katzman, G. H., 59
keratinocytes, 73
kernicterus, 87
Klisic, P. J., 142
knee hyperextension, 166–67
Knowles, R., 60

L
Laplace's law, 41
Lavender, T., 77
left ventricular dilatation, **58**
leukocoria, 114, **114**, 117, 118
lithium, 18
lower GI obstruction, 126–27
lung development, 32–34, **33**

M
maternal booking history, 4
maternal medical records evaluation, 4–10, **9**
MCADD, 176–77
McDonald, S., 222
meconium ileus, 126–27
meconium-stained liquor, 9
melanocytes, 73–74, 82
Mercer, J. S., 40, 41
metabolic disease screening, 11, 26
metatarsus adductus, 160–161, **161**
methadone withdrawal, 14
midwifery generally, xi–xii, 213–16, 224–25
milia, 78, **78**
miliaria (prickly heat), 78
Miller–Dieker syndrome, **51**
Mongolian blue spot, 74, **74**, 82
Moore, M., 17
Moro reflex, 94, **95**
mosaicism, 172
Mowat–Wilson syndrome, 190–191
mutation, 172

N
naevus flammeus (port wine stain), 84, **85**
naevus simplex (salmon patch haemangioma,
    stork marks), 83–84
nasolacrimal duct obstruction, 120
necrotising enterocolitis, 127–28
Neisseria gonorrhoea, 117
neonatal abstinence syndrome (NAS), 14
Ness, M. J., 77
New Ballard Score, 92, **93–94**
newborn blood spot test, 175–77
NIPE Screening Programme, 2, 214–15, 222, 223
NIPE SMART, xiii, 17, 221–22
NIPE Standards, xii–xiii, **16**
Noonan syndrome, **51**
NSC Antenatal Screening Programme, **5–7**, 10–14,
    18, 26
nuchal translucency screening, **6**
nucleotides, 172

O
Ohlsson, A., 10
oligohydramnios, 12
ophthalmia neonatorum, 117
opiates withdrawal, 14, 26
orchidopexy, 134
Ortolani test, 146
osteogenesis imperfecta, 186
ovaries. *see under* genital examination
'ox eye' (congenital glaucoma buphthalmos), 118,
    119

P
paroxetine, 18
Patau syndrome (trisomy 13), **51**, 183
patent ductus arteriosus (PDA), **45**, **51**
Pavlik harness, **150**, 150–151, **152**
penis. *see under* genital examination
persistent hyperplastic primary vitreous
    (PHPV), 117

persistent pulmonary hypertension of the
    newborn (PPHN), 44
petechiae, 77
phenylketonuria, 176
phototherapy, 91
pigmented naevi, 82–83, **83**
plagiocephaly, **105**
pneumothorax, 64
point mutation, 172
polydactyly, 163–64, **163–64**
polyhydramnios, 12
polysyndactyly, 164, **165**
Ponseti cast, 156–59, **157–60**, 166
port wine stain (naevus flammeus), 84, **85**
postnatal circulation, 38–39
Practice Development Groups, 224
Prader–Willi syndrome, 186
pregnancy
    amniotic fluid, 34
    complications risk factors, 8
    cord clamping, delayed, 39–40
    delivery mode alerts, 8–9
    history taking, 3
    renal pelvic dilatation monitoring, 12
prickly heat (miliaria), 78
professional issues
    case study, 225–26
    clinical effectiveness, 224
    The Code, 216–20
    competency framework initiatives, 213–15
    confidentiality, 218–20
    consent, 217–18
    education, competence, 222–23
    employer's role, 220
    policies and guidelines, local, 220–221
    practice recommendations, 223
    resources, 226
    risk management, 221–22
PROM, 10
psychosocial, safeguarding agenda, 17–20, **18**, **21**
Public Health England, xii
pulmonary atresia, **45**, **51**, **58**, 181
pulmonary stenosis, **45**, **51**
pulse oximetry, 53, 56, 59–61
PulseOx study, 60

Q
quadruple test, **6**

R
reflexes
    Babinski, 95, **96**
    grasp, 95, **95**
    Moro, 94, **95**
    rooting, sucking, 95–96, 207
    stepping, 96–97, **97**
    tonic neck, 96
Regulation of Health and Social Care Professionals,
    215
resources
    BCG vaccination, 26
    behavioural status, 210

resources (*continued*)
   cardiac screening, 65–66
   congenital heart defects, 65–66
   genital examination, 140
   hip dysplasia, 166–67
   history taking, 25–26
   jaundice, 100
   professional issues, 226
respiratory screening
   blood gases measurement, 64
   breathing movements, 34, 40–41, 52
   chest wall transillumination, 64
   cord clamping, delayed, 39–40
   examination generally, 44
   examination process, 62–65
   fetal circulation, 36–38, **37**
   hypoglycaemia/hypoxia/hypothermia impacts,
      42–44, **43**
   lung development, 32–34, **33**
   NIPE process map, 53, **54**
   overview, 32
   postnatal circulation, 38–39
   ultrasonography, 64–65
Resuscitation Council Guidelines, cord clamping,
   40
retinoblastoma, 116
retinopathy of prematurity, 110, 118
rhabdomyomata, **58**
rhesus status screening, **5**, 10–11
Richmond, S., 60
right atrial dilatation, **58**
right ventricular dilatation, **58**
risk management, 221–22
Romitti, P. A., 23
rooting reflex, 95–96, 207
Rosendahl, K., 143
rubella screening, **6**

S
Safeguarding, 17–20, **18**, **21**
salmon patch haemangioma (naevus simplex,
   stork marks), 83–84
scalded skin syndrome, 81, **81**
seborrhoeic dermatitis (cradle cap), 79, **79**
sensitivity, stress, 202–5, **203–5**
sex chromosome disorders, 172
sex determinants, 128–29, **129**
Shah, V. S., 10
shaken baby syndrome, 118
sickle cell disease, **5**, 174, 176
Simian crease, 178, **179**
single ventricle, **45**
skin
   acne (neonatal), 78–79, **79**
   assessment, 74–75, 99
   café-au-lait spots, 82
   Candida infection, 82
   care, 75–77
   cavernous haemangioma, 84
   colour, 74–75
   erythema toxicum neonatorum, 77, **78**
   herpes (neonatal), 81–82

   impetigo, 80, **81**
   jaundice (*see* jaundice)
   milia, 78, **78**
   miliaria (prickly heat), 78
   Mongolian blue spot, 74, **74**, 82
   pigmented naevi, 82–83, **83**
   pigment lesions, 82
   port wine stain (naevus flammeus), 84, **85**
   salmon patch haemangioma (naevus simplex,
      stork marks), 83–84
   scalded skin syndrome, 81, **81**
   seborrhoeic dermatitis (cradle cap), 79, **79**
   strawberry haemangioma, 84, **84**, 119, **119**
   sucking blisters, 79, **80**
   transient neonatal pustulosis, 79–80, **80**
   vascular birthmarks, 83
Skovgaard, R., 41
smiles, 202
smoking, 12–13, **21**
splintage, dynamic, **150**, 150–151, **152**
SSRIs, 18–19
standards, guidelines generally, xii–xiv, **5–7**,
   213–14, 220–221. *see also under specific topics*
Staphylococcus aureus, 80, 81
stepping reflex, 96–97, **97**
Stern, D., 194, 196
stethoscopes, 48–49, **49**
Stoeckle, J. D., 3
stork marks (salmon patch haemangioma, naevus
   simplex), 83–84
strabismus, 120
strawberry haemangioma, 84, **84**, 119, **119**
strawberry naevus (capillary haemangioma), 84,
   84, 119, **119**
Streptococcus pyogenes, 80
structure, function, 71–74, **72–73**
substance misuse, 13–14, **21**, 26
sucking blisters, 79, **80**
sucking reflex, 95–96, 207
sudden infant death syndrome (SIDS), 8, 13
swaddling, 199, **199–200**, 201
syndactyly, 164, **165**
syphilis screening, **5**

T
testes, undescended (cryptorchidism), **130**,
   130–134, **133**, 139–40
testes examination. *see under* genital examination
testicular torsion, 134, **135**
tetralogy of Fallot, **45**, **58**, 181, 186
thalassaemia screening, **5**, 174
Thangaratina, S., 60
tongue-tie (ankyloglossia), 109, 120–121
tonic neck reflex, 96
TORCH infections, 116–17
total anomalous pulmonary venous drainage
   (TAPVD), **45**
Toxocara, 116–17
Toxoplasmosis, 116
tracheo–oesophageal fistula, 126
transient neonatal pustulosis, 79–80, **80**
transposition of the great arteries (TGA), **45**, **58**

traumatic brain injury, 118
tricuspid atresia, **45**, **58**
tricyclic antidepressants (TCAs), 19
trisomy, 172
trisomy 13 (Patau syndrome), **51**, 183
trisomy 18 (Edward's syndrome), **51**, 183
trisomy 21 (Down's syndrome), **51**, 108, **115**,
     179–83, **181**
Trotter, S., 76
truncus arteriosus, 34, **35**, 36, **45**, **51**
Turner's syndrome, **51**, 183–86, **184–85**

U
UK National Screening Committee, xii–xiii
ultrasonography
     cardiac screening, 57–59, **58**
     genetic, chromosomal problems, 173–74
     hip dysplasia, 147–49
     history taking, **6–7**, 11
     respiratory screening, 64–65
umbilical vein, 36, **37**
undescended testes (cryptorchidism), **130**,
     130–134, **133**, 139–40
Ungerer, R. L. S., 10
uniparental disomy, 172
upper GI obstruction, 126

V
VACTERL syndrome, **51**
vagina. *see under* genital examination
valproate, 18
vascular birthmarks, 83
velocardiofacial syndrome, **51**, 186
ventricular septal defect, 36, **45**, 47, 48, **51**, **58**,
     65–66
vertical talus, congenital, 161–63, **162–63**
vomiting assessment, 124–25

W
Wilkinson, A. G., 149
William's syndrome, **51**
Winnicott, D., 193
Wolf–Hirschhorn syndrome, **51**
Wren, C., 45

X
X-linked inheritance, 173

Z
Zhao, Q.-M., 61